W0018596

A UNIFIED SYSTEM
FITNESS DESIGN

A Unified System Fitness Design proposes a new fitness framework that encompasses all fitness indicators in a holistic and comprehensive manner, striving to provide a comprehensive and inclusive definition of physical fitness, one that considers all attributes contributing to overall well-being, and crafting a flexible framework that can adapt to diverse contexts and purposes of physical fitness assessments. This new book is divided into three parts. Part I explores redefining and reconstructing the concepts of an inclusive and holistic fitness framework. In Part II, the reader is encouraged to embark on a journey to discover the interconnected system functions of physiological health, homeostasis, motor control, and energy regulation. Part III reinforces the role of wellness in the Unified Systems Fitness Design, guided by the principles of inclusion and equity, in the decision-making process. Finally, the perpetual complementation theory emerged from the design, making sense of the cyclical connection between the system functions for health and skill and strengthening the Health-Ability-Task Suitability (HATS) Framework. There are still many uncharted territories in the realm of fitness and wellness. *A Unified System Fitness Design* addresses these gaps in the literature and practice and seeks to inspire a transformative worldview that urges the reader to question the existing paradigms and explore innovative, inclusive approaches that cater to people with unique needs. In doing so, this exciting new volume aims to establish a common language for researchers and practitioners in the field, offering accurate and concise descriptions of each fitness component and its associated indicators in a universally understood terminology.

Nguyen Tra Giang, PhD is Dean, Institute of Sports Science and Management, University of Management and Technology Ho Chi Minh City, Cat Lai Ward, Thu Duc City, Ho Chi Minh City, Vietnam.

Oliver Napila Gomez, PhD is Deputy Head of the Sport Management Department of the Institute of Sports Science and Management, University of Management and Technology, Ho Chi Minh City, Vietnam.

A UNIFIED SYSTEM FITNESS DESIGN

Concepts of Holistic and Inclusive Fitness Framework

Nguyen Tra Giang and Oliver Napila Gomez

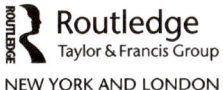
Routledge
Taylor & Francis Group

NEW YORK AND LONDON

Designed cover image: Oliver Napila Gomez

First published 2025
by Routledge
605 Third Avenue, New York, NY 10158

and by Routledge
4 Park Square, Milton Park, Abingdon, Oxon, OX14 4RN

Routledge is an imprint of the Taylor & Francis Group, an informa business

© 2025 Nguyen Tra Giang and Oliver Napila Gomez

The right of Nguyen Tra Giang and Oliver Napila Gomez to be identified
as authors of this work has been asserted in accordance with sections 77
and 78 of the Copyright, Designs and Patents Act 1988.

All rights reserved. No part of this book may be reprinted or reproduced
or utilised in any form or by any electronic, mechanical, or other means,
now known or hereafter invented, including photocopying and recording,
or in any information storage or retrieval system, without permission in
writing from the publishers.

Trademark notice: Product or corporate names may be trademarks
or registered trademarks, and are used only for identification and
explanation without intent to infringe.

ISBN: 978-1-032-82105-4 (hbk)
ISBN: 978-1-032-81745-3 (pbk)
ISBN: 978-1-003-50293-7 (ebk)

DOI: 10.4324/9781003502937

Typeset in Times New Roman
by Apex CoVantage, LLC

CONTENTS

FIGURES

TABLES

ABOUT THE AUTHORS

Dr. Nguyen Tra Giang is a well-known figure in the field of sports management, with over 15 years of teaching experience and an impressive academic background. She has made history as the first Vietnamese person to contribute to the Thailand men's ice hockey team and compete globally. Moreover, she was awarded the Erasmus Mundus Scholarship by the Council of Europe for her outstanding achievements in sports education, making her the first Vietnamese recipient of this prestigious scholarship. Dr. Nguyen's passion for sports education goes beyond academics. She believes sports and physical activity can be powerful tools for social change. As the Vice President of the Vietnam Chess Federation in 2023, she advocated for the role of sports in shaping gender norms, promoting unity, and addressing critical issues such as conflict resolution, reproductive health, and gender-based violence. In 2018, Dr. Nguyen collaborated with the US Department of State, the University of Tennessee, and ESPNW, USA, on a groundbreaking project called "Stay Active, Happy Her, Happy Us." The project aimed to inspire and empower female university students to actively engage in sports and physical activity. This innovative project exemplifies her commitment to promoting change and empowerment through sports. Dr. Nguyen is also the founder of the Chess and Physical Activities class for underprivileged children in difficult circumstances in Vietnam. This project aims to allow children to develop intellectually, physically, and spiritually, regardless of their social status. The project also offers a safe space for children to play and be happy, reflecting Dr. Nguyen's unwavering commitment to creating positive change through sports.

Dr. Nguyen Tra Giang
Dean, Institute of Sports Science and Management
University of Management and Technology, Ho Chi Minh City
Vietnam

Dr. Gomez is a transformative academic and specialist in research, pedagogy, and teaching innovation within physical education, fitness, wellness, sports, and dance. His extensive experience extends to curriculum development and instructional material design consultancy across Southeast Asia. Beyond his inaugural work, the 2017 publication "Physical EducASEAN Educator's Manual," he has made remarkable contributions by formulating teacher education curricula for Physical Education and Life Skills under UNESCO Myanmar. Dr. Gomez's repertoire includes the authorship of 12 student-teacher textbooks and 12 teacher-educator guides in partnership with the Ministry of Education in Myanmar, achieved through a collaborative effort with the Australian Council for Educational Research (ACER) and UNESCO. Dr. Gomez holds the esteemed position of deputy head of the sport management department at the Institute of Sports Science and Management, University of Management and Technology in Ho Chi Minh City, Vietnam. In addition, he serves as an adjunct faculty at Lourdes College Graduate School in Cagayan de Oro City, Philippines, imparting his insights to aspiring scholars. Dr. Gomez's multifaceted expertise and unyielding commitment to enhancing education and wellness make him a visionary in academic fitness and sports.

Dr. Oliver Napila Gomez
Deputy Head of Sport Management Department,
Institute of Sports Science and Management
University of Management and Technology, Ho Chi Minh City
Vietnam

ACKNOWLEDGMENTS

When we share our ideas with our friends worldwide, they listen to us, inspiring us to continue what we have started. It brings us joy to know that PE teachers, scholars, researchers, and professionals are fascinated with what we are building as innovators of 21st-century fitness. More so, our friends' input and feedback contributed to the growth and evolution of the Unified Systems Fitness Design concept as a holistic and inclusive framework.

We thank Ma'am Jessica Esparrago, Sir Julie Castillon, and the Higher Ed Department of Physical Education faculty at Xavier Ateneo, Cagayan de Oro City, Philippines. We also thank Dr. Wenna Balaido-Damulo, a teacher at Lower Yukon School District, Alaska, USA. When we consulted her, she was still with the Commission on Higher Education (CHED) in the Caraga Administrative Region.

We appreciate Sir Ricardo Roxas, a PE teacher from Central Mindanao University, Bukidnon, Philippines. His insights on academic writing and our discussion relating the concepts to real-world contexts reminded us to keep the concepts of the USFD as pragmatic as possible, supported by relevant literature and studies.

Ma'am Rita Gulac, a faculty at Lourdes College Graduate School, Cagayan de Oro City, Philippines, provided feedback on the measurement and evaluation aspect of the USFD Framework, which will be featured in the second book. We felt that we needed to thank her ahead of time because of her invaluable contribution to our work.

We thank the graduate students taking the Master of Arts in Education major in Teaching Physical Education from Lourdes College Graduate School in Cagayan de Oro City for their active participation in providing valuable feedback to enhance the content and quality of the USFD Framework. Through our lively focus group discussion, they were the first critics of the USFD concepts.

We thank the College of Sports, Physical Education, and Recreation (College of SPEAR) at the MSU Marawi Campus for allowing the USFD research team to conduct piloting. We also thank Dr. Hendely Arreza Adlawan, Dean of the College of SPEAR; Sir Nasroding Bashier, Chairperson of the Department of Athletics; Dr. Visminda Detalla, Chairperson of the Department of Research and Extension; college faculty, staff, and students who participated in our research.

We thank our friends from Sri Lanka, Indonesia, Thailand, Vietnam, the Philippines, and worldwide. We are grateful for your support of our work and welcome proposals, partnerships, and collaboration for future academic endeavors.

We appreciate your support.

– Dr. Oliver and Dr. Jane

PREFACE

Dr. Jane and I met in Davao City, Philippines, at an international conference in 2017. Then, we reunited in Bangkok, Thailand, in 2019 at another international conference. Since then, we have teamed up in our joint advocacy to promote exercise, physical activity participation, and sports, considering diversity, inclusion, and women's empowerment. We are kicking it off with our debut – the Unified Systems Fitness Design, the concept of a holistic and inclusive fitness framework.

It started as a start-up project to publish a book about health promotion, exercise, and participation in physical activity during the pandemic in Bangkok, Thailand. Little by little, we discovered uncharted territories in fitness concepts as we read recent books and articles. What started as a simple book plan grew in scope and complexity as we began questioning what we know about physical fitness.

While writing the book, Dr. Jane moved to Vietnam to spearhead the Institute of Sports Science and Management at the University of Management and Technology, Ho Chi Minh City. At this university, they pioneered the institute's Bachelor of Sport Management program, tailored uniquely for Vietnamese learners. One exciting highlight of the program is its strong emphasis on the role of physical fitness and health in sports.

In 2023, I moved to Ho Chi Minh City to work with Dr. Jane. The book's writing continued as the ideas about a new perspective of fitness exploded. We encountered so many gaps during this time and needed to discuss them. Eventually, our ideas began to fall into place as we made sense of the patterns in the literature. We are amazed with the framework we developed because it makes so much sense for us now.

In addition, we talked to physical educators, health professionals, and education policymakers to get their responses about the USFD Framework. We have initially presented our concept to our friends in Sri Lanka. Our conversations with them highlight that we share the same sentiments and must evolve our understanding of the fitness concepts we once knew.

We developed the USFD Framework to empower people with knowledge they can relate to. The USFD is more than a context-based framework. It is a holistic approach that can be adapted in various settings.

Lastly, publishing the book is just the beginning. Dr. Jane and I at the University of Management and Technology, Ho Chi Minh City, will continue writing books and presenting new perspectives that support our profession's transformative needs.

– Dr. Oliver Napila Gomez

DECLARATION OF AI USAGE IN SCHOLARLY ENDEAVORS

The authors hereby declare their utilization of artificial intelligence, specifically ChatGPT, Consensus.app, and Grammarly, for the following explicit purposes:

1. Facilitating the creation of precise and productive language composition
2. Enhancing the metacognitive process of the authors involved in the conceptualization of theoretical constructs
3. Assessing the relevance and applicability of referenced sources, and
4. Assistance in crafting Alt texts

In adherence to academic integrity and rigorous scholarship principles, the authors explicitly confirm that AI was not employed to generate substantive content or academic literature within this work. We emphasize our unwavering commitment to the conscientious and ethical application of technology, ensuring the augmentation of the quality of our research while preserving the genuine and authentic nature of our academic contributions.

INTRODUCTION

Unified Systems Fitness Design (USFD) is a fitness framework that promotes equity, inclusion, and a holistic approach to health and wellness. It integrates up-to-date fitness paradigms with scientific principles. The USFD Framework breaks down traditional boundaries to include a comprehensive, inclusive fitness concept, believing that physical fitness should be meaningful and accessible to everyone.

As sports managers and physical education teachers, the authors found it fascinating that their employers require a medical certificate to validate their *"physically fit to work"* status. They contended that a medical certificate's emphasis on physiological biomarkers and the absence of disease makes it inadequate to measure an individual's capacity to perform specific job-related tasks. On the other hand, psychomotor domains such as cardiovascular efficiency, muscular strength, endurance, flexibility, and skill-related fitness components like agility, balance, and coordination are fully considered.

Given the prevalence of medical certification as a measure of occupational readiness, the authors set out to investigate fitness concepts in different settings. The writers approached the problem with an open mind and a critical eye, realizing that physical fitness is highly relevant and operationalized as competencies and performance in the workplace in an occupational context. It cannot be contained in physical education and sports science settings. To understand fitness concepts, they investigated them in the academic literature, looked at empirical evidence, and did some reflective practice. The US Fitness Model (USFD) results from this conceptual and practical rethinking of fitness, its evaluation, and its impacts on health and work performance.

Physiological health, homeostasis, motor control, and energy regulation are the interrelated system functions thoroughly examined in Part II of the introduction to the USFD Framework. Part I reinterprets and rebuilds the pre-USFD concepts into a comprehensive and inclusive fitness framework, considering the context of the 21st century. Beginning with a definition of contemporary physical fitness and progressing to the identification of obstacles to perpetual complementarity – a theory developed by the writers to demonstrate their understanding of current physical fitness – each chapter adds to the overall knowledge of the USFD Framework.

Chapter 1 probes the most recent definition of fitness in *"The fitness puzzle,"* highlighting how fitness should encompass more than physical health and skill performance. It stresses the importance of fitness about a person's goals and the criteria needed to accomplish tasks efficiently. Readers are encouraged to exercise critical thinking and reevaluate their pre-USFD fitness knowledge as Chapter 2 explores the intriguing labyrinth of pre-USFD concepts. Chapter 3 encourages a paradigm shift, a 180-degree turn away from the previous sport-saturated context of fitness toward a holistic and inclusive approach, considering the philosophical and theoretical foundations of the transformative shift. In Chapter 4, learn the complex mechanisms of the human body and their fundamental mechanisms that allow us to live healthy lives and work on our physical tasks. The USFD Framework, a profound idea, is introduced in Chapter 5, which systematically introduces the collective functions of the systems when paired or grouped.

One all-encompassing method for studying and improving physical fitness is the Unified Systems Fitness Design (USFD). It emphasizes coordination, the bedrock of motor control that extends beyond simple eye–hand or eye–foot control. A valuable skill in athletics and everyday life, coordination results from the brain's communication with environmental factors.

The USFD Framework investigates all aspects of physical fitness in its comprehensive form, including homeostasis, mobility, energy regulation, and physiological health. It also gives rise to the perpetual complementarity theory, which connects system functions to physical activity, sports, exercise, and other everyday life.

Next, the book explores the function of wellness within the USFD Framework, covering topics such as the theory of perpetual complementarity and its obstacles. The subject of Chapter 8 is the nervous and endocrine systems' control of the different physiological processes, including growth, hormones, reproduction, and metabolism. Chapter 9 covers total energy expenditure and basal metabolic rate and regulates a balance between energy inputs and outputs through metabolic processes. In Chapter 10, we dive into aerobic control, which controls how the heart and lungs work together to ensure your muscles get oxygen.

Chapter 11 introduces motor control as a system that oversees movement production, regulation, and honing for different objectives. Focusing on controlling speed and agility, it addresses balance, speed, agility, reaction time, and flexibility. Chapter 12 examines how the human body's various compositions can be understood using compartment models, a system function that arose from pairing two systems.

Chapter 13 explores energy production and utilization, specifically the relationship between various energy systems, strength, power, and endurance, and how muscles generate force according to the sliding filament theory. Chapter 14 explores wellness, discussing how crucial it is to be aware and make decisions that align with the USFD Framework.

Chapter 15 examines the topic of perpetual complementation theory, explaining how the health support system functions for skills and vice versa. Taking care of physical health in preparation for physical activity improves physiological health and vice versa. The brake mechanisms that slow down the perpetual complementation cycle are also discussed. Diseases and injuries, which interfere with the system's ability to maintain health and acquire new skills, are examples of brake mechanisms of perpetual complementation. Understanding these ideas is essential for physical fitness to triumph over these challenges.

Coordination, homeostasis, movement, energy regulation, and physiological health are the cornerstones of the USFD Framework, which provides a holistic view of physical fitness and how to enhance it. In a world where harmony, balance, and health are the norm, readers can rediscover what it means to be physically fit by deciphering the intricate web of relationships within the system.

PART I

A new perspective on physical fitness

Redefining and reconstructing concepts of an inclusive and holistic fitness framework

1

THE FITNESS PUZZLE

Nguyen Tra Giang and Oliver Napila Gomez

This chapter aims to explore the concept of fitness and its evolution over time. Originally, fitness was exclusively based on biology, but with societal transformations, fitness also evolved. Comprehending the definition of fitness is essential because it goes beyond physical health to include the capability to adjust to different situations. Gaining fitness demands a delicate balance between the physical and social environments that are constantly changing. The authors share their insights on this interplay, using the Health-Ability-Task Suitability (HATS) Framework as a guide. They emphasize the positive impact that physical fitness can have on a person's overall health and functioning. The chapter concludes by stating that fitness is all about health, ability, and task suitability, and, therefore, it should be examined from different perspectives. To ensure that fitness remains a pertinent and comprehensive concept, the authors recommend reexamining its meaning with an open and fluid perspective, addressing confusion and issues, and considering the latest research and industry shifts.

Outcomes

By the end of this chapter, you will be able to

- demonstrate an understanding of how the concept of fitness encompasses physical well-being, mental health, and societal perspectives, recognizing its multifaceted nature
- define the core concepts of fitness and appreciate how these concepts underpin the broader understanding of fitness

DOI: 10.4324/9781003502937-2

- recognize the interdependence and overlapping nature of health-related and skill-related fitness components and appreciate the complexity of their classification
- critically analyze the operational and conceptual definitions of physical fitness and understand how emphasizing one definition over the other can impact understanding of the concept
- explore and evaluate new perspectives in fitness and understand how these perspectives contribute to a comprehensive view of fitness

What is fitness?

As a result of societal shifts in emphasis on the importance of mental health, technological progress, and overall physical health, the term "fitness" has now expanded beyond its biological roots to encompass a broader range of concepts. Nonetheless, returning to the first definition is crucial within the context of this work. If we want to understand the complexities of fitness, we need to grasp its essential meaning.

"Fit" can mean many things depending on context, including adaptability, appropriateness, acceptability, and propriety (Dictionary, 2020). When used as a verb, it denotes being appropriate for a given situation, item, or goal. This simple explanation captures the concept of alignment, highlighting how fitness is about being in perfect harmony with one another.

Several sites also provide brief explanations of fitness. Fitness is defined as optimal health and physical strength for humans (Cambridge University Press, 2023). Similarly, fit as alignment with a specific aim and appropriateness are emphasized (Cambridge University Press, 2023). Because of its duality, it necessitates combining the physical and compatibility aspects. These definitions are also echoed by Oxford University Press, which emphasizes health and the ability to adapt to different situations (Oxford University Press, n.d.).

Fitness has a dual meaning when seen through the prism of health and strength. According to Sozen (2016), it is the capacity for physical engagement and the amount to which the body can manage physical demands. This definition emphasizes the need for appropriate physiological functions. Meanwhile, fitness goes beyond just physical health, according to Hackfort and Klöppel (2020), and it reflects how well the human biopsychosocial system adjusts to different environments. This perspective highlights the complex relationship between a person's physical, mental, and social environments and their fitness level, illuminating the mutual influence of these factors.

Looking at fitness from a different angle, the part about how well it fits the job hits home. A state of complete mental, emotional, and physical health that enables people to carry out activities competently and safely is described by Gaikwad and colleagues (2017) as fitness. In addition to physical strength, this expanded definition recognizes the importance of mental and emotional resilience. Aside from having the physical skills necessary to be fit for work, training the mind and emotions to handle the stresses of the job are imperative. A person's fitness level is defined by their ability to face obstacles, physical abilities, and emotional resilience to adapt and succeed.

Thus, fitness is the trifecta of health, skills, and task suitability. This fundamental idea, which encompasses both the physical and compatibility dimensions, serves as a springboard for exploring the many facets of fitness. To emphasize our theory's interrelated and all-encompassing character, we refer to it in this book as the Health-Ability-Task Suitability (HATS) Framework. This name reflects the three key ideas – health, skills, and task suitability – shown graphically in Figure 1.1.

Various aspects of health can be seen in this diagram, which recognizes everyone's uniqueness and that some are healthier than others. Skills (strength), symbolized by the arrows, indicate a person's ability to move and successfully meet tasks. It should be noted that tasks require suitability with health profiles and the distinct contours of individuals' condition, as seen in the illustration of suitability, which features an aperture decorated with diverse shapes. This mutualistic relationship emphasizes the importance of health and compatibility in the context of fitness by showcasing their essential interaction.

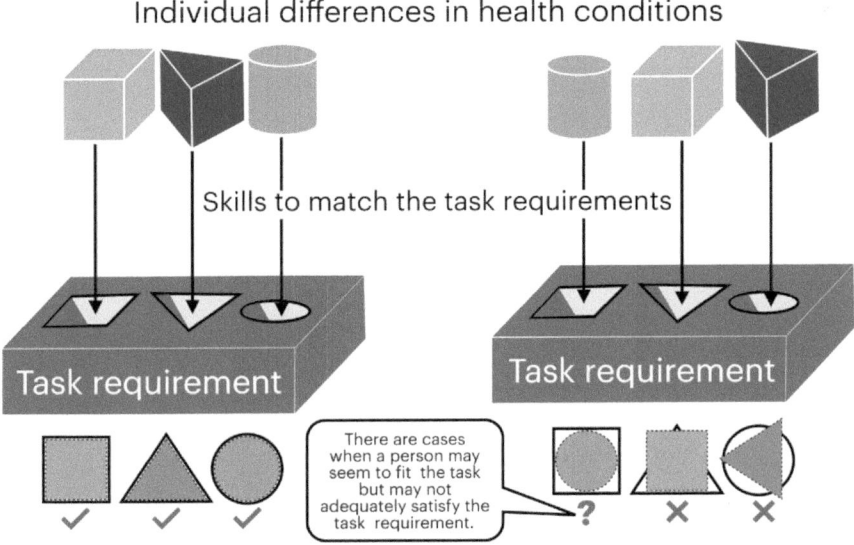

FIGURE 1.1   Health, skill, and task suitability aspects of fitness

Figure 1.1 depicts the interdependence of health, skill, and task suitability. To illustrate this point, let us use Alex, a college student, as an example. The variety of individual well-being is reflected in Alex's ebb and flow of health, which might range from enthusiastic to stressful days. Their skills, developed via training and experience, are like the diagram's arrow; they show they can do particular activities. A task's needs are reflected in its suitability, like a puzzle piece with a distinct shape. When Alex's abilities and mindset are in sync with the requirements of the task at hand, success may result. Misalignment, on the other hand, might lead to difficulties when elements like exhaustion are to blame. This highlights the dynamic interaction between health, skills, and task suitability and how individuals can maximize their performance by making educated adjustments when they grasp this synergy.

Physical fitness

Several studies have shown that being physically fit is an essential indicator of a person's health and happiness in today's culture (Dobosz et al., 2015; Iryanti et al., 2015; Korniloff, 2013; Rodrígues Bezerra, 2017). There is no universally accepted definition of physical fitness, but it does include the ability to do the things we do every day with ease and efficiency. Being physically fit, in a nutshell, entails being able to do things without becoming exhausted, coping with the physical demands of daily life, and being prepared for both anticipated and unforeseen events (Aboshkair et al., 2012; Devi & Kumari, 2014; Hasan & Wulandari, 2020; Hoeger & Hoeger, 2013; Powell, 2010; Salman & Nandiyanto, 2022; Sepriadi et al., 2022).

Physical fitness encompasses many skills that contribute to optimal bodily function and health. Physical fitness is like a squad of abilities that help our bodies do what they do best – keep us healthy (Corbin & Le Masurier, 2014). Both Fahey and colleagues (2015) and Corbin and his team (2008) state that it is about having optimum physical abilities, helping us live well and perform at our best in all areas of life, whether planning or dealing with the unexpected.

These experts try to convey that being physically fit is like having the tools to face life's challenges with strength, health, and preparedness. Having the stamina to go through the day, maintain good health, and savor every moment is just as important as having a powerful physique.

In today's society, being physically active is seen as a crucial sign of well-being and standard of living (Dobosz et al., 2015; Iryanti et al., 2015; Korniloff, 2013; Rodrígues Bezerra, 2017). However, the common understanding of physical fitness is that it pertains to a person's capacity to carry out tasks and work without becoming overly exhausted, to adjust to the physical demands of everyday life, to react appropriately in times of crisis, and to have sufficient energy to enjoy leisure activities (Aboshkair et al., 2012; Devi & Kumari, 2014; Hasan &

Wulandari, 2020; Hoeger & Hoeger, 2013; Powell, 2010; Salman & Nandiyanto, 2022; Sepriadi et al., 2022). Let us not forget that physical fitness is a construct (Baumgartner et al., 2015), a concept that gives a name and theoretical basis to a complex combination of characteristics (McCloskey, 2015). The more widely used a concept is among academics, the more it simplifies reality by becoming an objectified interpretation of shared observations (Wood, 2017).

While some constructs, like height or strength, are tangible and accessible to see, others, like fitness, motivation, or attitude, are intangible and difficult to quantify (Baumgartner et al., 2015). When a construct has been conceptualized, the next step is to operationalize it, which entails turning theoretical or abstract ideas into quantifiable quantities (Haucke et al., 2021; Miller et al., 2009; Bhattacherjee, 2012). Due to the restricted direct observability of constructs, this step is essential. It involves attaching the construct definition to specific indicators, which could be questions on a questionnaire or survey (Smith, 2020) or performance measures, depending on the nature of the construct. In physical fitness, specific indicators were previously called the fitness components.

According to the Institute of Medicine (2012) and Baumgartner and colleagues (2015), physical fitness is a condition or collection of traits representing the capacity to carry out physical activities and other tasks associated with present and future health results. The intangible concept of a "collection of traits" is emphasized, reflecting the capacity to perform the observable and quantifiable variable associated with physical fitness.

Furthermore, it is essential to employ an indirect strategy when measuring constructs (Baumgartner et al., 2015). Meanwhile, quantifying intangible and indirectly observable constructs requires the use of specific indicators (Rebellon, 2021). Operational definitions come in handy as they help assess the construct. In physical fitness, for example, the operational definition relates the attributes used to define physical fitness to an indirectly observable ability to perform physical activity (Baumgartner et al., 2015).

Consequently, the ability to do tasks becomes the focal point of physical fitness when operationally defined as a construct related to performance (Baumgartner et al., 2015). While physical fitness is conceptually defined as a set of attributes that are affected by exercise and regular physical activity (Frontera, 2018; Malar & Maniazhagu, 2020), the operational definition emphasizes performance context (Devi & Kumari, 2014; Salman & Nandiyanto, 2022; Sepriadi et al., 2022; Hasan & Wulandari, 2020). Unsurprisingly, this operationalization made physical fitness a phenomenon in the sports and exercise context.

Implications for practitioners and confusion about the construct's meaning might arise when the operational definition takes precedence over the conceptual one, leading to ambiguity and definitional issues (Ridley et al., 2021; Halpern, 2014). For example, the concept of physical fitness has been interpreted differently because it has been given several practical definitions by various writers

(Caspersen et al., 1985; Corbin & Le Masurier, 2014; Delaney, 2015; Hoeger & Hoeger, 2013; Karuppiah, 2017; Powell, 2010). As an example, Karuppiah (2017) defined it as physical fitness encompassing two notions: general fitness, which refers to general health and wellness, and specific fitness, which is concerned with the capacity to carry out specific duties associated with sports or jobs. Others have referred to it as health-related or skill-related fitness components (e.g., Corbin & Le Masurier, 2014; Hoeger & Hoeger, 2013).

In this book, we prefer the conceptual definition of physical fitness, which emphasizes a person's capacity to carry out daily tasks and activities and their overall risk of acquiring health problems (Tangen, 2020). The ability to engage in physical activities, a measure of fitness level, is encompassed in this conceptual definition (Institute of Medicine, 2012; Baumgartner et al., 2015). By focusing on physical fitness's conceptual definition instead of its measurement and evaluation-based operational definition, we are off to a good start, reducing the ambiguity caused by the latter and making it relevant for practitioners.

To sum up, while performance-based indicators were crucial to the operational definition of physical fitness, they should not be considered instead of the core components of the construct. These components include the capacity to carry out physical activities and tasks, the risk of developing health problems at an early stage, and the ability to sustain an individual's physiological functions for health reasons. People should only use the operational definition to define the construct in a quantitative and quantifiable fashion; it gives a clear and measurable description, but it should always be distinct from the fundamental substance of the construct. So, the operational definition based on performance alone should not supplant the conceptual definition of physical fitness as a multifaceted collection of qualities indicating the capacities to support an individual's overall health and enjoyment of life.

The fitness component dilemma

There are two common ways to categorize physical fitness: health-related and skill-related fitness components (Nikolaidis & Knechtle, 2022; Corbin et al., 2008; Caspersen et al., 1985). Other words that have been used that are comparable to the health- and skill-related concept include general fitness, which means a state of health and welfare, and specific fitness, which is a task-oriented description based on the ability to perform specific components of sports or jobs (Delaney, 2015; Caspersen et al., 1985; Karuppiah, 2017; Powell, 2010). Body composition, cardiorespiratory fitness, flexibility, strength, and endurance are all parts of health-related fitness (HRF). Skill-related fitness (SRF) measures include power, speed, agility, balance, and reaction time.

When solving the problems of indirect indicators and the absence of rational consistency in fitness, the HRF–SRF model was a giant leap forward. By

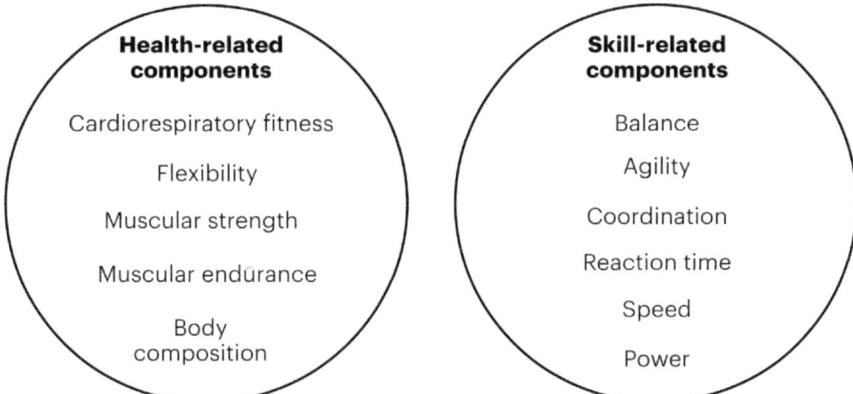

FIGURE 1.2   Two distinct fitness components – each with its own set of attributes and contexts

categorizing the many aspects of fitness according to their respective contexts, the model has provided the field with much needed clarity and structure (e.g., conceptual vs. operational, attribute vs. performance, and health vs. skill). A direct method of gauging physical fitness has been developed by creating classes of build indicators known as fitness components. Educators, practitioners, and academics have all embraced the paradigm, which has contributed to developing an all-encompassing strategy for physical fitness.

This leads many to classify fitness in terms of health-related aspects and fitness in terms of skill-related aspects, with the two groups having unique characteristics and applications (see Figure 1.2). Professionals and individuals can benefit from this differential by better comprehending the complex nature of physical fitness and adapting their training and evaluations appropriately.

Despite the complicated overlap of concepts (commonly ignored in the practical sense), fitness components have long been categorized as health-related or skill-related. This categorization technique has never been challenged. For example, most people agree that exercise activities focusing on health and wellness improve health and quality of life. Cardiorespiratory fitness, on the other hand, is just as crucial for long-distance running events and swimming. Gymnastics and rhythmic exercises also emphasize strength, flexibility, and muscular endurance. Sports that demand a similar amount of muscle mass, like many combat sports, can emphasize body composition. Conversely, health is tied to all aspects of fitness that pertain to skills.

According to Baumgartner and colleagues (2015, pp. 284–285), "because some components of performance-related fitness tests and health-related fitness tests overlap, the operational definitions are similar in some degree." This overlap is shown in Figure 1.3, a Venn diagram representation. We argue that

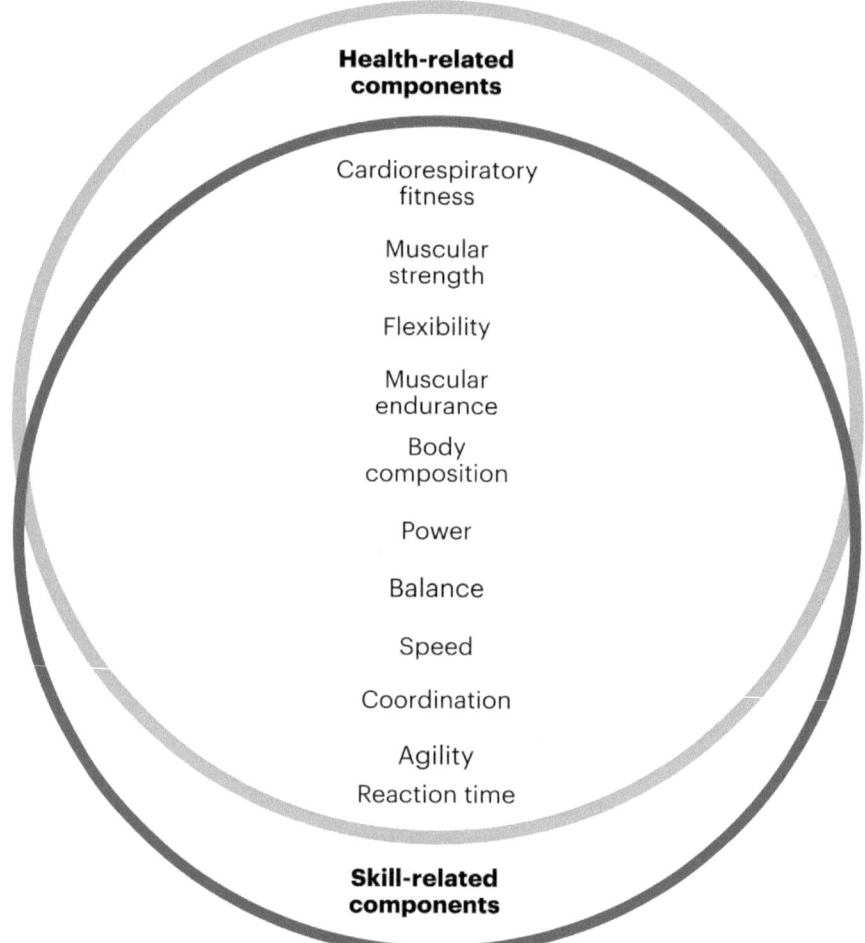

FIGURE 1.3   The overlapping concept of health- and skill-related fitness

whether a component is considered health- or skill-related depends on the sur-rounding circumstances. Such skills include balance and coordination, essential for success in many sports and general well-being. Children, the elderly, and those suffering from vertigo or dizziness are likely to fall, negatively affecting their health. Combat sports also require a certain level of health-related fitness.

In another example, boxing matches involve weighing the fighters to ensure that neither fighter has an unfair edge due to their body composition. In addition, players in different sports keep track of their body composition to perform at their best. These instances demonstrate how skill-related fitness is essential for promoting health and wellness and how health-related fitness fits nicely with performance-related contexts.

We take the overlapping of various fitness components as a severe problem. At best, there is no way to categorize or organize the components, and the lines between them must be clarified. This haziness allows us to pinpoint many other issues with defining physical fitness. We get that many on the ground are content with the status quo and would prefer it remain that way. Nevertheless, our expertise may be used in this area, incorporating 21st century agendas, such as inclusion and equity.

Although some of these issues are either entirely unknown or have yet to be addressed by researchers despite the numerous gaps in the literature, we will explain them in the next chapter, along with the flaws and challenges we discovered while teaching and practicing fitness. Furthermore, we will examine the significance of maintaining a well-rounded and comprehensive approach to physical fitness. This approach should consider the interconnectedness of all aspects, individual objectives, and circumstances, as well as the relative weight of each component.

Considering new fitness perspectives

New, innovative minds are cropping up in the fitness industry. The utilization of visual, vestibular, and proprioceptive inputs by the central nervous system to synchronize muscular action and generate a perception of balance was documented by Okudur and Sanioğlu (2012). Han and colleagues (2015) elaborated upon the need for these sensory inputs for spatial movement, which depends on body position and gravity. Since the eyes are visual extensions of the brain, visual information processing is also essential for balance (Melcher & Morrone, 2015).

These are only a few recent discoveries about balance, one of the skill-related fitness components in the previous model. A deluge of recent research on physical fitness has been released. However, the synthesis of their results has yet to be released.

In continuation, all these things (Okudur & Sanioğlu, 2012; Han et al., 2015; Melcher & Morrone, 2015) point to the idea that *balance + coordination* is the best way to describe the intricate process of maintaining equilibrium while also describing the interplay between senses and the skeletal muscular system. Training for better balance is integral to any fitness or sports program because it helps athletes perform better and lessens the likelihood of injuries to the lower extremities (Han et al., 2015). Maintaining equilibrium and avoiding falls are signs of good balance (Shoeb et al., 2020).

Another viewpoint is for hand–eye coordination. Several systems, including vision, perception, cognition, and muscle control, are said to be involved in the intricate process of hand–eye coordination (Szabo et al., 2020). For an object to be recognized and identified, the perceptual system processes the visual system's information regarding the object's position, motion, and shape. The mental apparatus then directs the motor apparatus to coordinate motions to approach and seize the item. When doing a task like catching a ball, the brain uses visual information to control, direct, and lead the hands to finish the task (Wong et al., 2019). However, the muscle system provides the force and accuracy to do the job well.

A new viewpoint on reaction time has also evolved. Zhu (2022) states that because it quantifies how long it takes for a person to react to stimuli, reaction time can be considered a form of speed. Quickness of reaction is a measure of an athlete's physical condition that helps them deal with sudden changes in the game, like the ball's placement or the direction of play. Athletic performance is directly proportional to the athlete's reaction time. Responding quickly is fundamental to being swift and nimble in athletic pursuits.

Moreover, the ability to quickly generate a large amount of force is a critical component of power, and the new viewpoint emphasizes speed–strength as a measure of fitness (Bianco et al., 2015). Athletes use it to improve their athletic prowess by performing sprinting, jumping, and throwing with velocity and explosive power.

According to another view, agility and change of direction speed (Rayner & Young, 2015) are distinct physical attributes that call for distinct kinds of motion. Unlike the quick whole-body reactions required for agility, swift directional changes do not necessitate a mental reaction. However, there needs to be more literature on agility because old classifications did not capture the essence of the physical trait.

The articles we mentioned are only a few new perspectives that make fitness dynamic, suggesting that staying current is essential. Due to increased studies and new perspectives, more than the conventional thinking on fitness components may be needed today. In light of new technologies, changing lives, and rising health challenges, exercise must be rethought to stay relevant. Moreover, new fitness component research and ideas suggest that their interaction is more essential than any single component. The speed–strength fitness characteristic integrates the two ideas to take a comprehensive picture of health. Complex physical traits, such as agility versus swiftness, must be defined to change directions. More studies and new perspectives on fitness components emphasize the need to reassess physical fitness regularly. Keeping fitness relevant in a changing environment takes an open mind and willingness to try new things.

Summary

A complex construct involving strength and health, fitness also incorporates mental health, technology improvements, and overall physical well-being. To complete tasks, people must be aware of how their physical skills interact with their emotional and mental resilience. With an emphasis on the conceptual rather than the operational definition of fitness, the Health-Ability-Task Suitability (HATS) Framework offers a primary platform for investigating the many facets of fitness.

There are two main categories of physical fitness: health-related and skill-related. Balance, coordination, reaction time, agility, speed, and power are all components of skill-related fitness (SRF). In contrast, cardiorespiratory fitness (HRF) encompasses these and the muscles' flexibility, strength, and endurance. By contextually grouping various fitness components, the HRF–SRF model solves the problems of indirect indications and physical fitness's lack of logical coherence.

However, the current definition of fitness has issues because several aspects overlap. A comprehensive perspective on physical fitness considers the weight of each factor, how they all work together, and the interconnectedness of personal objectives and environmental factors. This strategy can benefit both individuals and experts, as it improves understanding and measurement of the complex nature of physical fitness.

Various new viewpoints on health-related fitness have emerged, including speed–strength, agility, balance, hand–eye coordination, reaction time, and change-of-direction speed. Because fitness is a dynamic and ever-changing subject, tried-and-true methods may not cut it in the modern day. Rather than focusing on the parts themselves, new viewpoints argue that their interplay is crucial.

Review questions

1. In the context of this work, what is the most basic definition of "fitness"?
2. What does fitness mean in the HATS (Health-Ability-Task Suitability) Framework?
3. What are the two different meanings of fitness when you look at it through the lens of health and strength?
4. According to the new definitions, explain how fitness includes physical and mental health.
5. According to the research, what are the most critical parts of being physically fit?
6. How is physical fitness operationalized so that it can be measured?
7. Discuss how health-related fitness (HRF) and skill-related fitness (SRF) differ.
8. Why is it important to highlight the overlapping of health-related and skill-related fitness components?
9. Explain how new research has changed our understanding of fitness factors like balance, coordination, and reaction time.
10. Why is it essential to re-evaluate the definition and components of physical fitness?

Discussion questions

1. Should we think about changing or reassessing the conventional method of fitness component classification in light of the fuzziness and overlap between health-related and skill-related fitness?
2. Can we still provide a precise and quantifiable operational description while retaining the core ideas from the conceptual definition?
3. How can we integrate things like emotional well-being, diet, and amount of sleep when we think about fitness?
4. The chapter briefly discusses modern ideas like equity in fitness and inclusivity. How can we ensure that fitness evaluations and definitions are fair and inclusive?
5. How do you think fitness education will evolve in response to new shifting perspectives in physical fitness?

References

Aboshkair, K. A., Amri, S. B., Yee, K. L., & Samah, B. B. A. (2012). Factors affecting levels of health-related physical fitness in secondary school students in Selangor, Malaysia. *Journal of Basic & Applied Sciences, 8*(1), 202–216. http://www.life scienceglobal.com/images/Journal_articles/JBASV8N1A32-Aboshkair.pdf

Baumgartner, T. A., Jackson, A. S., Mahar, M. T., & Rowe, D. A. (2015). *Measurement for evaluation in kinesiology.* Jones & Bartlett Publishers.

Bhattacherjee, A. (2012). *Social science research: Principles, methods, and practices.* University of South Florida. http://scholarcommons.usf.edu/oa_textbooks/3/

Bianco, A., Jemni, M., Thomas, E., Patti, A., Paoli, A., Roque, J. R., Palma, A., Mammina, C., & Tabacchi, G. (2015). A systematic review to determine reliability and usefulness of the field-based test batteries for the assessment of physical fitness in adolescents-the ASSO project. *International Journal of Occupational Medicine and Environmental Health, 28*(3), 445. http://dx.doi.org/10.13075/ijomeh.1896.00393

Cambridge University Press. (2023). Fitness. In *Cambridge academic content dictionary.* https://dictionary.cambridge.org/dictionary/english/fitness?q=Fitness

Caspersen, C. J., Powell, K. E., & Christenson, G. M. (1985). Physical activity, exercise, and physical fitness: Definitions and distinctions for health-related research. *Public Health Reports, 100*(2), 126. https://www.ncbi.nlm.nih.gov/pmc/articles/PMC1424733/

Corbin, C. B., & Le Masurier, G. C. (2014). *Fitness for life* (6th ed.). Human Kinetics.

Corbin, C. B., Welk, G. J., Corbin, W. R., & Welk, K. A. (2008). *Concepts of physical fitness, Active lifestyles for wellness* (14th ed.). McGraw-Hill.

Delaney, L. (2015). *Project SPRAOI: A strategy to improve nutrition and increase physical activity in primary school children* [Master's thesis]. https://sword.cit.ie/hummas/1

Devi, S., & Kumari, S. (2014). Physical fitness status of female college athletes. *Research Journal of Physical Education Sciences, 2*(6), 5–7. https://bit.ly/3Y1mH85

Dictionary. (2020). Fit. *Dictionary.com.* https://www.dictionary.com/browse/fit

Dobosz, J., Mayorga-Vega, D., & Viciana, J. (2015). Percentile values of physical fitness levels among polish children aged 7 to 19 years-a population-based study. *Central European Journal of Public Health, 23*(4), 340. https://cejph.szu.cz/pdfs/cjp/2015/04/11.pdf

Fahey, T. D., Insel, P., Roth, W. T., & Insel, C. (2015). *Fit & well: Core concepts and labs in physical fitness and wellness* (11th ed.). McGraw-Hill Education.

Frontera, W. R. (2018). Physical activity and rehabilitation in elderly. In *Rehabilitation medicine for elderly patients*. Practical Issues in Geriatrics. Springer. https://doi.org/10.1007/978-3-319-57406-6_1

Gaikwad, J. S., Jaywant, S. S., & Pai, A. V. (2017). Retrospective analysis of work fitness in municipal corporation employees. *The Indian Journal of Occupational Therapy*, *49*(3), 85–90. https://aiota.org/temp/ijotpdf/ibat17i3p85.pdf

Hackfort, D., & Klöppel, Y. P. (2020). Mental fitness. In *The Routledge international encyclopedia of sport and exercise psychology* (pp. 249–267). Routledge.

Halpern, D. F. (2014). *Thought and knowledge: An introduction to critical thinking* (5th ed.). Taylor & Francis.

Han, J., Anson, J., Waddington, G., Adams, R., & Liu, Y. (2015). The role of ankle proprioception for balance control in relation to sports performance and injury. *BioMed Research International*, *2015*. https://doi.org/10.1155/2015/842804

Hasan, A., & Wulandari, I. (2020, August). Overview of students' physical fitness in Padang. In *1st international conference of physical education (ICPE 2019)* (pp. 35–37). Atlantis Press. https://doi.org/10.2991/assehr.k.200805.012

Haucke, M., Hoekstra, R., & van Ravenzwaaij, D. (2021). When numbers fail: Do researchers agree on operationalization of published research? *Royal Society Open Science*, *8*(9), 191354. https://doi.org/10.1098/rsos.191354

Hoeger, W. W., & Hoeger, S. A. (2013). *Principles and labs for physical fitness*. Cengage Learning.

Institute of Medicine. (2012). *Fitness measures and health outcomes in youth*. The National Academies Press.

Iryanti, N. P., Rustiningsih, S. K. M., & Wahyuni, S. (2015). *Hubungan status gizi dan kejadian anemia dengan kesegaran jasmani pada remaja putri kelas X dan XI di SMA Muhammadiyah 1 Surakarta* [Doctoral dissertation, Universitas Muhammadiyah Surakarta]. http://eprints.ums.ac.id/id/eprint/34593

Karuppiah, L. (2017). Isolated and combined influence of weight training and ladder training on selected physical physiological and performance variables among men kabaddi players. *International Journal of Scientific Research and Modern Education*, *2*(1), 24–29. http://ijsrme.rdmodernresearch.com/wp-content/uploads/2017/02/147.pdf

Korniloff, K. (2013). Interrelationships of physical activity and depressive symptoms with cardiometabolic risk factors. *Studies in Sport, Physical Education and Health*, *193*. https://jyx.jyu.fi/bitstream/handle/123456789/41435/1/978-951-39-5193-1_vaitos18052013.pdf

Malar, S., & Maniazhagu, D. (2020). Effects of integrative neuromuscular training combined with yoga and stretching exercises on abdominal strength endurance of primary school children. *Indian Journal of Public Health Research & Development*, *11*(3), 899–903. http://dx.doi.org/10.5958/2278-795X.2019.00017.1

McCloskey, M. W. (2015). What is transformational leadership. *People Bethel Education*. https://bit.ly/3YX4nOC

Melcher, D., & Morrone, M. C. (2015). Nonretinotopic visual processing in the brain. *Visual Neuroscience*, *32*, e017. https://doi.org/10.1017/S095252381500019X

Miller, V. A., Reynolds, W. W., Ittenbach, R. F., Luce, M. F., Beauchamp, T. L., & Nelson, R. M. (2009). Challenges in measuring a new construct: Perception of voluntariness for research and treatment decision making. *Journal of Empirical Research on Human Research Ethics: JERHRE*, *4*(3), 21–31. https://doi.org/10.1525/jer.2009.4.3.21

Nikolaidis, P. T., & Knechtle, B. (2022). Participation and performance characteristics in half-marathon run: A brief narrative review. *Journal of Muscle Research and Cell Motility*, 1–8. https://doi.org/10.1007/s10974-022-09633-1

Okudur, A., & Sanioğlu, A. (2012). The relationship between balance and agility performance in tennis players aged 12. *Selçuk University Journal of Physical and Sport*

Science, 14(2), 165–170. https://www.acarindex.com/dosyalar/makale/acarindex-1423931792.pdf

Oxford University Press. (n.d.). Fitness. In *Oxford learner's dictionaries*. https://www.oxfordlearnersdictionaries.com/definition/english/fitness?q=fitness

Powell, M. A. (2010). *Physical fitness: Training, effects, and maintaining*. RS Publications.

Rayner, R., & Young, W. (2015). Correlations between attacking agility, defensive agility, change of direction speed and reactive strength in Australian footballers. *Journal of Australian Strength and Conditioning, 23*, 108–111.

Rebellon, C. J. (2021). Construct validity. *The Encyclopedia of Research Methods in Criminology and Criminal Justice, 1*, 17–19. https://doi.org/10.1002/9781119111931.ch4

Ridley, C. R., Mollen, D., Console, K., & Yin, C. (2021). Multicultural counseling competence: A construct in search of operationalization. *The Counseling Psychologist, 49*(4), 504–533. https://doi.org/10.1177/0011000020988110

Rodrígues Bezerra, D. (2017). *Análisis de la condición física en el periodo de cinco años en los escolares de Ilhabela Litoral de Sao Paulo*. http://hdl.handle.net/11371/1306

Salman, Z. M., & Nandiyanto, A. B. D. (2022). Literature about maintaining physical fitness through digital in community. *International Journal of Research and Applied Technology (INJURATECH), 2*(1), 124–131. https://doi.org/10.34010/injuratech.v2i1.6732

Sepriadi, S., Syafruddin, S., Khairuddin, K., Ihsan, N., & Liza, L. (2022). Contribution of motor ability to physical fitness of elementary school students. *Jurnal MensSana, 7*(2), 126–134. https://doi.org/10.24036/MensSana.07022022.17

Shoeb, M., Mishra, A., Yadav, K. K., Kumar, S., & Yadav, S. (2020). Effect of BAPS board versus Frenkel exercise on balance in stroke patient's – a pilot study. *International Journal for Research in Applied Science & Engineering Technology, 8*(11). http://doi.org/10.22214/ijraset.2020.6397

Smith, M. C. (2020). *Using psychometric models to measure social and emotional learning constructs* (Order No. 28093391). ProQuest Central (2455786933). https://www.proquest.com/dissertations-theses/using-psychometric-models-measure-social/docview/2455786933/se-2

Sozen, H. (Ed.). (2016). *Fitness medicine*. BoD-Books on Demand.

Szabo, D. A., Neagu, N., Teodorescu, S., & Sopa, I. S. (2020). Eye-hand relationship of proprioceptive motor control and coordination in children 10–11 years old. *Health, Sports & Rehabilitation Medicine, 21*(3), 185–191. https://doi.org/10.26659/pm3.2020.21.3.185

Tangen, E. M. (2020). *Is there an association between total physical activity level and VO2max among fitness club members? A prospective one-year follow-up study* [Master's thesis]. https://hdl.handle.net/11250/2728091

Wong, T. K., Ma, A. W., Liu, K. P., Chung, L. M., Bae, Y. H., Fong, S. S., Ganesan, B., & Wang, H. K. (2019). Balance control, agility, eye-hand coordination, and sport performance of amateur badminton players: A cross-sectional study. *Medicine, 98*(2). https://doi.org/10.1097%2FMD.0000000000014134

Wood, M. S. (2017). Misgivings about dismantling the opportunity construct. *Journal of Business Venturing Insights, 7*, 21–25. https://doi.org/10.1016/j.jbvi.2017.01.001

Zhu, Q. (2022). Classification and optimization of basketball players' training effect based on particle swarm optimization. *Journal of Healthcare Engineering, 2022*. https://doi.org/10.1155/2022/2120206

2

COMPLEXITIES OF FITNESS

Oliver Napila Gomez and Nguyen Tra Giang

Modern fitness concepts face several obstacles, including a need for consensus on operationalizing the concept, a subjective definition of fitness, and an uneven emphasis on different aspects of fitness. Emphasizing the need for a composite understanding across age groups, this chapter explores the ambiguity surrounding the definition of physical fitness. Also discussed is the necessity for a comprehensive strategy, the fact that fitness definitions are subjective, and that health and skill-related factors are interdependent. In addition to criticizing the focus on optimal fitness levels, this chapter argues for a comprehensive view that considers specific goals and task requirements. Finally, it stresses the need for a balanced approach to physical education programs that promote overall physical development and lifelong physical activity, warning against programs that place too much emphasis on health-related components.

Outcomes

By the end of this chapter, you will be able to

- identify the current challenges and limitations of physical fitness and its components
- examine the confusion surrounding physical fitness and its components, which leads to multiple interpretations and measurement issues
- explain how fitness is subjective and context-dependent, depending on goals and activity or sport needs
- examine the issue of the traditional idea that health-related fitness (HRF) components are prerequisites for skill-related fitness (SRF)

DOI: 10.4324/9781003502937-3

- reflect on the importance of a holistic approach to physical fitness that prioritizes specific components based on fitness components, individual goals, contextual factors, and challenges.

Challenges in contemporary fitness concepts

The fact that the various aspects of fitness share concepts introduces a degree of difficulty. The components need clarity and differentiation regarding their classification, organization, and relationship.

We can see that there are a lot of other problems with our current understanding of physical fitness due to this ambiguity. Even though we recognize that many educators and practitioners have reached a consensus regarding their contemporary understanding of physical fitness and its components and that they do not wish for the contemporary concepts to be contested, we are not content with the concepts that were presented to us, particularly about the incorporation of 21st-century concepts such as fairness and inclusion. Although many researchers in the field have remained silent, this does not change the fact that there are problems.

We will present the problems and limitations of the contemporary fitness components model, although these issues either need to be heard of or are straightforward. No researcher has dared to discuss them despite the numerous gaps in the literature. This section will also examine the importance of taking a balanced and holistic approach to physical fitness, which considers the interdependence of each component, an individual's goals and context, and the relative importance of each component.

Fitness lacks clarity in its operationalization

One of the physical fitness construct's significant limitations is clarity in operationalizing it. This lack of clarity has resulted in various authors offering multiple interpretations. Unfortunately, the developmental history of the health-related fitness (HRF) and skill-related fitness (SRF) model, which seeks to categorize the construct into various fitness components, is still unknown. This needs to be further investigated through research.

Consequently, it has become challenging to measure physical fitness directly as a multifaceted concept, as it has been reduced to a collection of indirect indicators. Utesch and colleagues (2017) pointed out that current fitness assessments, especially for children, have a one-dimensional structure due to differences in theoretical assumptions and practical implications. The need for a sophisticated comprehension of the components of physical fitness across various age groups is highlighted by this variation. In addition, Santana and colleagues (2017) point out that it is not easy to measure physical fitness comprehensively because of the many facets of fitness and its effects on health and cognitive outcomes. Due to this ambiguity, there is a lack of logical cohesion among the various components of fitness, which has further contributed to the confusion. Consequently, the response to the question "How fit are you?" continues to be complicated. No answer can be considered simply straightforward.

The theoretical frameworks for understanding and promoting physical activity behavior have evolved and diversified (Rhodes et al., 2019). However, to gain a deeper comprehension of the concept and how it is operationalized, it is recommended that future research concentrate on investigating the historical development of fitness as a construct and further illustrating its complexity. This may assist in developing an all-encompassing definition of physical fitness and a direct measurement of the construct as a multifaceted idea.

Fitness is subjective

The HRF–SRF model of fitness components is widely used in physical fitness, even with the need to learn further about the history of its development. We looked for records of how the contemporary components were explored and how the indicators were validated through various methods of validation studies. We also searched for the origin and development of the physical fitness construct. Despite this, we were unable to locate anything. Despite this obstacle, the HRF–SRF model has significantly contributed to our understanding of physical fitness. This is because it has made it possible to identify particular characteristics and capabilities contributing to an individual's overall health and well-being.

According to Čuprika et al. (2019), individuals can interpret and provide their definition of fitness based on their abilities and knowledge. Consequently, there is no universally accepted definition of fitness despite its widespread appeal, even though, as stated by Čuprika and colleagues (2019), the concept of fitness is frequently defined as that of sport competitive fitness, as the implementation of a healthy lifestyle, and as physical fitness or health-oriented physical fitness.

In this context, we acknowledge that the interpretation of fitness components is highly subjective, heavily dependent on the context in which they are being used, and varies depending on the activity, sport, or situation in which they are being utilized. In situations where the context shifts, such as when dealing with special populations or older people, the HRF–SRF model inevitably loses its applicability.

Developing skill-related fitness components like speed, agility, and coordination enhances athletic performance. However, these components can only be used as comprehensive indicators of physical fitness considering the context of the activity, sport, or situation. The concept of speed, agility, and coordination in sports must be modified to apply to senior citizens' specific circumstances.

The use of the terms health-related and skill-related further demonstrates that the components are perceived in two different contexts. However, due to the subjective nature of the classification of physical fitness, these terminologies require optimization to be effective.

The term "subjective" indicates that the definition depends on the knowledge and experience of the individual using the term or phrase. On the other hand, the health-related and skill-related components are so well established that even a slight modification to the classification of another component could spark a debate. People can only associate health-related components with health because of their perceived importance to health rather than their athletic abilities. This is an example of subjectivity (Eshun, 2021).

When people only associate balance, which is considered to be skill-related, with sports and skills, they miss the perspective that balance is also essential in health-related contexts, particularly among older people and people who are taking medication. This is as a result of the example given previously. In addition, it is essential to know that the context of balance in sports, which is related to skills, is not the same as the context of balance among older people (health-related).

In light of this, the categorization of fitness components should not solely be determined by the context in which they are performed or by their association with either health or skills. Components of fitness are subjective and interconnected with one another. Suppose a person sees a fitness component as connected with a skill-related context. Another person may see it as having a connection with a health-related context. The solution to this problem is yet to be something we are aware of now. On the other hand, we will undoubtedly discuss it in this book.

HRF is not a prerequisite for SRF

Teenage athletes have nutritional health requirements for their daily training and competition, according to Sports Dietitians Australia (SDA). These requirements are in addition to the demands of growth and development that they face (Desbrow et al., 2014). As a result, we can reach a consensus that athletic participation requires a healthy body and proper nutrition (Pate et al., 2000). The fact that HRF components like flexibility, cardiorespiratory endurance, muscular strength, and muscular endurance are considered, by some practitioners, to be prerequisites for sports and physical activity is something that we find challenging to comprehend. This is because these components are involved in the processes related to skill-related fitness. Regarding the HRF–SRF model, we came across an unwritten understanding from a few practitioners, which needs to be considered.

According to our understanding, the nervous system, particularly the brain, is the first prerequisite for skill-related fitness. This is because, with motor control, both gross and fine movements would be possible to accomplish. The nervous system controls movement, regulates bodily processes, prevents individuals from becoming fatigued, increases their tolerance to exercise, and enables them to exercise without exhaustion (Mustafa et al., 2019). Through the coordination and regulation of movement, it is responsible for regulating movement, balance, coordination, thoughts, feelings, and memory, and it even controls respiration, digestion, and heartbeat (Driskell, 2022; Healthdirect, 2021). The brain monitors and controls all of the body's organs by receiving and processing impulses from both the inside and outside (Lavanya et al., 2022; Namazi, 2017). The coordination of muscle forces that results in movement is accomplished by sharing synaptic inputs between clusters of motoneurons. In addition, the central nervous system filters synaptic noise by adjusting the relative strengths of these inputs, enabling precisely controlled movement (Farina et al., 2016). Although some muscles may function independently, most vertebrates' muscles are controlled by their nervous systems (Hardy, 2023).

We conclude that flexibility, cardiorespiratory endurance, muscular strength, and muscular endurance are not prerequisites for skill-related fitness; they are used in conjunction with skill-related fitness. Physical activities and exercise can strengthen these HRF and SRF components.

If an athlete experiences dizziness, for example, they would not be able to stand in the playing area because they would not have the ability to maintain their balance, which is classified as SRF. The development of motor skills, the reduction of the risk of falling, and the increase in participation in a wide range of physical activities are all factors that contribute to the importance of balance in skill-related fitness (Jahanbakhsh et al., 2020). Supplying a solid foundation for movement execution and ensuring that the body is in the best possible alignment helps to improve performance in activities that require coordination, agility, and accuracy. The fear of falling or getting hurt is reduced when balance is improved, leading to increased participation in physical activities and improved functional capacities for a lifestyle high in physical activity (Stanmore et al., 2019).

As a compelling illustration of the crucial "prerequisite" role that balance plays as an essential fitness component, the case of stroke patients serves as an essential example. A cerebral vascular accident (CVA) victim may experience a loss of function that is either temporary or permanent as a result of damage to brain tissue. Stroke is a common nervous system illness caused by irregular blood circulation in the brain (Chen, 2022). When someone has a stroke, the muscles in their trunk are affected in addition to the muscles in their limbs. Motor paralysis of the limb muscles on one side of the body results from hemiplegia, which occurs after a stroke. However, trunk muscles on the body's ipsilateral and contralateral sides are also weakened (Samal et al., 2021). Recovery from a stroke requires a variety of skills, including the ability to grasp a variety of objects and the ability to perform vital daily chores independently. Even the recovery of functional sitting balance may be critical. Regaining control of the trunk has consequently been one of the primary focuses of stroke therapy (Jeong & Chung, 2023).

Balance is also dependent on the visual and auditory channels of the brain, and it is an essential component in maintaining equilibrium throughout static and dynamic activity (Bednarczuk et al., 2021; Teaford et al., 2023). A diminished capacity for balance can lead to a fear of falling, significantly impacting the quality of life and decreasing the ability to carry out routine activities (Roberts et al., 2022). A steady support base is essential for adequately executing activities (Sitthiracha et al., 2021). Evaluating and assisting in improving balance is essential because poor balance increases the risk of falling and disrupts a person's ability to stand and walk. Balance is essential in such activities (Soleimani et al., 2022; Stanmore et al., 2019).

Participation in sports or other forms of physical activity does not necessarily require HRF components despite these components being essential for overall health and well-being. Contributing to developing SRF components through participation in sports and physical activity can benefit health. On the other hand, the assumption that HRF components' development comes before SRF components in sports environments is only partially founded on proven facts. Although HRF components like cardiorespiratory fitness and muscular endurance are essential for overall health and well-being, it is possible that these components are not the only factors that determine health, success in sports, or success in some other physical activities.

Despite having suboptimal levels of specific health-related fitness components, many athletes have been discovered to excel in their respective sports. A powerlifter, for instance, might have a high level of muscular strength, but they might not necessarily have optimal levels of cardiorespiratory fitness like other athletes. Similarly, a sprinter might have exceptional speed and power but need optimal muscle endurance or flexibility.

As an additional point of interest, the relationship between HRF and SRF components is intricate and ever-changing. It is possible that improving SRF components like agility, balance, coordination, and reaction time will also have a positive impact on HRF components like strengthening the cardiovascular system and increasing muscular endurance. It is also essential to remember that the relationship between HRF and SRF components can change depending on the individual's intended outcomes and the particular demands of the sport or physical activity. For instance, a professional marathon runner might need to prioritize cardiorespiratory fitness and endurance, whereas a gymnast might need to prioritize balance, coordination, and flexibility. Both of these are essential elements of physical fitness.

One of two possibilities exists: either the notion that HRF comes before SRF is incorrect or our comprehension of the situation needs to be revised somehow. We agree that being in the best possible health condition is a precondition for carrying out daily activities effectively and efficiently. Because of this, before beginning an exercise program, we make it a habit to conduct regular assessments of the student's health conditions and determine whether or not they are prepared to participate in physical activity. On the other hand, HRF would not be beneficial in this setting.

The optimum health condition, which includes a healthy body composition, normal body functions, and a condition known as homeostasis, is that which we consider to be the prerequisite rather than HRF. It is necessary to revise our current understanding of physical fitness, which should consider that healthy body condition, which is an entirely different set of components, comes before high-resistance fitness (HRF) for the first time. Despite this, these are merely our presumptions, which can be researched in academic settings to gain a deeper comprehension of the complexities of the construct.

Imbalanced health and skill components

We brought up that our understanding of physical fitness needs to be revised to reflect that a healthy body condition is a prerequisite for performing well in physical activity. This is indicated in a study (Gu et al., 2016) that shows that the benefits of PA on physical and mental health are associated with four fitness measures.

In the meantime, the current fitness concept grouped flexibility, muscular strength, endurance, and body composition to form the health-related suite. This was done to better understand the relationship between these factors and health. According to what we have discussed, these components are shared by both skill-related and health-related fitness (Figure 1.3).

Significant research has been conducted to establish a correlation between the remaining components and health to justify their "health-relatedness." For instance, Smith and colleagues (2014) discovered that muscle fitness positively correlates with bone health, self-esteem, and perceived sports competence and negatively correlates with adiposity. This finding emphasizes the health benefits of muscular strength, which makes the component health related. Motor competence is positively associated with cardiorespiratory and musculoskeletal fitness, and there is strong evidence that it is inversely related to body weight status (Cattuzzo et al., 2016). However, this does not conceal the fact that the components are still based on performance.

The performance aspect of physical fitness is given more weight than the other aspects, resulting in an imbalance between the concepts under consideration. Among all the other components presented by the HRF–SRF component, body composition is the only one that can theoretically be considered a direct health component based on anthropometry, not performance. In contrast, ten other components are only related to health. However, the irony is that some negatively correlate with adiposity and body weight status (Smith et al., 2014; Cattuzzo et al., 2016).

High emphasis on optimum levels and disregarding
personal goals and task requirements

In our observation, classifying fitness components into HRF or SRF components does not consider an individual's goals or the context in which the tasks are performed. There is a tendency to concentrate solely on a particular aspect of physical fitness, which may neglect other equally important aspects.

Swann and colleagues (2020) found that unstructured goals in physical activity can be more psychologically beneficial than SMART or do-your-best goals. They suggested that fitness goals must be adaptable and aligned with individual preferences to boost engagement and performance. This indicates that it is unnecessary to emphasize optimum physical fitness levels.

The definition of physical fitness as a performance indicator explicitly mentions the ability to perform tasks effectively and efficiently. On the other hand, the requirements for effective and efficient tasks have yet to be mainly described. Because the primary criterion is optimum levels and performance, we are curious about the terms or criteria used for effectiveness and efficiency. This objective is not attainable even though it is essential to achieve optimal fitness levels.

For instance, experienced endurance athletes' effort distribution and performance changed without commonly available task-related feedback, highlighting the importance of realistic and activity-specific fitness programs (Smits et al., 2016). Experienced athletes can get comparable results by using data about their bodies and environments, highlighting the need for task-specific training and the possibility of using different pacing strategies based on the data.

The task requirement should serve as the basis for determining the effectiveness and efficiency of performance. In sprint racing competitions, achieving the highest possible speed is essential. On the other hand, controlled speed is helpful in other sports, which require coordination of several different motor control components and speed control. Additionally, we do not believe that individuals who participate in Zumba® Parties do so to reach their maximum heart rate or make the most of their maximum oxygen uptake capacities. Instead, they want to keep a close eye on their breathing and heart rate to ensure they can stay long and enjoy the exercise party without any risks.

Although we advocate for optimal training and enhancement of fitness components, fitness should be realistic and flexible, considering both personal goals and the requirements of the task at hand. Rather than focusing on reaching a certain level of physical fitness, Warburton and Bredin (2017) argue that people would benefit from just increasing their level of physical activity. Fitness is not a competition to achieve the highest possible level; instead, it is about enhancing the quality of life.

Isolated fitness components

A person's level of physical fitness can be better understood by breaking down the concept of physical fitness into its parts, often broken down into separate categories. Historically, the various aspects of physical fitness (Kolimechkov, 2017) have been considered in isolation rather than understood as a cohesive and interdependent whole. Using this method, an individual's performance level in each fitness component, such as cardiovascular endurance, muscular strength, muscular endurance, flexibility, and body composition, is evaluated separately. The results of this evaluation are then used to determine the individual's overall level of physical fitness. While providing valuable information about an individual's physical abilities, this approach has limitations in understanding an individual's overall physical fitness. Because these components are interdependent, it is possible that a comprehensive picture of an individual's overall physical fitness cannot be obtained by examining them separately.

It is possible to obtain valuable information about an individual's level of performance in each area of fitness by evaluating each component of fitness separately, but this approach does not take into account the fitness component separately; however, neither does this approach consider the interdependence of these components. For instance, an individual's capacity to perform strength and flexibility exercises is likely to be influenced by their cardiovascular endurance. Similarly, an individual's muscular strength will likely impact their capacity to exercise their cardiovascular endurance. Due to the interdependence of these components, it is possible that evaluating them separately will provide a partial picture of an individual's overall physical fitness.

In addition, evaluating the components of physical fitness on an individual basis yields valuable information, but it ignores the context and goals of the individual. The importance of each fitness component is determined by several factors, including age, gender, lifestyle, and genetics, which all play a role in determining fitness. For instance, the requirements for physical fitness are different for individuals who are sedentary and those who are athletes. The requirements of a particular occupation or sport are distinct from those of general health. For instance, a firefighter is expected to have a higher endurance level than an office worker. Components being evaluated in isolation without considering the goals and context can result in misleading assessments. The optimization of physical fitness programs for overall health, wellness, and performance can be accomplished through the utilization of an all-encompassing assessment strategy.

In a holistic approach to physical fitness, these components would be viewed as interconnected and interdependent, with the understanding that optimal performance in one area is likely to be influenced by performance in other areas. For instance, a person with a high level of muscular strength and endurance is likely also to possess a higher level of cardiovascular endurance and flexibility.

When we take a holistic approach to physical fitness, we can better understand an individual's overall physical capabilities and their potential for improvement. This can also lead to a comprehensive approach to programming physical fitness, in which each component is addressed to optimize overall physical fitness rather than focusing solely on specific areas of strength or weakness.

Prioritization of specific components over others

The fitness components model may give specific components more weight than others, which may result in neglecting other equally important components. It is necessary to simultaneously improve cardiovascular endurance and muscular strength (Bjarnason-Wehrens, 2019). However, putting cardiovascular endurance ahead of muscular strength may result in attention to strength training, leading to muscular imbalances and an increased risk of injury. Placing a higher priority on muscular strength and endurance might neglect cardiovascular exercise, resulting in an increased risk of cardiovascular disease.

Additionally, some people are solely concerned with selected fitness components. They may overlook other essential aspects of their physical health. For instance, there is a tendency to concentrate solely on developing muscular strength within the context of health-related fitness (HRF) while ignoring balance and coordination, which are considered part of the separate context of skill-related fitness (SRF). Taking this approach may result in an imbalance in physical fitness, the neglect of essential SRF components, and an increase in the likelihood of experiencing an injury (Cadore et al., 2014).

In addition, the relative importance of each component may differ from person to person depending on the individual's necessities and objectives. An endurance athlete, for instance, might prioritize cardiovascular endurance more than muscular strength, whereas a powerlifter might put more emphasis on muscular strength than cardiovascular endurance. Nevertheless, even in these circumstances, it is essential to balance all aspects of fitness to guarantee overall health and reduce the likelihood of injuries (Milanović et al., 2015).

To achieve overall health and fitness, it is essential to acknowledge that every aspect of fitness is interconnected and contributes to overall fitness. A balanced approach to fitness components is essential to minimize the risk of injury and maximize overall physical fitness (Karatrantou et al., 2016). Neglecting one or many of the components can have negative consequences, so it is essential to use a balanced approach.

When it comes to physical fitness, it is essential to take a holistic approach that considers the interdependence of all aspects of fitness, as well as the particular objectives and requirements of the individual (Esteban-Cornejo et al., 2014). It is possible to achieve optimal health, well-being, and performance in particular activities or sports by adopting a well-rounded approach to physical fitness that considers health and skill components equally important.

The danger of strong HRF component emphasis in the PE curriculum

In recent years, health and fitness have taken precedence over the traditional goals of improving students' power, speed, agility, balance, and coordination in physical education (PE) programs. The growing public consciousness surrounding the interconnected nature of obesity, cardiovascular disease, and diabetes has most likely contributed to a resurgence of interest in health and fitness-related activities. According to DeMet and Wahl-Alexander (2019), there is a need to improve physical education (PE) curricula because skill-related components should be standard in PE. However, they are not currently utilized in most PE programs.

There is a danger that physical education programs will place too much emphasis on health-related fitness and not enough on skill-related fitness. The latter is crucial for developing motor skills, success in athletic pursuits, and overall physical literacy. Due to this disparity, students may not learn the fundamental motor skills and movement patterns required to participate in various physical activities. Myer and colleagues (2015) state that the existing recommendations for children's physical activity put too much emphasis on the quantitative components of exercise and specific health-related features of fitness and not enough on the critical role of early motor skill development.

Physical education programs that do not focus on skill development have repercussions for kids of all ages. When kids and teens do not have enough time to work on their motor skills – which include things like balance, coordination, agility, power, and speed – it can be hard for them to get moving, play sports, and learn about physical fitness. Thus, as these people age, they may become less active and sedentary. Falling and related injuries are already common among the senior population, and ignoring these factors can make their physical function decline even worse. Faigenbaum and colleagues (2015) demonstrate that using strength and skill-based training in primary school physical education improves children's aerobic capacity and muscular fitness, highlighting the importance of a balanced approach that includes both health- and skill-related fitness components.

Finally, while health-related fitness is critical for addressing public health issues, a balanced physical education program that emphasizes both skill-related and health-related components is essential for promoting overall physical development and encouraging physical activity forever. A holistic view will allow us to mitigate the effects of a health-centric curriculum while providing individuals with the necessary resources to lead active, healthy lifestyles.

Summary

Contemporary fitness concepts face several challenges, including clarity regarding classification, organization, and the relationship between fitness components.

The operationalization of the health-related fitness (HRF) and skill-related fitness (SRF) model needs to be clarified, resulting in various authors offering several interpretations. Because of this ambiguity, there is confusion and a lack of logical cohesion among the various components of fitness, making it challenging to measure physical fitness directly.

Fitness is a subjective concept, and despite its widespread popularity, only some definitions of fitness are universally recognized and accepted. The HRF–SRF model has significantly influenced our understanding of physical fitness; however, the interpretation of this model is highly subjective and heavily dependent on the context in which it is used. The emergence of skill-related fitness components, such as speed, agility, and coordination, is essential for improving athletic performance; however, these components can only be used as comprehensive indicators if they consider the context of the activity, sport, or situation.

Due to the subjective nature of physical fitness classification, the terms health-related and skill-related require optimization to be effective. It is important to note that the relationship between HRF and SRF components is intricate and fluid. The former is necessary for achievement in sports or other forms of physical activity. The conventional understanding of physical fitness needs to be revised to consider that a healthy body condition is a precondition for performing physical activity levels.

In order to gain a better understanding of an individual's level of fitness, it is common practice to dissect physical fitness into its parts, which include cardiovascular endurance, muscular strength, muscular endurance, flexibility, and body composition. Because fitness is influenced by age, gender, lifestyle, and genetics, evaluating each component separately may not consider the individual's goals and the context in which they are being evaluated. In a holistic approach to physical fitness, these components would be viewed as interconnected and interdependent, with the understanding that optimal performance in one area is likely to be influenced by performance in other areas. It is essential to balance all aspects of fitness to optimize overall health and reduce the likelihood of experiencing an injury.

Review questions

1. What are some difficulties in classifying and arranging the fitness components covered in this chapter?
2. Why is the interdependence of fitness components viewed as a significant issue in modern understanding?
3. How do the issues with the existing concept of physical fitness relate to the 21st-century principles of inclusion and equity?
4. Why must the problems and restrictions be addressed with the contemporary HRF–SRF fitness components model?

5. How does the need for clarity in operationalizing physical fitness components impact our capacity to assess fitness effectively?
6. How are fitness components classified when their interpretation is subjective?
7. What role does context play in categorizing fitness components, and why is it crucial to consider this?
8. Why is it questioned in this chapter that health-related fitness (HRF) is a requirement for skill-related fitness (SRF)?
9. How is emphasizing optimum levels of physical fitness different from emphasizing normal levels?
10. What are the effects of favoring some fitness elements over others, and why is it crucial to have a balanced approach to fitness?

Discussion questions

1. How may the difficulties and ambiguities in categorizing fitness components be addressed to develop a comprehensive and helpful physical fitness model?
2. To what extent do the inclusiveness and fairness ideals of the 21st century affect how we define and assess physical fitness, and how may these ideals be included in fitness models?
3. How can the arbitrary interpretation of fitness components be improved to maintain consistency in evaluation and comprehension across various contexts?
4. How should the presumption that health-related fitness is required for skill-related fitness be reevaluated and possibly revised to reflect the complexity of physical fitness accurately?
5. What methods and tactics may be used to prioritize a fair and comprehensive picture of physical fitness that considers the interconnectedness of all fitness-related elements, personal objectives, and environmental factors?

References

Bednarczuk, G., Wiszomirska, I., Rutkowska, I., & Skowroński, W. (2021). Role of vision in static balance in persons with and without visual impairments. *European Journal of Physical and Rehabilitation Medicine, 57*(4), 593–599. https://doi.org/10.23736/S1973-9087.21.06425-X

Bjarnason-Wehrens, B. (2019). Recommendations for resistance exercise in cardiac rehabilitation: Do they need reconsideration? *European Journal of Preventive Cardiology, 26*, 1479–1482. https://doi.org/10.1177/2047487319856124

Cadore, E., Pinto, R., Bottaro, M., & Izquierdo, M. (2014). Strength and endurance training prescription in healthy and frail elderly. *Aging and Disease, 5*(3), 183–195. https://doi.org/10.14336/AD.2014.0500183

Cattuzzo, M., Henrique, R., Ré, A., Oliveira, I., Melo, B., Moura, M., Araújo, R., & Stodden, D. (2016). Motor competence and health related physical fitness in youth: A systematic review. *Journal of Science and Medicine in Sport, 19*(2), 123–129. https://doi.org/10.1016/j.jsams.2014.12.004

Chen, Y. (2022). Disturbed cerebral circulation and metabolism matters: A preface to the special issue "Stroke and Energy Metabolism". *Journal of Neurochemistry, 160*(1), 10–12. https://doi.org/10.1111/jnc.15552

Čuprika, A., Fernāte, A., & Čupriks, L. (2019). Essential characteristics of the fitness concept and the area of fitness in Latvia and the world. *Society Integration Education Proceedings of the International Scientific Conference* (Vol. 4, pp. 91–100). http://dx.doi.org/10.17770/sie2019vol4.3997

DeMet, T., & Wahl-Alexander, Z. (2019). Integrating skill-related components of fitness into physical education. *Strategies, 32*(5), 10–17. https://doi.org/10.1080/08924562.2019.1637315

Desbrow, B., McCormack, J., Burke, L. M., Cox, G. R., Fallon, K., Hislop, M., Logan, R., Marino, N., Sawyer, S. M., Shaw, G., Star, A., Vidgen, H., & Leveritt, M. (2014). Sports dietitians Australia position statement: Sports nutrition for the adolescent athlete. *International Journal of Sports Nutrition and Exercise Metabolism, 24*(5), 570–584.

Driskell, J. (2022). Introduction to the nervous system. In *All about anxiety: An introductory guide to neuroscience, assessment, and intervention*. https://pressbooks.pub/allaboutanxiety/chapter/chapter-2-introduction-to-the-nervous-system/

Eshun, A. K. (2021). *Effect of twelve week skill related fitness intervention on shooting accuracy among high school basketball players in the Cape Coast Metropolis, Ghana* [Doctoral dissertation, University of Cape Coast]. https://ir.ucc.edu.gh/xmlui/bitstream/handle/123456789/6456/ESHUN%2c%202021.pdf?sequence=1&isAllowed=y

Esteban-Cornejo, I., Tejero-González, C. M., Martinez-Gomez, D., del-Campo, J., González-Galo, A., Padilla-Moledo, C., Sallis, J. F., & Veiga, O. L. (2014). Independent and combined influence of the components of physical fitness on academic performance in youth. *The Journal of Pediatrics, 165*(2), 306–312.e2. https://doi.org/10.1016/j.jpeds.2014.04.044

Faigenbaum, A. D., Bush, J. A., McLoone, R. P., Kreckel, M. C., Farrell, A., Ratamess, N. A., & Kang, J. (2015). Benefits of strength and skill-based training during primary school physical education. *The Journal of Strength & Conditioning Research, 29*(5), 1255–1262. https://doi.org/10.1519/JSC.0000000000000812

Farina, D., Negro, F., Muceli, S., & Enoka, R. M. (2016). Principles of motor unit physiology evolve with advances in technology. *Physiology, 31*(2), 83–94. https://doi.org/10.1152/physiol.00040.2015

Gu, X., Chang, M., & Solmon, M. (2016). Physical activity, physical fitness, and health-related quality of life in school-aged children. *Journal of Teaching in Physical Education, 35*, 117–126. https://doi.org/10.1123/JTPE.2015-0110

Hardy, G. (2023). Exploring the muscular tissue and its types in human body. *Black Sea Scientific Journal Of Academic Research, 60*(1), 1–2. http://doi.org/10.36962/GBSSJAR/60.1.001

Healthdirect. (2021). *Nervous system*. https://www.healthdirect.gov.au/nervous-system

Jahanbakhsh, H., Sohrabi, M., Kakhki, A., & Khodashenas, E. (2020). The effect of task-specific balance training program in dual-task and single-task conditions on balance performance in children with developmental coordination disorder. *Acta Gymnica, 50*(1), 28–37. https://doi.org/10.5507/ag.2020.003Jeong, S., & Chung, Y. (2023, December). Task-oriented training with abdominal drawing-in maneuver in sitting position for trunk control, balance, and activities of daily living in patients with stroke: A pilot randomized controlled trial. In *Healthcare* (Vol. 11, No. 23, p. 3092). MDPI. https://doi.org/10.3390/healthcare11233092Karatrantou, K., Gerodimos, V., Häkkinen, K., & Zafeiridis, A. (2016). health-promoting effects of serial vs. integrated combined strength and aerobic training. *International Journal of Sports Medicine, 38*, 55–64. https://doi.org/10.1055/s-0042-116495

Kolimechkov, S. (2017). Physical fitness assessment in children and adolescents: A systematic review. *European Journal of Physical Education and Sport Science, 3*(4). https://doi.org/10.5281/zenodo.495725

Lavanya, V. K., Kumar, A., Nagaraj, S., & Kumar, N. (2022). Critical understanding of Shiras Shareeram from perspective of nervous system. *RGUHS Journal of AYUSH Sciences, 9*(1). http://doi.org/10.26715/rjas.9_1_6

Milanović, Z., Sporiš, G., & Weston, M. (2015). Effectiveness of high-intensity interval training (hit) and continuous endurance training for vo2max improvements: A systematic review and meta-analysis of controlled trials. *Sports Medicine, 45*, 1469–1481. https://doi.org/10.1007/s40279-015-0365-0

Mustafa, M. S., Li Yin Ong, M., Ab Hamid, S. A., & Kuan, G. (2019, September). Transcranial direct current stimulation enhances skill-related fitness among the under-15 football players. In *International conference on movement, health and exercise* (pp. 511–518). Springer. https://doi.org/10.1007/978-981-15-3270-2_52

Myer, G. D., Faigenbaum, A. D., Edwards, N. M., Clark, J. F., Best, T. M., & Sallis, R. E. (2015). Sixty minutes of what? A developing brain perspective for activating children with an integrative exercise approach. *British Journal of Sports Medicine, 49*(23), 1510–1516. https://doi.org/10.1136/bjsports-2014-093661

Namazi, H. (2017). Can we study the correlation between human brain signal and other biological signals? *Journal of Neuroscience, 2*(2), 1–3. http://dx.doi.org/10.20431/2456-057X.0202003

Pate, R. R., Trost, S. G., Levin, S., & Dowda, M. (2000). Sports participation and health-related behaviors among US youth. *Archives of Pediatrics & Adolescent Medicine, 154*(9), 904–911. http://doi.org/10.1001/archpedi.154.9.904

Rhodes, R., McEwan, D., & Rebar, A. (2019). Theories of physical activity behaviour change: A history and synthesis of approaches. *Psychology of Sport and Exercise, 42*, 100–109. https://doi.org/10.1016/j.psychsport.2018.11.010

Roberts, H. J., Johnson, K. M., Sullivan, J. E., & Hoppes, C. W. (2022). Fear of falling avoidance behavior is associated with balance and dynamic gait performance in community-dwelling older adults: a cross-sectional study. *Journal of Geriatric Physical Therapy, 46*(1), 82–89. https://doi.org/10.1519/JPT.0000000000000349

Samal, S. N., Samal, S. S., Ingale, N., Chaudhary, S., & Gawande, V. (2021). Efficacy of core strengthening exercises on Swissball versus conventional exercises for improving trunk balance in hemiplegic patients following stroke. *International Journal of Research in Pharmaceutical Sciences, 12*, 889–893. https://doi.org/10.26452/IJRPS.V12I1.4219

Santana, C., Azevedo, L., Cattuzzo, M., Hill, J., Andrade, L., & Prado, W. (2017). Physical fitness and academic performance in youth: A systematic review. *Scandinavian Journal of Medicine & Science in Sports, 27*. https://doi.org/10.1111/sms.12773

Sitthiracha, P., Eungpinichpong, W., & Chatchawan, U. (2021). Effect of progressive step marching exercise on balance ability in the elderly: A cluster randomized clinical trial. *International Journal of Environmental Research and Public Health, 18*(6), 3146. https://doi.org/10.3390/ijerph18063146

Smith, J., Eather, N., Morgan, P., Plotnikoff, R., Faigenbaum, A., & Lubans, D. (2014). The health benefits of muscular fitness for children and adolescents: A systematic review and meta-analysis. *Sports Medicine, 44*, 1209–1223. https://doi.org/10.1007/s40279-014-0196-4

Smits, B., Polman, R., Otten, B., Pepping, G., & Hettinga, F. (2016). Cycling in the absence of task-related feedback: Effects on pacing and performance. *Frontiers in Physiology, 7.* https://doi.org/10.3389/fphys.2016.00348

Soleimani, R., Alvandi, H., Azari, N., Mobasheri, M., Hasanzadeh, A., & Bagherikholenjani, F. (2022). Impact of balance training on fear of falling and fall rate in older women. *Journal of Education and Community Health*, *9*(3), 155–161. https://doi.org/10.34172/jech.2022.23

Stanmore, E. K., Mavroeidi, A., de Jong, L. D., Skelton, D. A., Sutton, C. J., Benedetto, V., Munford, L. A., Meekes, W., Bell, V., & Todd, C. (2019). The effectiveness and cost-effectiveness of strength and balance Exergames to reduce falls risk for people aged 55 years and older in UK assisted living facilities: A multi-centre, cluster randomised controlled trial. *BMC Medicine, 17*(1), 49. https://doi.org/10.1186/s12916-019-1278-9

Swann, C., Hooper, A., Schweickle, M., Peoples, G., Mullan, J., Hutto, D., Allen, M., & Vella, S. (2020). Comparing the effects of goal types in a walking session with healthy adults: Preliminary evidence for open goals in physical activity. *Psychology of Sport and Exercise*, *47*, 101475. https://doi.org/10.1016/J.PSYCHSPORT.2019.01.003 Teaford, M., Mularczyk, Z. J., Gernon, A., Cannon, S., Kobel, M., & Merfeld, D. M. (2023). Joint contributions of auditory, proprioceptive and visual cues on human balance. *Multisensory Research*, *36*(8), 865–890. https://doi.org/10.1163/22134808-bja10113 Utesch, T., Dreiskämper, D., Strauss, B., & Naul, R. (2017). The development of the physical fitness construct across childhood. *Scandinavian Journal of Medicine & Science in Sports*, *28*, 212–219. https://doi.org/10.1111/sms.12889

Warburton, D., & Bredin, S. (2017). Health benefits of physical activity: A systematic review of current systematic reviews. *Current Opinion in Cardiology*, *32*, 541–556. https://doi.org/10.1097/HCO.0000000000000437

3

THEORETICAL FRAMEWORK

Nguyen Tra Giang and Oliver Napila Gomez

This chapter aims to simplify the understanding of physical fitness by presenting the proponents' positionality, advocacy, and theoretical perspectives. It advocates for a holistic and inclusive framework for physical fitness, addressing the fragmented understanding of health-related fitness (HRF) and skill-related fitness (SRF) components. The chapter acknowledges the complexity of fitness as a multifaceted construct and emphasizes the need for inclusive and accessible fitness assessment and discourse. Existing fitness models often involve separate, interconnected components, questioning the preeminence of HRF components over SRF components. It emphasizes the importance of balance, traditionally classified as SRF components, for health, especially in the older population. A paradigm shift towards a holistic fitness model aligned with transformative worldviews and systems theory is needed, reflecting the dynamic interplay of various body systems and their interaction with the environment. The chapter calls for a unified fitness framework that redefines physical fitness to encompass all aspects of health and skill-matching task requirements. It advocates for social justice, accommodates diverse populations, and facilitates communication between practitioners, making fitness evaluation and improvement a goal accessible to everyone.

Outcome

By the end of this chapter, you will be able to

- evaluate the reflexivity, leading to improved clarity in terminology and contributing to inclusive fitness assessments

DOI: 10.4324/9781003502937-4

- analyze how various body systems interact to support physical activity and overall well-being, using this knowledge to design personalized fitness plans
- investigate how skill-related fitness components are linked to enhanced health, well-being, and disease prevention
- explore how the transformative worldview and systems theory can help organize and integrate various fitness components, ensuring a comprehensive evaluation of an individual's overall fitness

A holistic approach to physical fitness

This chapter investigates the multifaceted nature of physical fitness and its implications for individuals looking to improve their overall health and wellness. The importance of unifying the concept of physical fitness and its evaluation through physiological fitness is emphasized, as is the advocacy for holistic methodologies that maintain the essence of fitness. Additionally, the enhancement of clarity through terminology revisions and attribute-based categorization for inclusive assessments is done.

The chapter also investigates physiological fitness's role in health-related fitness, particularly emphasizing the morphologic, muscular, cardiorespiratory, motor, and metabolic dimensions. This article highlights the significance of skill-related fitness components, such as power, speed, reaction time, hand–eye coordination, agility, joint flexibility, and cardiorespiratory fitness, as well as the significance of balance as a health-related fitness indicator, particularly for the older population.

In addition, the chapter delves into the transformative worldview and systems theory, both of which raise questions about the established power dynamics and social structures. These theories advocate for inclusive, equitable, and holistic fitness practices. This chapter aims to support social justice and inclusion in fitness practices, propose a unified fitness framework, provide a comprehensive definition of physical fitness, and design a common language for researchers and practitioners.

Our reflexivity

The foundation of our work is based on our awareness of the following: (1) the necessity of unifying the concept of physical fitness and evaluation through physiological fitness; (2) the importance of taking a holistic approach and preserving the essence of physical fitness; (3) the possibility of improving the clarity of terms, revising terminology, and categorizing individuals based on attributes to facilitate inclusive evaluation.

Unifying concepts and assessments through physiological fitness

One of the most recent developments in the field of fitness is a concept that encompasses the effective operation of all of the body's systems, including the anatomical, muscular, circulatory, nervous, and glandular systems (Singh & Trikha, 2022). In the context of physical activity, physiological fitness refers to how organ-level systems, such as the musculoskeletal, cardiovascular, and neurological systems, collaborate to facilitate physical activity (Stewart, 2003; Weening-Dijksterhuis, 2014). In order to achieve the highest possible level of physical fitness, it is necessary for all of these systems, including the muscles and bones, the heart and blood vessels, the brain and nerves, to operate effectively. For instance, muscle strength and cardiovascular fitness are essential attributes for day-to-day activities and overall health. In order to achieve coordinated movement, it is also essential to have effective neurological coordination. Individuals can concentrate on particular aspects of their physiological fitness to achieve optimal health when they better understand the significance of these systems. However, there is a need for published material on physiological fitness, and no framework that uses the idea of physiological fitness has been developed.

On the other hand, physical fitness refers to morphological characteristics such as body mass, height, percentage of body fat, and body composition (Gumieniak, 2017). Physiological fitness is an essential unifying concept for overall physical fitness, although it has yet to be widely known in many students' educational institutions.

There has been a shift toward a comprehensive and multidimensional approach to measuring health-related fitness. This shift has occurred in addition to incorporating physiological fitness from the previous approach. Frehlich and colleagues (2022) have revised the traditional five health-related fitness components to include morphologic, muscular, cardiorespiratory, motor, and metabolic components. This update was made regarding the traditional five components. Body composition and flexibility are included in the morphologic component, whereas grip strength and endurance are included in the muscular component. The cardiorespiratory component measures both the maximum oxygen consumption and the sustained cardiorespiratory capacity. The metabolic component (Corbin et al., 2008) measures blood lipid and glucose levels, while the motor component measures balance and proprioceptive activity. Both components are used to assess performance. This multidimensional approach can obtain a comprehensive picture of overall health-related fitness.

This shift toward a comprehensive and multidimensional approach is essential because it acknowledges that health-related fitness is not only about physical appearance or cardiovascular endurance but also includes a variety of other factors, such as muscle strength, flexibility, and balance. By adopting a holistic approach to health-related fitness, it is possible to better understand the various aspects of fitness, including how they interact with one another and contribute to overall health.

Other performance-based indicators, born out of operationalization, are also essential for overall health, even though HRF fitness components are essential for health and wellness. One such component of fitness that needs to be addressed is skill-related fitness, which is not typically taught in physical education and is infrequently evaluated in general health and fitness evaluations (DeMet & Wahl-Alexander, 2019; Spaniol et al., 2013). On the other hand, skill-related fitness has been associated with improved cardiovascular health (Parsons, 2017), highlighting the necessity of considering it when evaluating health-related fitness.

Balance is another essential aspect frequently overlooked in aging, even though it is linked to accidents, disability, and even death (Blodgett et al., 2020). Poor balance is the primary independent factor contributing to accidental falls, particularly among elderly individuals (Gong, 2020; Casaña et al., 2021). This highlights the significance of evaluating balance as a health-related fitness indicator.

Performance-based indicators, such as power, speed, reaction time, hand–eye coordination, and agility, are also essential for overall health. These indicators include skill-related fitness and balance, which are equally important (Bianco et al., 2015). Additionally, joint flexibility is one of the most critical factors in determining athletic performance in sprinters and endurance runners (Suga et al., 2021). This highlights the importance of considering joint flexibility as a skill-based fitness indicator. Like the previous example, cardiorespiratory fitness has been linked to increased muscular mass and improved balance (Lintu et al., 2016), highlighting the significance of evaluating it as a skill-based fitness indicator.

Therefore, to provide a comprehensive evaluation of an individual's overall fitness, it is necessary to take a unified approach to the concepts utilized in fitness. Suppose individuals consider the interconnectedness of these fitness components. In that case, they can identify areas where they can improve their fitness and achieve optimal physical fitness and overall health.

- Physical fitness is a multifaceted construct that involves attributes and abilities to support an individual's physiological functions for health purposes.
- Unifying fitness components provides a comprehensive and multidimensional approach to measuring health and skill components.
- Physiological fitness is an essential unifying fitness concept for overall physical fitness.
- A unified approach to health and performance-related fitness concepts is needed to comprehensively evaluate an individual's overall fitness.

Holistic approach and the essence preservation of physical fitness

Physical fitness is a multifaceted construct involving attributes and abilities related to a person's ability to perform exercises and functions, with implications for their current and future health outcomes. In Chapter 1, we discussed the concept of physical fitness and the distinction between its conceptual and operational definitions. We also emphasized that physical fitness is a multifaceted construct. The performance-based indicators used to indirectly evaluate the concept of physical fitness are the primary focus of the operational definition of physical fitness (Baumgartner et al., 2015). On the other hand, ambiguity and definitional problems may arise because the operational definition is becoming more prevalent than the conceptual definition.

In our argument, we advocated for the conceptual definition of physical fitness to be brought to the forefront. This definition encompasses a comprehensive understanding of the construct (holistic approach) and its connection to overall health and risk factors. Taking a holistic approach to fitness is essential because it emphasizes a comprehensive and all-encompassing perspective on physical fitness. This approach considers the individual in their entirety and acknowledges the interconnectedness of numerous factors relevant to health and skills. We can preserve the essence of physical fitness, implying that physical fitness can become a more valuable tool for practitioners and eliminate confusion caused by different interpretations if we prioritize the conceptual rather than the operational definition.

- The traditional approach to physical fitness has limitations, and a more holistic approach is necessary.
- Performance-based indicators can measure physical fitness, but the operational definition should differ from the construct's essence.

Clarity improvement of terms, terminology revisions, and attribute-based categorization for inclusive assessment

Those who need to become familiar with the terminology used in sports or athletics may need help comprehending performance-based terminology currently utilized in fitness models. Confusion and incorrect interpretation of fitness components are possible outcomes, particularly for individuals just starting their journey toward a healthy lifestyle.

Suppose the terminology that is used for fitness indicators were to be revised so that it reflected the physical fitness construct rather than a particular skill. In that case, it might provide a precise and concise method for classifying and measuring the various components of fitness. This is another approach that could be taken to unify the components of fitness to guarantee that all physical fitness components are unified indicators of overall physical fitness.

Employing attributes-based terminology makes it possible to shift the focus away from particular skills or movements and toward the qualities being measured or evaluated. This information may help individuals better understand the components of physical fitness and how they relate to their overall health and well-being.

A term that reflects physical fitness as an attribute, which has the potential to reflect a skill, can make it easy to measure and compare fitness components across different populations, such as athletes and nonathletes. This ease of measurement and comparison can be a significant benefit. The current skill-based terminology in fitness models is frequently geared toward athletes and sports performance. As a result, it is not easy to compare the fitness levels of individuals from different athletic backgrounds. Utilizing terminology based on attributes allows for measuring and comparing fitness components based on qualities such as strength, endurance, and flexibility. These qualities are relevant to athletes and individuals who do not participate in athletics. Regardless of an individual's athletic background or skill level, this can provide an inclusive and accurate method of evaluating physical fitness for all individuals.

The authors have identified some challenges in the realm of physical fitness, and the purpose of this book is to address those challenges and present potential solutions to make the concepts applicable to the context of the 21st century. Through their interpretation of "inter-related components," the authors hope to clarify the concepts of physical fitness. This interpretation may be difficult to understand for some individuals due to the numerous fitness components and models that are currently available. The authors hope that by presenting their proposed solutions, they will assist readers in gaining a better understanding of physical fitness and how it can be established in today's world. Individuals interested in enhancing their physical fitness in a manner that is pertinent and applicable to their lives are the target audience for this book, which aims to provide advice and practical insights to those individuals.

- The current performance-based terminology in fitness models can be challenging to understand, leading to confusion and misinterpreting fitness components.
- Revising the terminology for fitness indicators can provide a straightforward and concise way to contextualize and measure fitness components.
- Attribute-based terminology can shift the focus towards the qualities being measured, providing an inclusive and accurate way to assess physical fitness for all individuals.
- All fitness components are crucial for a person's fitness, regardless of the context (health or skill), and should be considered in physical fitness assessments.

Our theoretical perspective

A theoretical perspective offers a worldview that guides the development of the unified fitness model. This enables the authors to systematically organize and integrate the various fitness components and indicators. Because this viewpoint ensures that all aspects of physical fitness are considered and accounted for, it can comprehensively evaluate an individual's overall fitness.

To add insult to injury, the theoretical perspective also serves as a common language for researchers and practitioners in physical fitness. This helps ensure that the terminology used to describe fitness components and indicators is consistent and clear. If individuals use this common language, they will quickly understand their fitness assessments and identify areas where they can improve, which can help reduce confusion and misinterpretation of fitness components.

Transformative worldview

To begin, we used the transformative worldview as a foundation for our ideas to promote holistic thinking among fitness professionals and practitioners. The transformative worldview is a critical research approach addressing social justice, discrimination, and oppression (Mertens, 2021). It does this by challenging unequal power dynamics and social structures, which ultimately results in the reconstruction of knowledge and society in an equitable and just manner (Nieminen et al., 2023). Research grounded in this worldview strongly emphasizes social justice and inclusion, resulting in child-centered and child-inclusive research (Canosa et al., 2019).

In the same way that it seeks to challenge and transform unequal power dynamics and social structures, which may affect the accessibility and inclusivity of physical fitness practices and assessments, the transformative worldview is a research approach that aligns with the authors' assumptions. A critical–transformative approach to physical fitness could center on promoting social justice and inclusion and advocate for a comprehensive and holistic evaluation of an individual's overall fitness. This evaluation would include physiological and performance-related fitness components, and it would be grounded in attribute-based terminology that is both understandable and accessible to all individuals.

The authors advocate for adopting a transformative worldview in physical fitness, which aligns with their aim to challenge unequal power dynamics, promote social justice and inclusion, and develop a comprehensive and accessible approach to evaluating individual fitness that includes physiological and performance-related components.

Systems theory

In addition, our theoretical perspective is founded on the systems theory, which was initially developed and established in the 1940s by Ludwig von Bertalanffy. Subsequently, W. Ross Ashby and George Bateson further developed this theory (Wilkinson, 2011). The theory investigates various kinds of systems and the interdependencies that exist between them. It focuses on the dynamic relationships that exist between components, the hierarchical ordering of those components, and how those components interact with the environment through a variety of mechanisms, such as feedback, negative entropy, and new emergence (Lai & Huili Lin, 2017; Stichweh, 2011). Throughout infancy, every individual possesses a dynamical system that is interconnected and composed of significant subsystems that develop at different rates. These subsystems include cognitive, sensory, emotional, perceptual, and control systems (Myer et al., 2015).

We were led to the realization by the systems theory that the components of fitness are characteristics of the various systems that make up the body, such as the nervous system, the musculoskeletal system, the cardiorespiratory system, and the endocrine system. In light of this, we acknowledge that the human body is a complex system that is made up of a variety of components that are interdependent with one another. This is a fundamental concept in the field of systems theory. In addition to being an essential concept in systems theory, the various fitness components that make up each body system collaborate to keep the body in a state of equilibrium and adapt to its surroundings.

Furthermore, we acknowledge the hierarchical ordering of components within the body, an essential aspect of systems theory. In addition to being components of the extensive human body system, the nervous system, musculoskeletal system, cardiorespiratory system, and endocrine system are all components of the human body. Each of these systems possesses its own set of distinctive qualities and functions that contribute to the overall health and fitness of the individual.

Last, we acknowledge that the body experiences interactions with its surroundings through various mechanisms, a fundamental idea in systems theory. In order to preserve equilibrium and ensure survival, the body must continually adjust to the environment in which it finds itself. Feedback mechanisms, negative entropy, and emergence are all mechanisms described in systems theory. This adaptation involves all of these mechanisms.

The authors employ systems theory to conceptualize fitness components as attributes of the body's interdependent subsystems, emphasizing the dynamic relationships, hierarchical ordering, and environmental interactions among these components, aligning with the fundamental principles of systems theory.

Our objectives

Based on our positionality and theoretical perspective, we aim to propose a unified fitness framework that considers all fitness components and indicators holistically and comprehensively. This framework will also include a definition of physical fitness that is both comprehensive and inclusive, taking into account all components and attributes that contribute to overall well-being. In order to accommodate a wide variety of situations and objectives for physical fitness evaluations, we developed a framework that is also sufficiently adaptable. A common language was also developed for researchers and practitioners working in the field of physical fitness. This language includes a description that is both accurate and concise of each fitness component and the indicators that are associated with it. Additionally, this language makes use of common language or terminology.

In addition, we promote social justice and inclusion in physical fitness practices and assessments by utilizing a transformative worldview. This involves considering individual differences, cultural norms, a variety of lifestyles, and geographical locations. While preserving equilibrium and adjusting to the surrounding environment, we know the hierarchical ordering and interdependencies between the body's various components.

Summary

Within the scope of this chapter, the multifaceted nature of physical fitness and its implications for individuals looking to improve their overall health and wellness are discussed. The importance of unifying the concept of physical fitness and its evaluation through physiological fitness is emphasized, as is the advocacy for holistic methodologies that maintain the essence of fitness. Additionally, the enhancement of clarity through terminology revisions and attribute-based categorization for inclusive assessments is done. In addition, the chapter emphasizes the significance of physiological fitness in health-related fitness, with particular attention paid to the morphologic, muscular, cardiorespiratory, motor, and metabolic dimensions.

In addition, the chapter delves into the transformative worldview and systems theory, both of which raise questions about the established power dynamics and social structures. These theories advocate for inclusive, equitable, and holistic fitness practices. This chapter aims to advocate for social justice and inclusion in fitness practices, propose a unified fitness framework, provide a comprehensive definition of physical fitness, and design a common language for researchers and practitioners.

Physiological fitness is a relatively new concept in fitness that encompasses the efficient functioning of all of the body's systems, including the anatomical, muscular, circulatory, nervous, and glandular systems. It is an essential unifying concept for achieving overall physical fitness. Health-related fitness can be measured using a comprehensive and multidimensional approach. This approach acknowledges that different aspects of fitness can be better understood by examining how they interact and contribute to overall health.

A comprehensive evaluation of an individual's overall fitness requires a unified approach to fitness concepts. This is necessary in order to provide such an evaluation. Suppose individuals consider the interconnectedness of these fitness components. In that case, they can better identify areas where they can improve their fitness and achieve optimal physical fitness and overall health.

This chapter advocates for a holistic definition of physical fitness. This definition would involve a comprehensive understanding of physical fitness (holistic approach) and its connection to overall health and risk factors. Let us give the conceptual definition more weight than the operational definition. We can preserve the essence of physical fitness, make it a valuable tool for practitioners, and eliminate the confusion caused by different interpretations.

The current performance-based terminology used in fitness models can perplex individuals who need to become familiar with the terminology used in sports or athletics. This can result in confusion and a misunderstanding of the components that make up fitness. By revising the terminology to reflect the physical fitness construct rather than a particular skill, it may be possible to provide a precise and concise method for classifying and measuring the various components of fitness. Using terminology based on attributes shifts the focus away from specific skills or movements and toward the measured qualities. Measuring and comparing different aspects of fitness across different populations, such as athletes and nonathletes, is much simpler.

The purpose of this book is to discuss the difficulties associated with physical fitness and offer potential solutions that will make it applicable to the context of the 21st century. The purpose of the authors is to provide clarity on the concepts of physical fitness through their interpretation of "interrelated components," which can be confusing for some individuals due to the numerous fitness components and models that are currently available. They propose a unified fitness framework that considers all fitness components and indicators holistically and in an all-encompassing way. This framework also includes a definition of physical fitness that is all-encompassing and all-inclusive, taking into account all the components and attributes that contribute to overall well-being.

The transformative worldview, founded on the systems theory, encourages holistic thinking among fitness professionals and practitioners. This approach seeks to challenge unequal power dynamics and social structures by promoting social justice and inclusion in physical fitness practices and evaluations. This book proposes a unified fitness framework that considers all fitness components and indicators holistically and comprehensively. Additionally, the book will include a definition of physical fitness that is both comprehensive and inclusive, taking into account all components and attributes that contribute to overall well-being.

Review questions

1. What are the three fundamental concepts upon which the authors' work in this chapter is built, and why are they essential for comprehending physical fitness?

2. Describe the idea of physiological fitness and the importance of it in terms of physical well-being.
3. Describe the multifaceted approach to fitness for health discussed in this chapter. What elements are part of this strategy, and why is it crucial?
4. How does the chapter highlight the significance of balance as a health-related fitness indicator, specifically in the context of aging?
5. Talk about skill-related fitness elements' contribution to overall health and fitness. Why are these factors frequently missed in conventional fitness tests?
6. What are the central tenets of transformative worldview, and how do they apply to fitness?
7. How can systems theory be used to better understand how the human body's complexity relates to fitness?
8. Why is it important for academics and practitioners in physical fitness to speak a common language?
9. How does the chapter suggest addressing the difficulties with physical fitness and improving its applicability to the 21st-century environment?
10. What are the chapter's main goals, and how do they relate to inclusiveness and holistic fitness?

Discussion questions

1. The idea of physiological fitness challenges what concepts of physical fitness? What effects might including organ-level systems in fitness evaluations have?
2. What are some advantages of a holistic approach to physical fitness, and how might it change fitness standards and evaluations? Is there a downside to giving the conceptual definition precedence over the operational definition?
3. Especially in light of aging, discuss the significance of balance as a health-related fitness indicator. How might exercise regimens for the elderly better address balance and lower their fall risk?
4. Examine the contribution of skill-related fitness components on overall fitness and health. How would our approach to fitness tests and training programs alter if these elements were included?
5. Consider the transformative worldview and systems theory from a theoretical standpoint as they relate to physical health. How might these viewpoints affect physical fitness's study, application, and inclusivity?

References

Baumgartner, T. A., Jackson, A. S., Mahar, M. T., & Rowe, D. A. (2015). *Measurement for evaluation in kinesiology*. Jones & Bartlett Publishers.

Bianco, A., Jemni, M., Thomas, E., Patti, A., Paoli, A., Ramos Roque, J., Antonio, P., Mammina, C., & Tabacchi, G. (2015). A systematic review to determine reliability and usefulness of the field-based test batteries for the assessment of physical fitness in adolescents–The ASSO Project. *International Journal of Occupational Medicine and Environmental Health*, *28*(3), 445–478. http://dx.doi.org/10.13075/ijomeh.1896.00393

Blodgett, J. M., Cooper, R., Davis, D. H., Kuh, D., & Hardy, R. (2020). Associations between factors across life and one-legged balance performance in mid and later life: Evidence from a British birth cohort study. *Frontiers in Sports and Active Living*, *2*, 28. https://doi.org/10.3389/fspor.2020.00028

Canosa, A., Graham, A., & Wilson, E. (2019). Progressing a child-centred research agenda in tourism studies. *Tourism Analysis*, *24*(1), 95–100. https://doi.org/10.3727/1 08354219X15458295632007

Casaña, J., Calatayud, J., Silvestre, A., Sánchez-Frutos, J., Andersen, L. L., Jakobsen, M. D., Ezzatvar, Y., & Alakhdar, Y. (2021). Knee extensor muscle strength is more important than postural balance for stair-climbing ability in elderly patients with severe knee osteoarthritis. *International Journal of Environmental Research and Public Health*, *18*(7), 3637. https://doi.org/10.3390/ijerph18073637

Corbin, C. B., Welk, G. J., Corbin, W. R., & Welk, K. A. (2008). *Concepts of physical fitness, active lifestyles for wellness* (14th ed.). McGraw-Hill.

DeMet, T., & Wahl-Alexander, Z. (2019). Integrating skill-related components of fitness into physical education. *Strategies*, *32*(5), 10–17. https://doi.org/10.1080/08924562.2019. 1637315

Frehlich, L., Christie, C. D., Ronksley, P. E., Turin, T. C., Doyle-Baker, P., & McCormack, G. R. (2022). The neighbourhood built environment and health-related fitness: A narrative systematic. *International Journal of Behavioral Nutrition and Physical Activity*, *19*(1), 1–19. https://doi.org/10.1186/s12966-022-01359-0

Gong, W. (2020). Effects of dynamic exercise utilizing PNF patterns on the balance of healthy adults. *Journal of Physical Therapy Science*, *32*(4), 260–264. https://doi.org/10.1589/jpts.32.260

Gumieniak, R. J. (2017). *Establishing a legally defensible physical employment standard for Canadian wildland fire fighters* [Doctoral dissertation]. http://hdl.handle.net/10315/33560

Lai, C. H., & Huili Lin, S. (2017). Systems theory. In C. R. Scott & L. Lewis (Eds.), *The international encyclopedia of organizational communication* (pp. 1–18). John Wiley & Sons, Inc. https://doir.org/10.1002/9781118955567.wbieoc203Lintu, N., Savonen, K., Viitasalo, A., Tompuri, T., Paananen, J., Tarvainen, M. P., & Lakka, T. (2016). Determinants of cardiorespiratory fitness in a population sample of girls and boys aged 6 to 8 years. *Journal of Physical Activity and Health*, *13*(11), 1149–1155. https://doi.org/10.1123/jpah.2015-0644

Mertens, D. M. (2021). Transformative research methods to increase social impact for vulnerable groups and cultural minorities. *International Journal of Qualitative Methods*, *20*. https://doi.org/10.1177/16094069211051563

Myer, G. D., Faigenbaum, A. D., Edwards, N. M., Clark, J. F., Best, T. M., & Sallis, R. E. (2015). Sixty minutes of what? A developing brain perspective for activating children with an integrative exercise approach. *British Journal of Sports Medicine*, *49*(23), 1510–1516. http://doi.org/10.1136/bjsports-2014-093661

Nieminen, J. H., Bearman, M., & Tai, J. (2023). How is theory used in assessment and feedback research? A critical review. *Assessment & Evaluation in Higher Education*, *48*(1), 77–94. https://doi.org/10.1080/02602938.2022.2047154

Parsons, S. L. (2017). *Assessing the physical fitness level of children with intellectual disability in the Grahamstown region of the eastern cape, and subsequently designing, implementing, and evaluating the efficacy of an exercise intervention* [Master's thesis, Rhodes University]. https://commons.ru.ac.za/vital/access/services/Download/vital:22478/SOURCE1

Singh, D., & Trikha, S. (2022). Physical and physiological effect of yoga. *Yoga in Modern Era*. https://www.sdcollegeambala.ac.in/wp-content/uploads/2022/08/yoga 2022-8.pdf

Spaniol, F. J., Jarrett, L. M., Ocker, L. B., Bonnette, R. A., & Melrose, D. R. (2013). Skill-related fitness of undergraduate kinesiology students. *The Physical Educator, 70*(3), 282–297.

Stewart, A. L. (2003). Conceptual challenges in linking physical activity and disability research. *American Journal of Preventive Medicine, 25*(3), 137–140. https://doi.org/10.1016/S0749-3797(03)00187-9

Stichweh, R. (2011). Systems theory. In B. Badie (Ed.), *International encyclopedia of political science*. Sage.

Suga, T., Terada, M., Tomoo, K., Miyake, Y., Tanaka, T., Ueno, H., Nagano, A., & Isaka, T. (2021). Association between plantar flexor muscle volume and dorsiflexion flexibility in healthy young males: Ultrasonography and magnetic resonance imaging studies. *BMC Sports Science, Medicine and Rehabilitation, 13*(1), 1–8. https://doi.org/10.1186/s13102-021-00233-z

Weening-Dijksterhuis, B. (2014). *Physical exercise to improve or maintain activities of daily living performance in frail institutionalized older persons*. Research Institute SHARE. https://research.hanze.nl/nl/publications/physical-exercise-to-improve-or-maintain-activities-of-daily-livi

Wilkinson, L. A. (2011). Systems theory. In S. Goldstein & J. A. Naglieri (Eds.), *Encyclopedia of child behavior and development*. Springer. https://doi.org/10.1007/978-0-387-79061-9_941

4

THE BUILDING BLOCK SYSTEMS OF FITNESS

Oliver Napila Gomez and Nguyen Tra Giang

This chapter defines physical fitness by outlining the body's interconnected functions and proposing a comprehensive fitness framework that considers health, skills, and task completion. It starts with systems theory, which states that people develop at different rates but are all part of an extensive, interconnected system. A systems-theory-based fitness framework is required to conform to the HATS Framework. Modern conceptions of fitness often divide various physiological processes into separate buckets, which ignores the interdependent nature of the body's systems. The authors acknowledge the limitations of traditional fitness paradigms and propose an all-encompassing model considering the endocrine, cardiovascular, musculoskeletal, and nervous systems and their interactions. Fitness is a collection of physical characteristics and the coordinated action of various bodily systems. All sorts of things, from the most ordinary to the most strenuous, rely on these systems to help people stay healthy, learn new physical skills, and get things done. A holistic approach to fitness evaluation and training methodologies is suggested, considering systemic functions for health, skills, and task completion. This strategy should be based on an in-depth knowledge of how the various systems in the body work together to enhance a person's physical abilities.

Outcome

By the end of this chapter, you will be able to:

- explore the complex role played by the central nervous system (CNS) in controlling several physiological processes

DOI: 10.4324/9781003502937-5

- recognize the importance of the musculoskeletal system in physical activity and its function in maintaining bodily functions
- discover how the cardiovascular and respiratory systems work together to support physical performance and overall health
- investigate the hormonal regulation of diverse biological activities and its consequences for physical fitness and body structure

The fundamental body systems in physical fitness

According to systems theory, every individual possesses a dynamic system that is interconnected and composed of significant subsystems that develop at different rates. To begin developing a holistic and inclusive fitness design, the proponents investigate the question, "Which body systems function for health, skills, and completing tasks?" The HATS framework, which embodies the definition of fitness, was aligned with identifying the systems by the systems theory.

Physical fitness relies on the harmonious interaction of four central body systems: the nervous system, musculoskeletal system, cardiorespiratory system, and endocrine system. Understanding these systems is critical for improving physical fitness and health since they regulate mobility, energy use, metabolic balance, and physiological processes, all influencing an individual's overall well-being and performance. A deep understanding of these systems empowers individuals to take proactive steps in maintaining their health and longevity, prioritizing regular physical activity, balanced nutrition, and overall wellness. Appreciating these systems may help individuals optimize their fitness journeys and lead healthy lives.

The nervous system – coordinating body functions and movements

The central nervous system (CNS) plays a significant role in controlling humans' physiologic and behavioral characteristics. It includes the brain, spinal cord, and nerves that extend to every inch of the skin and are responsible for controlling and regulating all processes occurring in the different systems of the human body, including body movements. As a central nervous system component, the brain influences human behavior, emotion, cognitive activities, and even imaginative tasks (Banerjee et al., 2022). In contrast, the spinal cord, a significant central nervous system, transmits impulses from the brain to organs and tissues, regulating the body's motor and sensory processes (Rasulova & Makhmudova, 2022).

The neurons of the CNS regulate consciousness and mental activity, while the spinal extensions of the central nervous system's neuron pathways control the operation of skeletal muscles and organs (Mănescu, 2013). This complicated interaction underscores the central nervous system's essential role in regulating body activities.

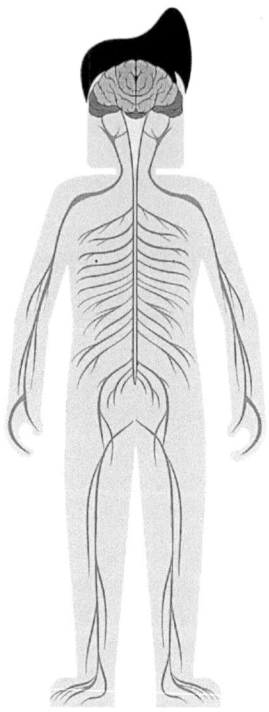

FIGURE 4.1   The nervous system

The CNS exerts extensive command over the body's operations (Satapathy et al., 2021). Multiple feedback loops enable the CNS to start actions and sustain regulatory processes (Schouten & Mugge, 2018). This complex system guarantees the smooth operation of several physiological systems.

The CNS also controls physiological activities such as energy metabolism, immunological response, reproduction, and development (Khrimian, 2017). The system affects sweat gland activation by releasing neurotransmitters into the autonomous neural system (Wohlrab et al., 2023) and regulates many secretory systems, highlighting its extensive regulatory potential (Hong et al., 2022).

In addition, the CNS plays a crucial role in essential biological functions, such as the whole body's metabolism, body temperature, and blood pressure (McDougall et al., 2015). It changes the metabolic state, consequently affecting the functioning of other systems and obtaining essential data from them (Polito et al., 2022). Another crucial role of the central nervous system is maintaining metabolic balance by regulating food intake (Roman et al., 2016).

In addition to these many activities, the CNS regulates the human musculo-skeletal system to ensure its coordinated operation (Goldfarb et al., 2013). The

CNS governs human force output by sequentially recruiting motor units in skeletal muscles and modulating their neuronal firing rate (Rohlén, 2021).

Furthermore, this book considers the CNS as the body's control system. The CNS receives sensory inputs from other systems involved in kinesthesia, which is the ability to sense body position and movements. The proprioceptive system in the muscles and joints, the vestibular system in the inner ear, and the visual system are all involved in kinesthesia. Together, these systems enable the body to perform complex movements, maintain balance, and navigate the environment, providing the brain with the necessary information to make decisions and coordinate movement. Kinesthesia is a crucial component of physical activity and is essential for everyday movements and complex movements involved in sports, dance, and other physical activities.

The brain is responsible for receiving messages from various sense organs of the body, including the classic external sense organs, such as sight, smell, hearing, taste, and touch. However, it also recognizes two internal sense organs, the proprioceptive and vestibular senses, which are relevant to kinesthetic fitness.

Proprioceptors are specialized sense organs located in soft tissues such as muscles, ligaments, and tendons, and their nerve endings send information to the nervous system. In other words, the proprioceptive system refers to the internal awareness and feeling of the movement of muscles, ligaments, and joints (Nissim et al., 2014). Proprioception is responsible for a person's awareness of body position and movement, allowing them to sense the location of different body parts, the position of the body, the required quality of movement for a particular action, and the properties of objects such as force, weight, rigidity, and thickness.

The vestibular system pertains to stability or operating within the gravitational pull (Wiebelhaus & Hanson, 2016). It comprises components inside the inner ear that sense movement and changes in head position (Erdönmez, 2020). In other words, the vestibular system contributes to a person's spatial awareness, posture, and sense of balance, which is crucial in maintaining balance during movement and changes in body position. Together, proprioception and the vestibular sense provide the necessary information for kinesthetic fitness, enabling the body to move accurately and precisely in space, improving overall physical health and performance.

The musculoskeletal system – supporting body structure and movements

The musculoskeletal system encompasses bones, muscles, cartilage, tendons, ligaments, joints, and connective tissue. It provides support, stability, and movement to the body while storing calcium and phosphorus and protecting vital organs (Park & Shin, 2016). The system consists of muscles connected to an internal skeleton essential for sophisticated human activity (Li et al., 2022).

It is common knowledge that the skeletal system is a critical human body component that provides a structural framework for movement and support. The 206 bones that comprise the skeletal system are essential for many bodily functions, including movement, protection of vital organs, and the production of red blood cells.

The primary role of the skeletal system is to create a foundation for the body, protect essential organs, and permit bodily mobility via the attachment of bone to other skeletal elements such as muscles, tendons, and ligaments (Davis & Hall, 2017; Ramcharan, 2015; Yen et al., 2020). The skeletal system gives mechanical support to the body, responds to external mechanical forces, and serves as a repository for regular mineral metabolism (Hiam et al., 2019). Bones can modify their shape and structure to fulfill their role and withstand stress (Phillips et al., 2015).

Without bones, the human body would be unable to maintain a stable shape or stand upright. The bones work together to form the body's structure and allow for various movements, such as walking, jumping, and bending. They also play a crucial role in maintaining posture and balance.

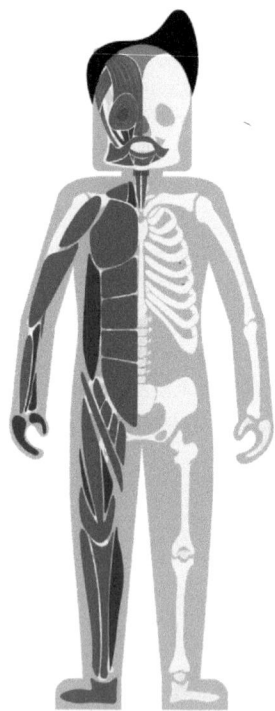

FIGURE 4.2 The musculoskeletal system

In addition to providing support and movement, the skeletal system protects vital organs (DiGirolamo et al., 2013; Elefteriou, 2018; Trainor & Merrill, 2014). For example, the skull protects the brain, while the rib cage protects the heart and lungs. The bones act as a protective shield that helps prevent damage to these critical organs during physical activities or accidents.

Another critical function of the skeletal system is the production of red blood cells (Pettiford, 2019). Red blood cells are essential for carrying oxygen throughout the body and are produced in the bone marrow. The bone marrow is a soft, spongy tissue found in the center of most bones in the body. It produces red blood cells, white blood cells, and platelets necessary for proper immune function.

Moreover, ligaments hold two long bone structures together to form a joint. A flexible connective tissue called cartilage provides additional cushioning between bone-to-bone structures to prevent bones from rubbing against each other. However, the bone and joint structures alone cannot move the body. The skeletal system needs the assistance of the muscular system to complete the body's system responsible for movements.

The skeletal muscles, which are attached to the bones and cover the skeletal system, are voluntary muscle tissues controlled by the brain. Tendons connect the opposite ends of skeletal muscles to the bones. Major skeletal muscles are typically attached to an immovable bone (origin) and a movable bone (insertion). When skeletal muscles contract, they shrink, pulling the insertion toward the origin (concentric muscle contraction). When skeletal muscles relax, they return to their regular length (eccentric muscle contraction).

The body performs tasks that engage the muscles, joints, and bones to move within a given range of motion and produce force. Tasks may involve carrying, lifting, pushing, pulling, or throwing objects from one point to another. When lifting heavy objects, the muscles shrink and stretch to produce force. This type of muscular contraction is called isotonic contraction. The contraction is called isometric contraction when the muscles contract without altering their length. Pushing and pulling are examples of such muscular contractions.

The cardiorespiratory system – facilitating energy production

The body's ability to engage in aerobic physical activity relies heavily on the cardiovascular and respiratory systems. The cardiovascular system includes the heart and blood arteries, responsible for pumping and carrying blood throughout the body (Hegardt, 2021). On the other hand, the respiratory system refers to the parts of the body that are involved with breathing (Flores et al., 2014; Hamrick-King & Sewell, 2017; Sewell, 2022), including the nose, mouth, pharynx, trachea, and lungs (Flores et al., 2014).

The function of the cardiorespiratory system is crucial on a motor and functional level in children and adults (Naranjo & Garnero, 2023). These two systems

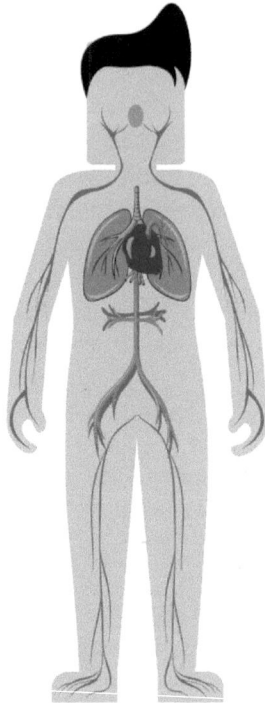

FIGURE 4.3   The cardiorespiratory system

transport oxygen and glucose to fuel aerobic respiration during physical activity. The circulatory system, which includes the heart, arteries, capillaries, and veins, transports the blood carrying oxygen and glucose needed for aerobic activities. This process is called cardiovascular endurance, which refers to the ability of the circulatory system to work effectively and efficiently to complement the extensive work of the engaged muscles.

The lungs breathe in oxygen and exhale carbon dioxide to facilitate aerobic respiration. As the intensity of aerobic activity increases, the circulatory system must deal with the muscles' demand for increased circulation to match the body's fuel and oxygen needs. The heart must be healthy and fit to pump blood, while the lungs should be fit to handle the physiological response of increased oxygen and carbon dioxide transport.

The endocrine system – regulating essential body functions and processes

The endocrine system is associated with body composition and structure, dieting, and physical activity. From a biological perspective, the overall activity of

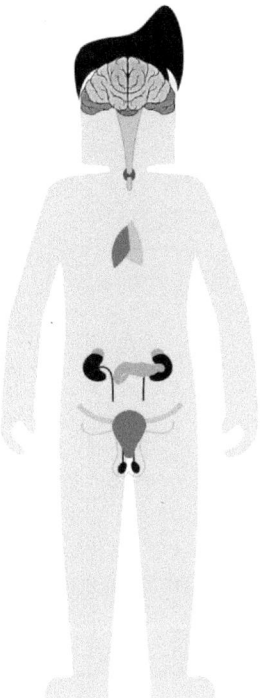

FIGURE 4.4   The endocrine system

the endocrine system, which includes the pineal gland, hypothalamus, pituitary gland, thyroid, parathyroid glands, thymus, pancreas, adrenal glands, ovary (in females), and testes (in males), contribute to the condition of the human body. For example, Charkoudian and Stachenfeld (2014) concluded that reproductive hormones significantly influence thermoregulatory mechanisms. This means that hormones involved in the reproductive system, such as estrogen, progestogens, and testosterone, play a notable role in regulating the body's ability to maintain a stable internal temperature. These hormones affect the body's response to heat and its ability to dissipate or conserve heat as needed. They can impact blood flow, sweating, and neural control systems involved in thermoregulation.

Moreover, internal metabolic processes regulate the functions and structures of the body. Hormones and glands are inherently responsible for energy production, growth, and development of tissues and response mechanisms. The activity of the hormones influences the body's structure. For example, Pirahanchi and colleagues (2022) explained how the thyroid influences many organ systems, including bone development and maturation and the central nervous system's (CNS) maturity. It enhances the synthesis of sodium ($Na+$)-potassium ($K+$)-ATPase, increasing oxygen consumption and generating heat. Encouraging glucose uptake, glycogenolysis, gluconeogenesis, lipolysis, protein synthesis, and degradation, the hormones also stimulate the metabolism (net catabolic effect).

Hypothyroidism occurs when the thyroid gland does not release enough thyroid hormones into the bloodstream, which can cause weight gain (Pirahanchi et al., 2022). Similarly, a high level of somatotropin, the growth hormone secreted by the pituitary gland, may cause gigantism, while a deficiency may result in dwarfism (Rathor et al., 2019; Sadiq & Tadi, 2022). Hence, body composition must be associated with the fitness of the endocrine system.

The fundamental functions

The exploration of the fundamental functions of fitness, which are based on the interaction of different body systems, has revealed a complex network essential for overall health, the acquisition of skills, and the performance of tasks. The biological and mechanical processes governed by the body's systems, specifically the nervous, musculoskeletal, cardiorespiratory, and endocrine systems, are intertwined with these functions, which can be broken down into health, skill, and task completion functions.

Functions for health

The cardiorespiratory and endocrine systems are primarily responsible for regulating functions for health. These systems are crucial in maintaining homeostasis, producing energy, and surviving. The coordination of oxygen delivery by the cardiorespiratory system and the regulation of metabolic processes and hormonal balances by the endocrine system are two of the most important aspects of maintaining life and facilitating the body's adaptive responses to various stimuli and stresses.

For instance, regular health checkups involve monitoring vital signs. Vital signs, such as heart rate and blood pressure, indicate the health of the cardiorespiratory system. Additionally, an individual's commitment to eating a balanced diet is essential for maintaining homeostasis and preventing chronic diseases such as hypertension and hyperlipidemia. This commitment helps the individual's endocrine system by correctly balancing the hormonal and metabolic functions.

Functions for skills

The nervous system and the musculoskeletal system are primarily responsible for managing functions related to skill. These systems collaborate to bring about movement control and coordination. The intricate network of neurons and synapses that make up the nervous system processes sensory information, which can then be used to control movement precisely. In the meantime, the musculoskeletal system provides the structural framework and the mechanics for movement. Muscles contract and relax in response to electrical stimulation from the nervous system.

The daily practice routine of a ballet dancer, for instance, is an excellent example of the refinement of movement and skill. For each performance, the dancer must have precise control over their movements. This necessitates a well-tuned nervous system for coordination and a robust musculoskeletal system, which is necessary for the strength and grace of each ballet pose and jump.

Functions for completing tasks

The integrative processes of the systems are included in the functions responsible for completing assigned tasks. The cardiovascular and respiratory systems provide energy, the endocrine system ensures that the body is in the best possible state internally, and the nervous system is responsible for coordination. The musculoskeletal system is responsible for carrying out tasks safely and efficiently. This all-encompassing operation guarantees that tasks are carried out with the necessary amount of energy, precision, and strength.

The nervous system is essential in coordinating the body's functions and movements. It performs the function of the command center, processing inputs from various sources to generate coordinated and interactive outputs. The fact that this system is responsible for everything from simple reflexes to complex cognitive functions highlights its critical role in maintaining adequate physical fitness.

The musculoskeletal system provides the necessary support and movement mechanisms, enabling the physical execution of tasks. Furthermore, it helps maintain the body's structure, makes movement possible, and engages in dynamic interactions with other systems to modulate strength, endurance, and flexibility.

The cardiorespiratory system plays an essential role in producing energy. Delivering oxygen and removing carbon dioxide support stamina and endurance, enabling aerobic activities to be sustained for extended periods and providing the foundation for endurance.

The endocrine system regulates functions and processes that are essential to the body. It modulates growth, metabolism, and adaptation to physical demands and influences body composition and capacity for activity and recovery.

As an illustration, a firefighter needs to possess the physical capability to meet the requirements of the job, which frequently include lifting heavy equipment, breaking through barriers, and rescuing individuals from dangerous environments. Their cardiorespiratory system needs to be trained to handle strenuous activity and smoke inhalation; their endocrine system needs to be able to manage stress responses effectively; their nervous system needs to be able to react quickly to changing circumstances; and their musculoskeletal system needs to be strong and flexible enough to move debris and carry weights. Their training guarantees that all of these systems are in the best possible condition to fulfill the requirements of the life-saving tasks they are responsible for.

In conclusion, the fundamental functions of the building block systems of fitness highlight the interconnectedness of the various systems that make up the body. To achieve a robust state of fitness, all these systems must work together in harmony. Each of these systems contributes to the preservation of health, the development of skills, and the capacity to carry out tasks. Not only is the interaction between these systems necessary for the individual components of fitness, but it is also necessary for the overall physical literacy of a person.

Summary

Physical fitness relies on the interaction of four central body systems: the nervous system, musculoskeletal system, cardiorespiratory system, and endocrine system. The nervous system, comprising the brain, spinal cord, and nerves, controls various physiological processes, including body movements. It influences human behavior, emotion, cognitive activities, and imaginative tasks. The spinal cord transmits impulses from the brain to organs and tissues, regulating the body's motor and sensory processes.

The CNS controls physiological activities such as energy metabolism, immunological response, reproduction, and development. It also regulates the human musculoskeletal system, ensuring its coordinated operation. The CNS receives sensory inputs from other systems involved in kinesthesia, which allows the body to perform complex movements, maintain balance, and navigate the environment.

The brain receives messages from various sense organs, including the proprioceptive and vestibular senses, which are relevant to kinesthetic fitness. Proprioception and the vestibular sense provide the necessary information for kinesthetic fitness, enabling the body to move accurately and precisely in space and improving overall physical health and performance. Understanding these systems is essential for maintaining health and longevity, prioritizing regular physical activity, balanced nutrition, and overall wellness.

The musculoskeletal system is a crucial human body component, consisting of bones, muscles, cartilage, tendons, ligaments, joints, and connective tissue. It provides support, stability, and movement to the body while storing calcium and phosphorus and protecting vital organs. The skeletal system is essential for maintaining posture and balance, providing mechanical support, responding to external forces, and serving as a repository for regular mineral metabolism.

The skeletal system is critical in producing red blood cells, essential for carrying oxygen throughout the body. The bone marrow, a soft, spongy tissue found in most bones, produces these cells. The skeletal system also includes the cardiorespiratory system, which transports oxygen and glucose to fuel aerobic respiration during physical activity.

The endocrine system, including the pineal gland, hypothalamus, pituitary gland, thyroid, parathyroid glands, thymus, pancreas, adrenal glands, ovary (in females), and testes, contributes to the condition of the human body. Hormones involved in the reproductive system, such as estrogen, progestogens, and testosterone, play a significant role in regulating the body's ability to maintain a stable internal temperature, impacting blood flow, sweating, and neural control systems involved in thermoregulation.

Internal metabolic processes regulate the body's functions and structures, with hormones and glands inherently responsible for energy production, growth, and development of tissues and response mechanisms. The thyroid gland, for example, influences various organ systems, such as bone development and maturation and the maturation of the central nervous system (CNS). Body composition must be associated with the fitness of the endocrine system, as it plays a crucial role in maintaining the body's structure and function.

Review questions

1. What are the main parts of the nervous system, and how do they affect how bodily activities are regulated?
2. Describe how the vestibular and proprioceptive systems contribute to kinesthetic fitness.
3. How does the musculoskeletal system support and facilitate physical activity and movement?
4. Describe the functions of bones aside from supporting the body structurally.
5. Why is cardiorespiratory endurance crucial for fitness, and what role does the cardiovascular system play in facilitating aerobic exercise?
6. What are the respiratory system's main parts, and how does it support the body during physical activity?
7. Talk about the endocrine system's role in controlling body weight, metabolism, and thermoregulation.
8. Give examples of how endocrine system hormones can affect an individual's physical fitness and general health.
9. Describe the interactions and cooperation of the four elemental bodily systems – nervous, musculoskeletal, cardiorespiratory, and endocrine – to promote physical fitness.
10. Why is it crucial for those who want to increase their physical fitness and general health to be thoroughly aware of various body systems?

Discussion questions

1. How does a person's attitude to exercise and movement training change due to learning about the nervous system? Give examples or personal stories.
2. Talk about how the nervous and musculoskeletal systems work together to enable coordinated movement. How might this information be used to enhance daily tasks or athletic performance?
3. Learn about cardiovascular endurance and the role it plays in physical fitness. What advantages may people expect from improving their cardiovascular fitness, and how can they do it?
4. How do endocrine system hormones affect body composition, metabolism, and general fitness? Discuss any particular diet or exercise regimens that help optimize hormonal balance.
5. Consider the chapter's holistic approach to physical training, emphasizing how the four body systems and their functions work together. How might this viewpoint influence fitness training plans and health advice for people of all ages and fitness levels?

References

Banerjee, A., Bhattacharya, D. K., & Dey, A. (2022). Effect of cognitive task on the central nervous system. In *Computational advancement in communication, circuits and systems: Proceedings of 3rd ICCACCS 2020* (pp. 259–269). Springer. https://doi.org/10.1007/978-981-16-4035-3_23

Charkoudian, N., & Stachenfeld, N. S. (2014). Reproductive hormone influences on thermoregulation in women. *Comprehensive Physiology, 4*(2), 793–804.

Davis, G., & Hall, M. (2017). *The makeup artist handbook: Techniques for film, television, photography, and theatre*. Taylor & Francis.

DiGirolamo, D. J., Kiel, D. P., & Esser, K. A. (2013). Bone and skeletal muscle: Neighbors with close ties. *Journal of Bone and Mineral Research, 28*(7), 1509–1518. https://doi.org/10.1002/jbmr.1969

Elefteriou, F. (2018). Impact of the autonomic nervous system on the skeleton. *Physiological Reviews, 98*(3), 1083–1112. https://doi.org/10.1152/physrev.00014.2017

Erdönmez, S. S. (2020). *NADI tangible tasks: A system to structure daily life based on personal preferences for people with autism spectrum disorder*. http://hdl.handle.net/10589/153788

Flores, C. M., Luxenberg, J. S., & Werdegar, D. (2014). Enhancing and managing client care. In *Long-term care administration and management: Effective practices and quality programs in eldercare*. Springer Publishing Company.

Goldfarb, M., Lawson, B. E., & Shultz, A. H. (2013). Realizing the promise of robotic leg prostheses. *Science Translational Medicine, 5*(210). https://doi.org/10.1126/scitranslmed.3007312

Hamrick-King, J. H. J., & Sewell, B. S. (2017). Review of the aging of physiological systems. *Gerontological Nursing: Competencies for Care, 67*.

Hegardt, F. (2021). *Optimization-based geometry correction of blood flow CFD simulations using 4D-flow data* [Doctoral dissertation, Lund University].

Hiam, D., Voisin, S., Yan, X., Landen, S., Jacques, M., Papadimitriou, I. D., Munson, F., Byrnes, E., Brennan-Speranza, T. C., Levinger, I., & Eynon, N. (2019). The association between bone mineral density gene variants and osteocalcin at baseline, and in response to exercise: The Gene SMART study. *Bone*, *123*, 23–27. https://doi.org/10.1016/j.bone.2019.03.015

Hong, Y., Zhang, L., Liu, N., Xu, X., Liu, D., & Tu, J. (2022). The central nervous mechanism of stress-promoting cancer progression. *International Journal of Molecular Sciences*, *23*(20), 12653. https://doi.org/10.3390/ijms232012653

Khrimian, L. N. (2017). *The role of osteocalcin in the regulation of brain development and functions* [Doctoral dissertation, Columbia University]. https://doi.org/10.7916/D8F76J62

Li, F., Adrien, N., & He, Y. (2022). Biomechanical risks associated with foot and ankle injuries in ballet dancers: A systematic review. *International Journal of Environmental Research and Public Health*, *19*(8), 4916. https://doi.org/10.3390/ijerph19084916

Mănescu, D. C. (2013). Solutions to fight against overtraining in bodybuilding routine. *Marathon*, *5*(2), 182–186. https://marathon.ase.ro/pdf/vol5/2/10ManescuD.pdf

McDougall, S. J., Münzberg, H., Derbenev, A. V., & Zsombok, A. (2015). Central control of autonomic functions in health and disease. *Frontiers in Neuroscience*, *8*, 440. https://doi.org/10.3389/fnins.2014.00440

Naranjo, F. J. R., & Garnero, J. L. (2023). Ergospirometry & body percussion: Case study based on BAPNE FIT method. *Retos: Nuevas Tendencias en Educación Física, Deporte y Recreación*, *48*, 674–683. https://dialnet.unirioja.es/descarga/articulo/8853159.pdf

Nissim, M., Ram-Tsur, R., Zion, M., Mevarech, Z., & Ben-Soussan, T. D. (2014). Effects of aquatic motor activities on early childhood cognitive and motor development. *Open Journal of Social Sciences*, *2*(12), 24.

Park, S., & Shin, S. Y. (2016). Manual therapy of shoulder musculoskeletal diseases when arms are lifted while spread straight. *International Information Institute (Tokyo). Information*, *19*(7A), 2761. http://dx.doi.org/10.14303/jmms.2015.092

Pettiford, R. (2019). *The skeletal system*. Bellwether Media.

Phillips, A. T., Villette, C. C., & Modenese, L. (2015). Femoral bone mesoscale structural architecture prediction using musculoskeletal and finite element modelling. *International Biomechanics*, *2*(1), 43–61. https://doi.org/10.1080/23335432.2015.1017609

Pirahanchi, Y., Toro, F., & Jialal, I. (2022). Physiology, thyroid stimulating hormone. In *StatPearls*. StatPearls Publishing. PMID: 29763025.

Polito, R., Valenzano, A., Monda, V., Cibelli, G., Monda, M., Messina, G., Villano, I., & Messina, A. (2022). Heart rate variability and sympathetic activity is modulated by very low-calorie ketogenic diet. *International Journal of Environmental Research and Public Health*, *19*(4), 2253. https://doi.org/10.3390/ijerph19042253

Ramcharan, M. A. (2015). *Development of functional interactions among cortical and trabecular traits during growth of the lumbar vertebral body*. City University of New York.

Rasulova, N., & Makhmudova, M. (2022). Neurological diseases as a social and hygienic problem. *Science and Innovation*, *1*(D5), 261–263. http://doi.org/10.5281/zenodo.7076133

Rathor, K. R., Mohanty, G., Lenka, S., & Katti, N. (2019). Growth hormone disorders and its oral manifestations. *Indian Journal of Public Health Research & Development*, *10*(11). https://doi.org/10.1038/nrendo.2018.22

Rohlén, R. (2021). *Identification of single motor units in ultrafast ultrasound image sequences of voluntary skeletal muscle contractions* [Doctoral dissertation, Umeå Universitet].

Roman, C. W., Derkach, V. A., & Palmiter, R. D. (2016). Genetically and functionally defined NTS to PBN brain circuits mediating anorexia. *Nature Communications*, *7*(1), 11905. https://doi.org/10.1038/ncomms11905

Sadiq, N. M., & Tadi, P. (2022). Physiology, pituitary hormones. In *StatPearls*. StatPearls Publishing. PMID: 32491488. https://europepmc.org/article/nbk/nbk557556

Satapathy, P., Hota, S., & Jena, S. K. (2021). Classification of brain magnetic resonance images using ICA-MLP. *International Research Journal on Advanced Science Hub, 3*, 27–29. https://doi.org/10.47392/irjash.2021.135

Schouten, A. C., & Mugge, W. (2018, October). Closed-loop identification to unravel the way the human nervous system controls bodily functions. In *International conference on neurorehabilitation* (pp. 617–621). Springer International Publishing. https://doi. org/10.1007/978-3-030-01845-0_123

Sewell, B. S. (2022). Review of the aging of physiological systems. *Gerontological Nursing: Competencies for Care, 75*.

Trainor, P. A., & Merrill, A. E. (2014). Ribosome biogenesis in skeletal development and the pathogenesis of skeletal disorders. *Biochimica et Biophysica Acta (BBA)-Molecular Basis of Disease, 1842*(6), 769–778. https://doi.org/10.1016/j.bbadis.2013.11.010

Wiebelhaus, S. E., & Hanson, M. F. (2016). Effects of classroom-based physical activities on off-task behaviors and attention: Kindergarten case study. *Qualitative Report, 21*(8). http://dx.doi.org/10.46743/2160-3715/2016.2448

Wohlrab, J., Bechara, F. G., Schick, C., & Naumann, M. (2023). Hyperhidrosis: A central nervous dysfunction of sweat secretion. *Dermatology and Therapy*, 1–11. https://doi. org/10.1007/s13555-022-00885-w

Yen, C. H., Hsu, C. M., Hsiao, S. Y., & Hsiao, H. H. (2020). Pathogenic mechanisms of myeloma bone disease and possible roles for nrf2. *International Journal of Molecular Sciences, 21*(18), 6723. https://doi.org/10.3390/ijms21186723

5

THE DESIGN OF THE FRAMEWORK

Nguyen Tra Giang and Oliver Napila Gomez

The Unified Systems Fitness Design (USFD) Framework offers a new way to apply systems theory to understand physical fitness. In particular, it zeroes in on the endocrine, nervous, cardiorespiratory, and musculoskeletal systems as they perform physical fitness. The intricate relationships between these systems are exposed by the USFD, which employs paired and grouped system operations to study their interdependence. Among the systems that collaborate to guarantee peak performance in different endeavors are the neurological, musculoskeletal, cardiorespiratory, and endocrine systems. The USFD introduces the pairing system functions that are the outcome of merging two systems. Six paired system functions are critical to physical performance and fitness measures. Aerobic control and motor control are two examples of such functions. Because of the interconnected nature of these processes, it is clear that fitness assessment and programming must consider a wide range of physiological systems.

Outcomes

By the end of this chapter, you will be able to

- explain the USFD Framework (Unified Systems Fitness Design) and its importance in viewing the body as a complex system with interrelated parts
- identify and define the nervous, musculoskeletal, cardiorespiratory, and endocrine systems and their essential roles in the USFD Framework
- analyze motor control, aerobic control, body function regulation, energy production and utilization, body composition, and metabolism as paired system functions and their roles in physical fitness

DOI: 10.4324/9781003502937-6

- discuss how the combination of three building block systems form movement, energy regulation, physiological health, and homeostasis functions, affecting fitness and health
- explore the Interconnected Functions Framework's paired and grouped system functions and their effect on an individual's physical well-being and performance

Introducing the Unified Systems Fitness Design framework

This chapter begins an in-depth examination of physical fitness, considering the intricate interconnections in our physiological systems. The USFD offers a fresh viewpoint on comprehending our bodies' inner workings and reactions to outside stimuli due to its solid foundation in systems theory. We will look at the nervous, musculoskeletal, cardiorespiratory, and endocrine systems, which are the building block systems of our physical fitness.

However, the USFD does something different and uses paired and grouped system operations to study these systems' interdependent nature, revealing the complex mechanisms that underpin our physical abilities to perform tasks. Therefore, by deciphering the interdependent systems in our bodies, we can make sense of the USFD and find ways to get in shape.

Functions of the primary systems

Our fitness design synthesizes the building block systems, with the primary systems serving as the foundation for all other interconnected physical fitness functions.

Figure 5.1 illustrates the essential functions of the building block systems. The nervous system regulates and coordinates the body's motions and functions by transferring chemical and electrical signals between neurons. The musculoskeletal system makes movement possible. Energy production is essential for all living things, and the cardiorespiratory system helps. Lastly, the endocrine system controls how various organs work using hormones.

Using electrical signal transmission, the nervous system regulates and controls the operations of various bodily systems. The skeletal system gives the body the framework it needs to move. Another vital role of the cardiorespiratory system is to help produce and use energy. On the other hand, the endocrine system uses hormones the body has to control how various organs work.

Since they are fundamental to the individual's survival and the body's general functioning to perform purposeful tasks, the building block systems form the basis of physical fitness. They coordinate their efforts to guarantee efficient and effective functioning, allowing for peak performance across various physical activities with varying intensities and durations.

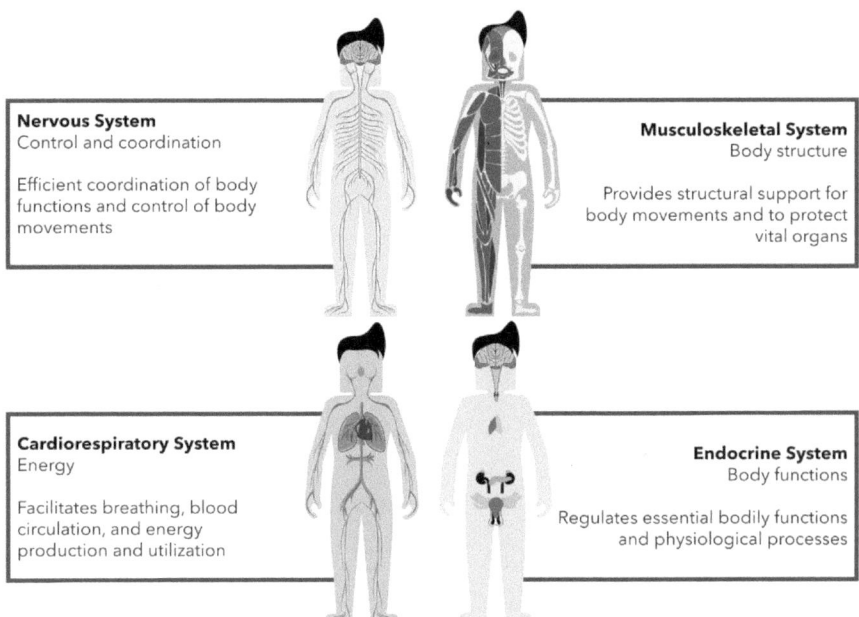

FIGURE 5.1   Functions of the primary systems, the building blocks of fitness

The paired systems matrix

The USFD acknowledges the interdependence of the building block systems. Pairing two systems together yields what are known as paired system functions. We created the paired systems matrix to determine the pairing and primary tasks of two combined systems of the body to pair the primary systems. Please note that we invented most of these terms to comprehend their purposes better. Six paired system functions were generated by combining the four systems that make up the body, as shown in Figure 5.2.

Motor control (NM)

The musculoskeletal system and the nervous system (which includes the peripheral and central nervous systems) collaborate to generate motion and control movement of the body. Motor control refers to coordinating movement concerning the surroundings, work, and tasks (Blackinton, 2017). The brain can control the position, speed, and acceleration of external organs and muscles (Bhattacharyya et al., 2021; Seifert, 2020). It also incorporates all the sensory and motor processes that contribute to spinal control, such as the mechanoreceptors and peripheral muscles, as well as the neural networks in the brain and spinal cord

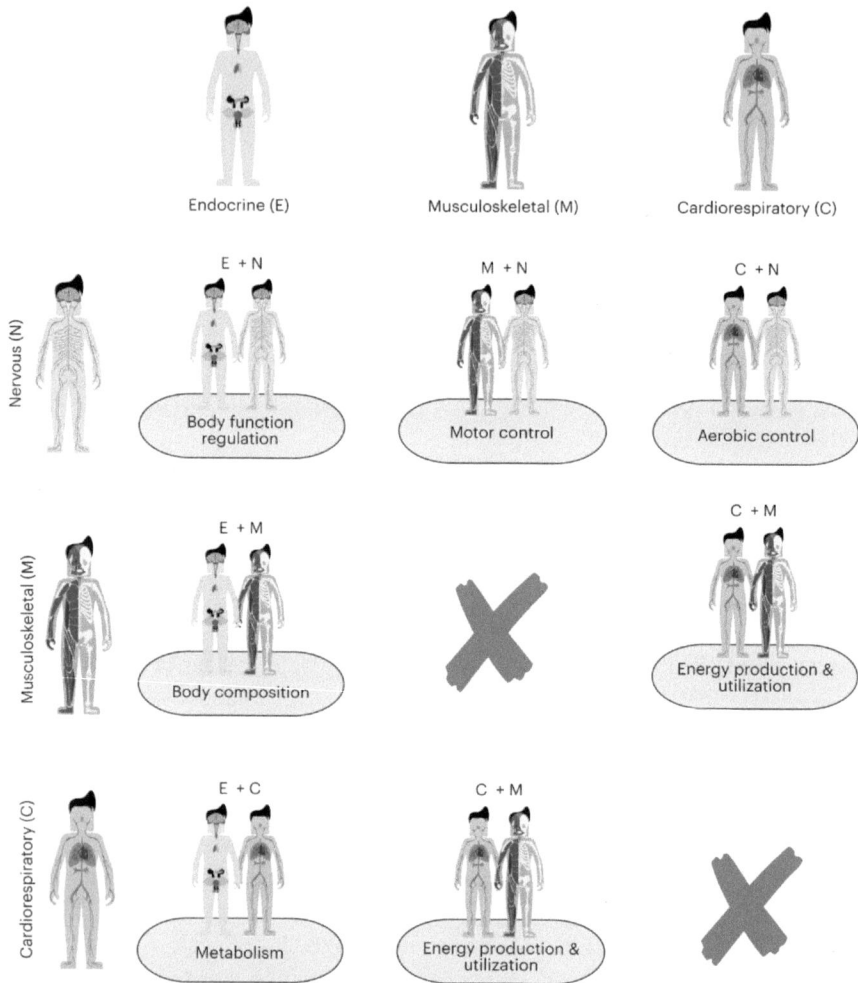

FIGURE 5.2   The USFD paired systems matrix

that coordinate the activation of muscles to meet the demands of spinal movement and impedance/stiffness (Hodges et al., 2019).

In addition, the ability to direct muscles to produce specific movements is known as motor control (Rice, 2021). Proper posture and balance, the ability to carry out routine tasks, and the ability to participate in physical activities and workouts all depend on motor control processes that include planning, programming, and execution.

The motor control function is already responsible for several fitness indicators in the HRF–SRF model. What we mean by **"kinesthetics"** is the ability to perceive the motion and location of limbs, which includes, broadly, the sensation of force (Mihelj et al., 2014; Wang et al., 2022). To rephrase, kinesthetics is the branch of neuroscience concerned with regulating movement in the skeletal muscles through the central nervous system.

When controlling and coordinating the body, space, and quality of movements, kinesthetics – also known as motor control – are crucial. Among these functions are maintaining balance, responding quickly, controlling speed, and being agile. The central nervous system integrates multimodal sensory data (from the surrounding environment and proprioception) to accomplish an activity. It activates muscles to control voluntary and involuntary movements (Bisi & Stagni, 2020).

Balance refers to the control in maintaining equilibrium while stationary or moving, which is essential for activities such as standing, walking, and running.

Reaction time is the time it takes to respond to a stimulus and is critical for sports such as tennis and basketball, where quick reactions can mean the difference between winning and losing.

Speed control is the control in modulating the speed of movement, which is essential for activities such as driving and playing musical instruments.

Agility is the ability to change direction quickly and efficiently, essential for sports such as soccer and football.

Flexibility refers to the range of motion in the joints, giving the body the fundamentals for a wide range of possible movements from simple to complex. Flexibility is the general range of motion all the joints can perform with the minimum force.

Motor control encompasses reflexes and various involuntary and voluntary motions controlled by the central nervous system to add flexibility to the concept. Motor control becomes adaptable when it uses sensory information to modify and activate muscles appropriately based on the task. This process is known as flexibility. Because of this flexibility, motions can be fine-tuned to meet the evolving demands of the work and the environment, guaranteeing optimal motor performance.

Aerobic control (NC)

The cardiovascular system is one of many that rely on the autonomic nervous system's functioning (Jänig, 2022). According to Russo and colleagues (2017), the sympathetic and parasympathetic branches of the autonomic nervous system regulate the cardiorespiratory system. The vagus nerve signals to the parasympathetic branch, releasing acetylcholine and slowing the heart rate. On the other hand, norepinephrine is released by the sympathetic branch, which speeds up the heart rate along with the sympathetic chain of nerves. When we are at rest, our parasympathetic nervous system is in overdrive, preventing the release of noradrenaline and quickly regulating our heart rate. Sympathetic activity is low at rest but increases in response to exertion or stress.

To rephrase, the regulation of breathing and heart rate is controlled by the neuronal and cardiorespiratory systems working together. Employing a feedback loop connecting the brain with the lungs, the cardiorespiratory control system modifies the cardiorespiratory system's operation. A new fitness indicator derived from these two systems is aerobic control, which is the capacity of the respiratory centers in the brainstem to control the heart rate at rest and during exercise. Aerobic capacity and endurance are indicators of the cardiorespiratory control system, which is essential for providing the body with enough oxygen for aerobic respiration.

Aerobic control reflects the body's ability to coordinate and control breathing and oxygen delivery to the working muscles during exercise. Physically fit individuals have low resting heart rates and high oxygen uptake, demonstrating effective breathing and heart rate monitoring during exercise. This is similar to the cardiorespiratory fitness in the HRF–SRF model but emphasizes controlling aerobic capacity and endurance for exercising safely, matching the intensity of the workout with the personal aerobic level.

Autonomic dysfunction, or dysautonomia, affects approximately 70 million people globally. It occurs when the brain cannot regulate the heart rate and breathing (Starling et al., 2021). This disorder affects digestion, respiration, blood pressure, and heart rate. Specifically, abnormal heart rate variability (HRV) values are associated with cardiac dysautonomia (de Faria Cardoso et al., 2022).

Body function regulation (NE)

The hypothalamus and other parts of the central nervous system control the secretion of hormones by the endocrine glands. Jänig (2014) states that the nervous system stimulates the pituitary gland and then secretes hormones that control the function of other endocrine glands. Furthermore, according to Jänig (2014), the sympathetic division of the autonomic nervous system, which initiates hormone secretion in reaction to stress or stimuli, is one neural input pathway via which the nervous system can directly control hormone secretion. The intricate interaction between the endocrine and neurological systems regulates numerous physiological processes.

Neuronal networks in the hypothalamus regulate hormones but also have essential roles in autonomic processes, sleep, aggression, and sexual behavior (Saper & Lowell, 2014). Its complex network allows for the precise regulation of essential biological processes.

Some studies show how the endocrine and neurological systems interact in various settings. For instance, Farr and colleagues (2016) pointed out that the endocrine system is under the nervous system's control via the numerous neuronal networks in the brain. An essential part of homeostatic regulation is the hypothalamus's work in controlling hunger and energy expenditure. One possible cause of obesity is how the brain's reward systems respond to food. People's attention and cognitive control systems govern their eating behavior, while emotional and memory processes impact their hunger. The human brain uses a complex network of neural circuits and mental operations to control food intake.

According to another study, the autonomic nervous system plays a vital role in controlling the body's glucose levels by regulating pancreatic islet cells, which include α-cells and β-cells. The secretion of insulin and glucagon is affected by glucose concentration, as stated by Thorens (2014). Insulin secretion is enhanced at high glucose levels, and glucagon secretion at low glucose levels. These cells' activity is influenced by the autonomic nervous system's sympathetic and parasympathetic branches; disorders involving this regulatory system can result in conditions like type 2 diabetes. However, additional research is needed to fully understand the interplay between the autonomic nervous system and brain cells that sense nutrients in order to manage glucose levels and diabetic dysfunctions, according to the authors.

Further research is required to fully comprehend the intricate web of relationships that regulates core body temperature via the neurological system's influence on the endocrine system (Tan & Knight, 2018). According to Tan and Knight (2018), sensory neurons in the nervous system detect changes in core body temperature and transmit signals to the brain, which regulates core body temperature. In order to regulate core body temperature, these signals are processed in the preoptic area of the brain. Sweating, shivering, and the relaxation or widening of blood vessels are all parts of the thermoregulatory system that work together to keep the body at a constant temperature. Moreover, a person's preference for a warmer or cooler environment regulates temperature.

Put another way, the endocrine and neurological systems collaborate to control how various bodily organs perform their duties. They keep the internal environment stable and guarantee proper bodily function. Body function control, the capacity of the system to regulate physiological processes, is a new fitness indicator coined by this systemic partnership (e.g., glucose levels, body temperature, and blood pressure).

Body function control is an involuntary control attribute that reflects the ability of the body to adjust the body functions to a state of homeostasis (internal balance) in response to internal and external stimuli. Indicators include typical vital signs (heart rate variability, blood pressure, and temperature), healthy weight, good stability and balance, good digestive health, restfulness, and stress response or mental health. For example, when blood pressure rises, the body controls the heart rate and constricts the blood vessels to sustain the organs with oxygen continuously. Keeping the body's functions controlled is essential for health and fitness. Conditions that disrupt body functions include diabetes, thyroid disorders, and autoimmune diseases. These conditions lead to a range of health problems.

Energy production and utilization (CM)

Integrating the cardiorespiratory and musculoskeletal systems makes energy production and utilization possible. During physical activity, the heart, blood vessels, and lungs supply the muscles with oxygen and nutrients through the cardiorespiratory system. Aerobic metabolism involves the conversion of carbohydrates and lipids into ATP, an energy-rich molecule, and this process cannot occur without oxygen (ATP). To meet the energy demands of exercise, the cardiorespiratory system enhances the absorption and distribution of oxygen (Plowman & Smith, 2017).

According to Badrić et al. (2021), cardiorespiratory fitness refers to the capacity of the respiratory and cardiovascular systems to sustain vigorous and rhythmic movements involving big muscle groups over an extended duration. A measure of this capacity to deliver oxygen to tissues during prolonged physical exertion, maximum oxygen consumption (VO_2 max), is typically used in incremental testing (Lu et al., 2018). Maintaining intense activity or exercise for an extended period without experiencing fatigue is a hallmark of cardiorespiratory fitness (Gao & Zhou, 2021).

Cardiorespiratory fitness refers to the body's ability to simultaneously produce energy through the energy system pathways and efficiently transport oxygen to the working muscles during physical activity.

A strong cardiorespiratory capacity is essential for energy synthesis and efficient oxygen delivery to the working muscles.

On the other hand, cardiorespiratory endurance refers to the body's ability to sustain physical activity for extended periods without fatigue. However, endurance also depends on other factors, such as muscle strength and efficiency, as well as mental and emotional factors, such as motivation and perseverance.

Muscles, bones, and joints comprise the musculoskeletal system, which generates motion and force. Our skeletal muscles contract when we lift heavy objects or push ourselves, producing mechanical effort. ATP, the energy source for contraction, powers muscular contraction and movement. This process involves the cross-bridge cycling of actin and myosin filaments (Standring, 2016).

So, the kinetic system – which includes the energy production and utilization system – supplies the energy needed to move and engage in physical activity. Energy production and utilization in the musculoskeletal and cardiorespiratory systems also retained specific indicators from the HRF–SRF model. These indicators included endurance, muscular strength, and cardiorespiratory fitness. Movement requires energy production and consumption, which is facilitated by the strength and endurance of the muscles.

A metabolic syndrome is a group of interrelated health problems that makes it hard for the body to produce and use energy. Metabolic illnesses include diabetes, obesity, cardiovascular disease, stroke, and type 2 diabetes.

Muscular strength. The demand for energy production increases as the intensity of a task or physical activity increases, demanding muscle fibers to work to produce force, a fitness indicator called muscular strength. This fitness indicator utilizes energy through the musculoskeletal system, producing the ability to lift heavy objects due to the force-production mechanism.

Muscular endurance. The duration of the physical activity demanding energy production and utilization is called muscular endurance. However, the musculoskeletal system adjusts muscle fiber recruitment depending on the task requirement (anaerobic or aerobic). Hence, we are coining the term "aerobic muscular endurance," which refers to the muscular endurance tasks that utilize energy produced from the aerobic energy system. We are also coining the term "anaerobic muscular endurance" to refer to the muscular endurance tasks that utilize energy produced from the anaerobic lactic energy system.

Body composition (ME)

The endocrine and musculoskeletal systems control the proportions of various tissues in the body, forming what is known as the body composition system. The endocrine system secretes hormones that influence metabolism and fat storage, while the musculoskeletal system establishes the groundwork for movement and energy expenditure. Resistance training, cardiovascular exercise, and a balanced diet can help maintain a healthy body composition, which is essential for health and fitness in general.

Hence, body composition, a fitness indicator in the HRF–SRF model, is kept. Also, remember that the endocrine system controls metabolism and fat mass, whereas the musculoskeletal system is called the fat-free mass.

Body composition refers to the relative proportion of lean mass with fat mass, consistent with the general definition of the term. In this framework, the emphasis is on the body structure provided by the musculoskeletal system (lean mass). Fat mass is added because of the integration of the endocrine system influenced by food intake, levels of physical activity, and metabolism. Obesity is a condition associated with body composition. An excessive fat mass characterizes this condition compared with the body's lean mass.

Metabolism (CE)

Metabolism, energy production, and utilization are regulated when the cardiorespiratory and endocrine systems collaborate. Hormones released by the endocrine system control metabolism; the cardiorespiratory system uses them to generate energy, and exercise raises metabolic rate both during and after the activity. As an example, the energy regulation of cells is greatly affected by thyroid hormones, which affect thermogenesis, lipid metabolism, appetite regulation, and critical peripheral targets like adipose tissue, liver, muscle, and pancreatic β-cells. This, in turn, affects different parts of the metabolic syndrome and, in the end, the control of body weight and blood pressure (Iwen et al., 2013).

Hence, the metabolic system, which integrates the endocrine and cardiorespiratory systems, is expanding its fitness indicator to include metabolic processes. The metabolic rate reveals how much energy an organism uses to maintain physiological functions like breathing, blood circulation, and temperature.

Metabolic rate refers to the amount of energy consumed to maintain a life phenomenon (Kim et al., 2018) and the amount of energy required per unit of time to sustain life (Lawler et al., 2019).

Metabolism is a measure of physical fitness because it shows how efficiently a person uses energy. The rate at which energy is produced and used can be explained by metabolic rate. An increased rate of energy expenditure, as measured by a higher metabolic rate, indicates an active state of the body. An active and efficient metabolism is often associated with endurance and intensity in physical activities, which could be a sign of that.

The grouped systems

Integrating these three foundational frameworks for physical fitness produces four grouped system functions, as shown in Figure 5.3. We also coined most of these terms to better understand how the grouped system works.

All four primary functions – control and coordination, energy, the body's structure, and the body's functions – are distinct and comprehensive. On the other hand, when we combine three systems, we can observe how they work together to form interdependent functions:

Movement (NMC)

Critical to movement and performance, this grouped system function encompasses NM, MC, and CN, all of which deal with energy production and utilization. Energy production and utilization fuel physical activity, while aerobic control allows working muscles to receive oxygen efficiently. With motor control, precise motions are possible, elevating the level of performance. Motor control, energy production and utilization, and aerobic control are the three paired system functions that make up this fitness-grouped system function, which reflects the body's ability to perform tasks effectively and efficiently.

Energy regulation (MCE)

The musculoskeletal, endocrine, and cardiorespiratory systems work together to control the body's energy during exercise and other forms of physical activity, all while keeping the body's composition in good shape. We refer to this set of operations as the energy regulation grouped system function since they generate and use movement-related energy. A person's body composition, energy production and utilization (MC), and metabolism (CE) all interact with one another (ME). Consequently, we are incorporating energy regulation, which manages the generation and consumption of energy for high-level physical activity, metabolism, and healthy body composition.

Physiological health (NME)

Healthy body composition is maintained through regulating energy for exercise and physical activity engagement by the grouped system function, which consists of the musculoskeletal, endocrine, and cardiorespiratory systems. Because they generate and use energy related to motion, we refer to this combination as the energy regulation grouped system function. Their interplay encompasses MC, CE, and body composition, all involved in metabolism (ME). In order to maintain healthy body composition, regulate metabolism, and engage in high-intensity physical activities, we are incorporating energy regulation.

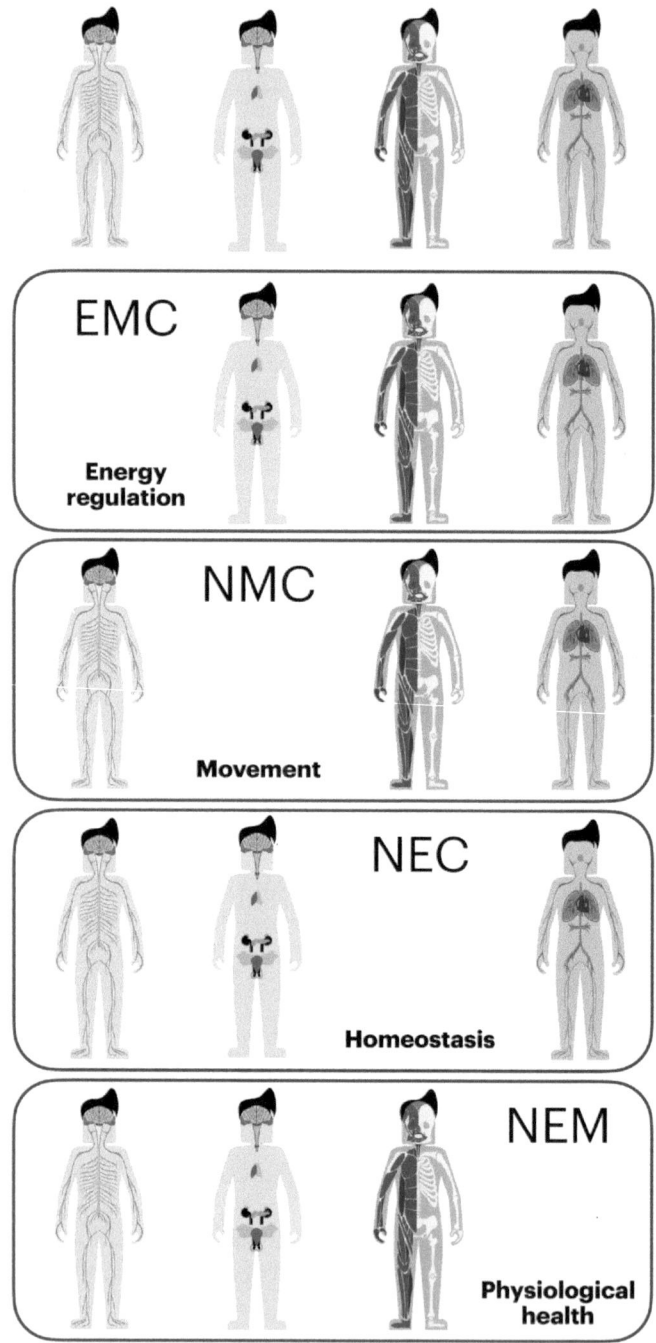

FIGURE 5.3   The USFD grouped system functions

Homeostasis (NCE)

Homeostasis is the capacity of the body to maintain a stable internal environment through regulation of breathing and respiration (NC), metabolism (CE), and energy production and utilization. This capacity is enhanced by the nervous system's integration with the combined functions of the endocrine and cardiorespiratory systems (NE). When many physiological variables, including heart rate, blood sugar, and blood pressure, are within normal ranges, we say that the body is in a state of homeostasis. For the body to adapt to various stresses, homeostasis keeps the internal environment stable despite the constant flow of external stimuli, such as those experienced during physical activity.

The body's optimal state is homeostasis. When homeostasis is disturbed, fever, irregular heart rate, unstable blood sugar levels, and fluid loss are all symptoms of an internal environment out of whack. Severe illnesses like heart disease, kidney disease, diabetes, and others can develop if the body is unable to maintain a balanced internal environment.

Organization of the paired system and grouped system functions

There are three connected system functions in every set. Figure 5.4 shows, for instance, that aerobic control, motor control, and energy production and utilization comprise the grouped system functions of movement.

The commonality of purpose between the two grouped systems, however, does reveal a pattern. System functions related to movement and physiological health, for instance, share the paired function of motor control (Figure 5.4). The interconnectedness of the body's functions is demonstrated here.

To further elaborate, we arranged the paired and grouped system functions in Figure 5.5 to demonstrate their interdependence. We developed the Interconnected Functions Framework model to illustrate the shared nature of the paired and grouped system functions.

A key concept in the Interconnected Functions Framework is the relationship between paired and grouped system functions. In the same way that systems theory investigates the ever-changing connections between parts of systems, these paired functions depict the linkages and interactions among the building block systems.

Summary

The Unified Systems Fitness Design (USFD) is a framework for understanding physical fitness based on systems theory. It identifies the body as a complex system with primary systems, including the nervous, musculoskeletal, cardiorespiratory, and endocrine systems. Each system has specific functions, such as

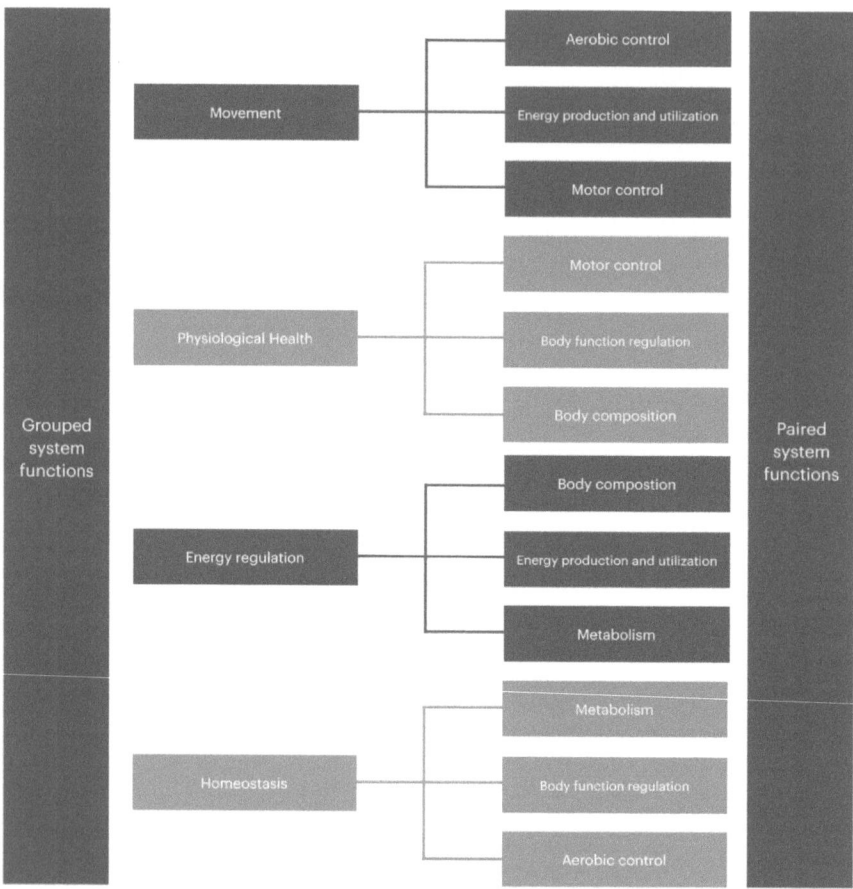

FIGURE 5.4   Grouped system functions and paired system functions

controlling body movements, generating force for physical activities, supporting energy production, and regulating body functions.

The USFD uses a paired systems matrix to identify relationships and main functions between these primary systems. Six paired system functions are identified: motor control, aerobic control, body function regulation, energy production and utilization, body composition, and metabolism.

The USFD also identifies four grouped system functions resulting from the combination of three primary systems: movement (NMC), energy regulation (MCE), physiological health (NME), and homeostasis (NCE). These functions reflect the body's ability to perform tasks effectively and efficiently, regulate energy production and utilization, maintain physiological health, and maintain internal environment stability.

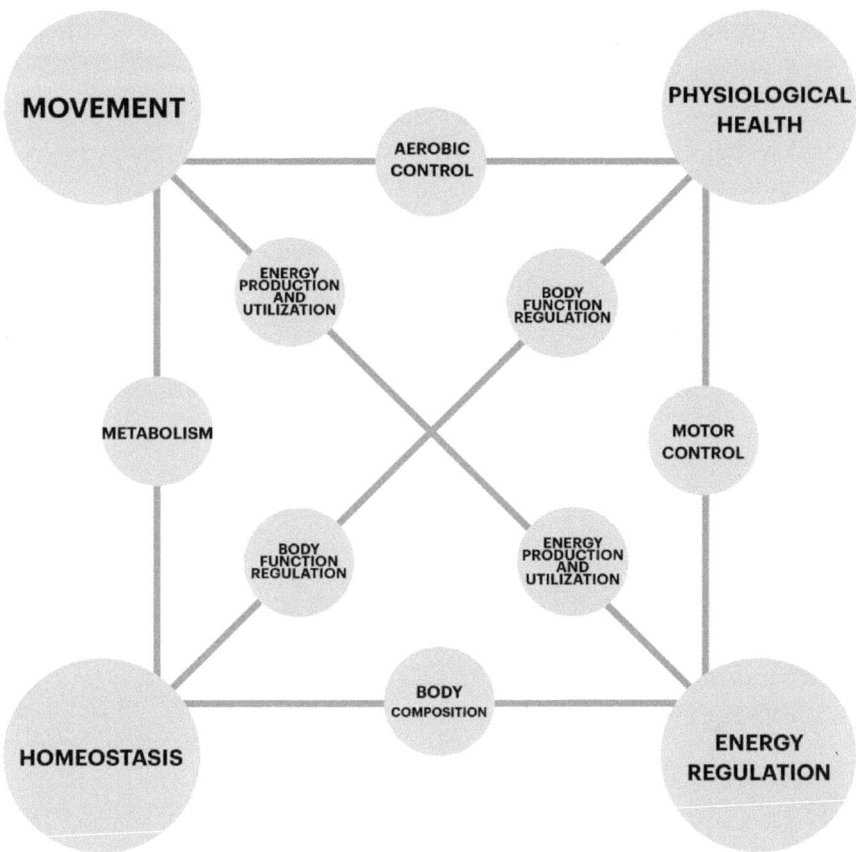

FIGURE 5.5   The interconnected functions framework

The Interconnected Functions Framework illustrates how paired system functions are shared by grouped system functions, highlighting the interdependencies and interactions between the primary systems. This framework demonstrates how the body's functions are interconnected, like systems theory, which explores dynamic relationships within systems.

Review questions

1. What is the USFD guiding principle, and how does it regard physical fitness?
2. Describe the four building block systems that the USFD identified. How do they improve a person's general fitness?
3. How does the USFD develop a framework for comprehending how these fundamental systems interact?

4. What role does the USFD's paired systems matrix play?
5. Describe *motor control* as a paired system function. How does it relate to total movement effectiveness and physical fitness?
6. What is *aerobic control,* and why is it crucial for physical fitness?
7. How do the endocrine and nervous systems perform *body function regulation*?
8. How do the musculoskeletal and cardiorespiratory systems work together to promote *energy production and utilization*?
9. How do the endocrine and musculoskeletal systems interact to control body composition?
10. What is *metabolism* as a paired system function, and what roles do the endocrine and cardiorespiratory systems play in controlling metabolic processes?

Discussion questions

1. How can a customized fitness plan be created based on the USFD principles to cater to a person's unique fitness demands and goals? Give examples of how the functions of each basic system may be modified to enhance fitness.
2. How might the paired systems matrix optimize workout regimens in real-world fitness training? Discuss practical ways to combine workouts that focus on various coupled system functions.
3. Discuss how diet and nutrition choices support the USFD-identified primary systems and paired system functions. What dietary changes can be made to improve overall fitness and energy balance?
4. Consider how the USFD can handle typical fitness issues, including weight control, muscle development, and cardiovascular endurance. How can people overcome these obstacles by understanding paired and grouped system functions?
5. Examine the significance of tracking and evaluating advancement in a workout regimen that adheres to the USFD Framework. How can one monitor changes in motor control, aerobic control, body composition, metabolism, and the regulation of bodily functions?

References

Badrić, M., Roca, L., & Prskalo, I. (2021, September). Differences in the level of cardiorespiratory fitness about nutrition status of children in primary education. In *9th international scientific conference on kinesiology* (p. 216). https://www.bib.irb.hr/1145397/download/1145397.9-Conference-Kinesiology-2021-Proceedings-_FINAL.pdf#page=218

Bhattacharyya, S., Konar, A., Raza, H., & Khasnobish, A. (2021). Brain-computer interfaces for perception, learning, and motor control. *Frontiers in Neuroscience, 15,* 1361. https://doi.org/10.3389/fnins.2021.758104

Bisi, M. C., & Stagni, R. (2020). Human motor control: Is a subject-specific quantitative assessment of its multiple characteristics possible? A demonstrative application on children' motor development. *Medical Engineering & Physics*, *85*, 27–34. https://doi.org/10.1016/j.medengphy.2020.09.002

Blackinton, M. T. (2017). *Learning a novel motor task helps students apply motor control principles to PT practice* [Podium Presentation]. https://nsuworks.nova.edu/hpers/2017/all_events/21/

de Faria Cardoso, C., Ohe, N. T., Bader, Y., Afify, N., Al-Homedi, Z., Alwedami, S. M., O'Sullivan, S., Campos, L. A., & Baltatu, O. C. (2022). Heart rate variability indices as possible biomarkers for the severity of post-traumatic stress disorder following pregnancy loss. *Frontiers in Psychiatry*, *12*, 700920. https://doi.org/10.3389/fpsyt.2021.700920

Farr, O. M., Chiang-Shan, R. L., & Mantzoros, C. S. (2016). Central nervous system regulation of eating: Insights from human brain imaging. *Metabolism*, *65*(5), 699–713.

Gao, H., & Zhou, C. (2021). Effects of cardiorespiratory fitness on cognitive function in middle school students: A systematic review. *Discobolul-Physical Education, Sport & Kinetotherapy Journal*, *60*. https://doi.org/10.35189/dpeskj.2021.60.s2

Hodges, P. W., Van Dieёn, J. H., & Cholewicki, J. (2019). Time to reflect on the role of motor control in low back pain. *Journal of Orthopaedic & Sports Physical Therapy*, *49*(6), 367–369. https://www.jospt.org/doi/10.2519/jospt.2019.010

Iwen, K. A., Schröder, E., & Brabant, G. (2013). Thyroid hormones and the metabolic syndrome. *European Thyroid Journal*, *2*(2), 83–92. https://doi.org/10.1159/000351249

Jänig, W. (2014). Sympathetic nervous system and inflammation: A conceptual view. *Autonomic Neuroscience*, *182*, 4–14. https://doi.org/10.1016/j.autneu.2014.01.004

Jänig, W. (2022). *The integrative action of the autonomic nervous system: Neurobiology of homeostasis*. Cambridge University Press.

Kim, M. C., Park, H. S., Paik, J. K., Jung, D. Y., & Lee, S. M. (2018). Changes in serum lipids according to the amount of exercise activity in middle-aged women. *Indian Journal of Public Health Research & Development*, *9*(12). http://dx.doi.org/10.5958/0976-5506.2018.02169.1

Lawler, K., Bell, I., Bryant, C., Pickering, S. H., Gillding, E. R., Rapley, S., & Rolfe, M. (2019). Jump distance of Monistria concinna in relation to metabolic rate and femur length: Mass ratio. *Field Studies in Ecology*, *2*(1). https://studentjournals.anu.edu.au/index.php/fse/article/view/224

Lu, Z., Woo, J., & Kwok, T. (2018). The effect of physical activity and cardiorespiratory fitness on all-cause mortality in Hong Kong Chinese older adults. *The Journals of Gerontology: Series A*, *73*(8), 1132–1137. https://doi.org/10.1093/gerona/glx180

Mihelj, M., Novak, D., & Begus, S. (2014). Haptic modality in virtual reality. In *Virtual reality technology and applications. Intelligent systems, control and automation: Science and engineering* (vol. 68). Springer. https://doi.org/10.1007/978-94-007-6910-6_7

Plowman, S. A., & Smith, D. L. (2017). *Exercise physiology for health, fitness, and performance* (4th ed.). Wolters Kluwer.

Rice, A. (2021). *Motor control-based assessment of therapy effects in individuals post-stroke: Implications for prediction of response and subject-specific modifications* [Doctoral dissertation, University of Tennessee]. https://trace.tennessee.edu/utk_graddiss/6648

Russo, M. A., Santarelli, D. M., & O'Rourke, D. (2017). The physiological effects of slow breathing in the healthy human. *Breathe*, *13*(4), 298–309. https://doi.org/10.1183/20734735.009817

Saper, C. B., & Lowell, B. B. (2014). The hypothalamus. *Current Biology*, *24*(23), R1111–R1116. https://doi.org/10.1016/j.tins.2012.12.008

Seifert, L. (2020). Motor control: Coordination and stroking parameters in young swimmers. In *High performance youth swimming* (pp. 171–189). Routledge. https://doi.org/10.4324/9780429465598

Standring, S. (Ed.). (2016). *Gray's Anatomy: The anatomical basis of clinical practice* (41st ed.). Elsevier.

Starling, C. T., Nguyen, Q. B. D., Butler, I. J., Numan, M. T., & Hebert, A. A. (2021). Cutaneous manifestations of orthostatic intolerance syndromes. *International Journal of Women's Dermatology*, *7*(4), 471–477. https://doi.org/10.1016/j.ijwd.2021.03.003

Tan, C. L., & Knight, Z. A. (2018). Regulation of body temperature by the nervous system. *Neuron*, *98*(1), 31–48. https://doi.org/10.1016/j.neuron.2018.02.022

Thorens, B. (2014). Neural regulation of pancreatic islet cell mass and function. *Diabetes, Obesity and Metabolism*, *16*(S1), 87–95. https://doi.org/10.1111/dom.12346

Wang, L. Y., Han, P. H., & Chan, L. (2022, February). Push-ups: Enhancing kinesthetic experience with shape-forming devices on the feet soles. In *Proceedings of the sixteenth international conference on tangible, embedded, and embodied interaction (TEI '22)* (pp. 1–8). Association for Computing Machinery. https://doi.org/10.1145/3490149.3501333

6

COORDINATION

The essence of motor control

Oliver Napila Gomez and Nguyen Tra Giang

In this chapter, emphasis has been placed on appreciating the worth of coordination in both sports and everyday life. The significance of visual input control toward efficient and accurate motor control is emphasized. This chapter highlights how the brain can combine sensory data, motor control elements, and other body parts. Coordination manifests itself in manipulative, non-locomotor, and locomotor movements. Concrete examples show the importance of coordination in professional contexts, daily lives, and sports activities. Influences that neurological disorders and impairments have on brain functions are shown, hence revealing a complicated relation between them. Gaining an insight into the complex aspects of coordination is vital for clinical practices when addressing coordination-related problems and advancing fitness levels and performance.

Outcomes

By the end of this chapter, you will be able to

- examine why the USFD hailed coordination as the essence of physical fitness, being the ability to coordinate movements to perform accurate and efficient movements in sports and daily activities
- elucidate the fundamental elements of coordination, including the body's parts, sensory inputs, and fitness elements
- explore the role of the nervous system in regulating sensory inputs and coordinating movements

DOI: 10.4324/9781003502937-7

- connect coordination to a variety of sports and real-world scenarios, comprehending its importance in a range of activities and assessing how different coordination elements interact in these operations
- survey the conditions that impact coordination, the challenges they pose, and how they affect a person's ability to perform daily tasks and engage in physical activity

Coordination: the core of skill and movement

The heart of athletic skill is precise and accurate bodily control in reaction to visual input (Rodrigues, 2020). For example, volleyball smash accuracy is based on leg muscle explosive force and hand–eye coordination (Yulianti, 2017). Hand–eye coordination also allows goal-directed use of the arm, hand, and fingers to create regulated, precise, and quick motions in badminton (Wong et al., 2019). Coordination is essential for these abilities, as it is the process through which eyes and brain work together to command hands or feet to do an action, such as catching or kicking a ball (Wong et al., 2019). Coordination integrates eyes, hands, and feet in a continuous process of the eyes directing body action while the athlete responds swiftly and correctly to the visual input (Rodrigues, 2020). Hand–eye coordination is essential in sports, daily life, and work (Szabo et al., 2020).

Elements of coordination

In this chapter, we highlight the role of the primary nervous system in coordinating and regulating the body – movement coordination results when various senses, body parts, and energy simultaneously accomplish a task. The elements of coordination involve the synchronization of these different factors. Figure 6.1 illustrates the elements of coordination.

The brain is the most sophisticated organ humans possess. It is responsible for transmitting commands to the body's conscious and unconscious activities (Albán et al., 2019). It is the center of consciousness and regulates all voluntary and involuntary physical movements and processes. Hence, its function must also be the most important for fitness.

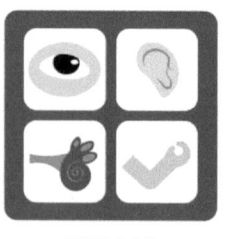
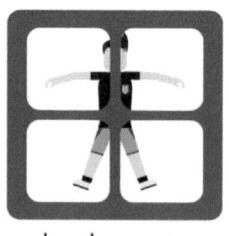
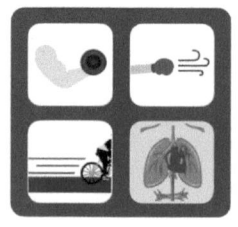

senses   body parts   energy regulation

FIGURE 6.1 Elements of coordination in the USFD Framework

We consider coordination the most crucial function for physical fitness. It involves using different body parts together smoothly and efficiently to perform a movement accurately and effectively. Without the brain's effective and efficient coordination and control of the body, including the autonomic functions, all other fitness indicators will cease to develop. It will be chaos internally and externally.

> ***Coordination,*** *whether voluntary or autonomic, is a fundamental component of human performance, showcasing the brain's remarkable capacity to seamlessly integrate diverse bodily functions, playing a pivotal role in fostering interconnectedness within group and paired systems across various domains, including movement, physiological health, energy regulation, and the maintenance of homeostasis.*

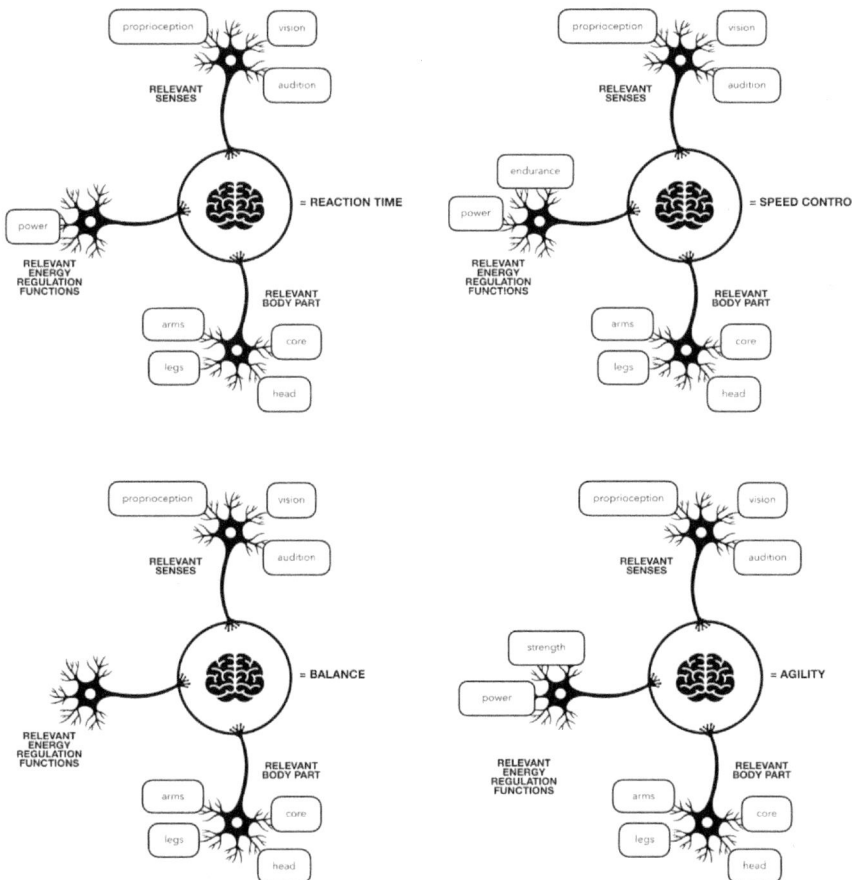

FIGURE 6.2   The brain's role is to coordinate and control

Coordination holds and synchronizes all the coordination elements. It reflects the ability to use different body parts together smoothly and efficiently to perform a movement accurately and effectively. These coordination elements work together simultaneously to achieve a particular task, and the nervous system plays a crucial role in coordinating these elements. The nervous system integrates sensory information from different senses, regulates energy, and ensures that movements are executed accurately and efficiently.

Coordination impairments are often caused by neurological illnesses that impact the brain, such as dementia, cerebellar disorders, and stroke (Andrews, 2014; McShane, 2023; Moore et al., 2023; Musaeus et al., 2023). In addition, Wilson and colleagues (2013) discovered that children with developmental coordination disorder (DCD) had severe difficulty with coordination, motor control, and cognitive processes. This shows that DCD may impact their ability to plan and regulate their movements and behaviors.

Coordination deficiencies result from brain-related illnesses or injuries, which might transpire as decreased balance, clumsiness, or difficulty performing exact motions. The occurrence of coordination deficits in these illnesses provides evidence that coordination is intimately related to brain function.

We postulate that coordination reflects the brain's ability to collect input from the sensory systems, process this information, regulate the required energy, and produce an outcome executed through the body parts. The brain can synchronize different elements of movement to produce an efficient and effective outcome. The process starts with the sensory systems, such as sight, hearing, balance, and proprioception, which collect information about the body's position, movement, and environment. The brain then processes this information, adjusts the right amount of force, and utilizes energy for movement necessary to accomplish the task, such as strength, power, or endurance. Finally, the brain produces an outcome executed through the body parts, such as hand–eye or foot–eye coordination, maintaining balance, or changing direction quickly. Thus, the outcome is often observed as motor control fitness indicators such as balance, reaction time, speed control, and agility.

The USFD perception of coordination involves integrating multiple elements to produce smooth and effective movement. It requires adjusting the level of movement based on the task's demands. Through coordinated movements, individuals can improve their physical performance and reduce the risk of injury.

In other words, coordination is crucial for activities that require precise and complex movements, such as sports, dance, and other physical activities. The nervous system controls the body parts in collaboration with the senses and other fitness components, regulating movements, speed, and force development. The nervous system receives sensory inputs from the sense organs and uses them to coordinate movements and adjust them to changing situations.

The most common examples of coordination are hand–eye and foot–eye coordination. With hand–eye coordination, the sense of sight and proprioception in the arm muscles and joints work together to accomplish tasks. One classic example is ball juggling. For foot–eye coordination, the sense of sight pairs with the sense of proprioception in the legs. A classic example from Vietnam is the game *da cau* or foot badminton. Players use their eyes and feet to control the direction of a shuttlecock.

Apart from hand–eye and foot–eye coordination, there are several other ways by which the brain synchronizes the elements of coordination. Several possible combinations are presented in the following table:

TABLE 6.1 Sample combinations of the elements of coordination

Elements of coordination	*Sample combinations*	*Examples*
Senses: • **sight** • **hearing** • **balance** • **proprioception**	sight and proprioception	In basketball, a player needs to use their eyes to track the ball while simultaneously using their hands to dribble or shoot the ball accurately.
	hearing and vestibular sense	Activities such as dance or gymnastics, where hearing the music and maintaining balance and stability are crucial for performance.
	touch and proprioception	Activities such as rock climbing, where the sense of touch and proprioception in the fingers and hands are crucial for maintaining grip and balance.
Body parts: • **left upper extremities** • **right upper extremities** • **left lower extremities** • **right lower extremities** • **core head**	left upper extremities and right lower extremities right upper extremities and left lower extremities	When walking, running, and swimming, the left upper extremities are in coordination with the right lower extremities and vice versa to accomplish well-coordinated locomotor movements.
	upper extremities and core	When throwing a ball or performing a push-up, the core is in coordination with the upper extremities to execute a well-coordinated movement.

(*Continued*)

TABLE 6.1 (Continued)

Elements of coordination	Sample combinations	Examples
Energy regulation functions: • **muscular strength** • **aerobic muscular endurance** • **anaerobic muscular endurance** • **power**	muscular strength and anaerobic muscular endurance	To get the most out of a circuit training program, muscle strength is required for high-intensity exercises like squats, push-ups, and lunges, and anaerobic muscular endurance to sustain through multiple rounds of these exercises without resting.
	muscular strength and power	In powerlifting, the athlete needs to have the strength to control the weight and the force to quickly extend the hips, knees, and ankles in order to drive the weight overhead when switching from the clean to the jerk.
	anaerobic muscular endurance and power	Combining high-intensity interval training with plyometric exercises like burpees or jump squats teaches the muscles to continue producing force even when they are fatigued, enhancing anaerobic endurance and power generation efficiency.
Senses and body parts: • **sight** • **hearing** • **vestibular sense** • **proprioception** • **left upper extremities** • **right upper extremities** • **left lower extremities** • **right lower extremities** • **head** • **core**	sight and left upper extremities sight and right upper extremities	When playing tennis, the player uses their sight to track the ball and their upper extremities, such as the left or right arm, to control the racquet and hit the ball. Another example is playing the guitar. The player uses their sight to read the music sheet or the chords on the guitar and their right upper extremities, such as the right arm and hand, to control the strings and produce the desired sound.

(*Continued*)

TABLE 6.1 (Continued)

Elements of coordination	Sample combinations	Examples
	vestibular sense and upper extremities	When performing a handstand, the vestibular sense maintains the body's position, while the upper extremities, such as the arms and shoulders, support the weight of the body and control the movement.
	vestibular sense, head, and upper extremities	When performing a headstand, the sense of balance is essential in maintaining the body's position, while the head and the upper extremities, such as the arms and shoulders, support the weight of the body and control the movement.
Senses and fitness components: • **sight** • **hearing** • **vestibular sense** • **proprioception** • **muscular strength** • **aerobic muscular endurance** • **anaerobic muscular endurance** • **power**	sight and muscular strength	Visual and muscular strength coordination are essential in archery. The archer needs clear, stable vision to focus on the target. The arms, shoulders, and core must be strong enough to draw the bow and propel the arrow accurately.
	hearing and aerobic muscular endurance	Hearing and aerobic muscular endurance are important in Zumba and spin classes. The intensity and pace of the exercise are determined by hearing the music's rhythm and tempo. Aerobic muscular endurance lets people move to the music for long periods.

(Continued)

TABLE 6.1 (Continued)

Elements of coordination	Sample combinations	Examples
	proprioception and anaerobic muscular endurance	Proprioception and anaerobic muscular endurance must be coordinated for rock climbing. To climb efficiently, climbers must be aware of their body, limbs, and muscles. Climbers can perform powerful moves, maintain grip strength, and sustain effort through difficult sections without oxygen.
	Vestibular sense and power	In vault and floor routines, gymnasts must coordinate their vestibular sense (which aids balance and spatial orientation) with power. Vestibular sense helps gymnasts balance during flips, spins, and jumps. Gymnasts need power for explosive movements and dynamic routines.
Body parts and fitness components: • **left upper extremities** • **right upper extremities** • **left lower extremities** • **right lower extremities** • **core** • **head** • **speed control** • **agility** • **coordination** • **balance** • **reaction time**	left and right lower extremities and speed control	When running or sprinting, the athlete uses both their left and right legs to move forward at different speeds based on the terrain, slope, and other factors.
	core and balance	When practicing yoga, the practitioner engages their core muscles to maintain balance and stability in various poses and movements.
	left and right upper extremities and strength	In weightlifting, the athlete uses their left and right arms to lift weights and build strength in their upper extremities.

(*Continued*)

TABLE 6.1 (Continued)

Elements of coordination	Sample combinations	Examples
Senses, body parts, and fitness components: • **sight** • **hearing** • **vestibular sense** • **proprioception** • **left upper extremities** • **right upper extremities** • **left lower extremities** • **right lower extremities** • **head** • **core** • **muscular strength** • **aerobic muscular endurance** • **anaerobic muscular endurance** • **power**	sight, right lower extremities, and muscular strength	Precision kicks in tae kwon do require sight, right lower extremities, and muscle strength. Sight helps the practitioner locate and measure distance. A powerful kick is then executed with the practitioner's dominant right lower extremity. Kicking requires leg muscle strength, especially quadriceps, hamstrings, and calves.
	vestibular sense, core, aerobic muscular endurance	Long-distance cycling requires vestibular, core, and aerobic muscle coordination. The vestibular sense aids balance and spatial orientation during turns and terrain changes. Core muscles stabilize and support the upper body, transferring power to the pedals efficiently. Aerobic muscular endurance lets cyclists use oxygen efficiently for long distances.
	proprioception, upper extremities, power	Climbers must coordinate proprioception, upper extremities, and power to perform dynos (dynamic moves in rock climbing), which involve jumping to a hold. Proprioception is needed to sense the body and limbs in space and jump at the right time. Power comes from the arms and shoulders to lift the body to the target hold. To overcome gravity and reach the desired height or distance, explosive power is essential.

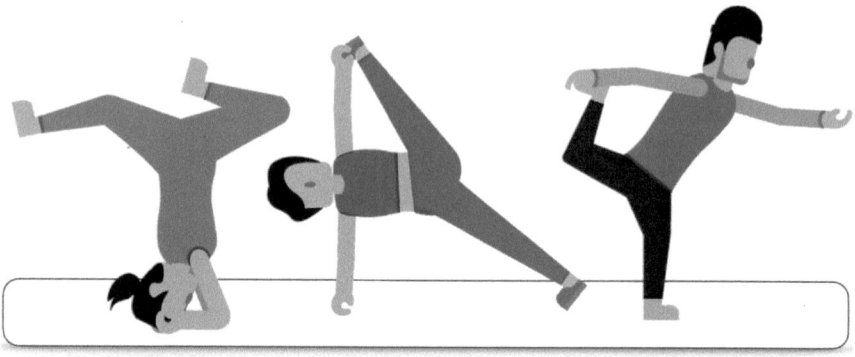

FIGURE 6.3 Different non-locomotor movements require the elements of coordination

Coordination and movement

When movement involves several elements executed simultaneously, however simple the movement may seem, coordination is at work. This fitness component can be observed in non-locomotor, locomotor, and manipulative movements.

Non-locomotor movements and coordination

Non-locomotor coordination involves the synchronization of body elements in place. Non-locomotor movements are performed in place without moving from one location to another. Coordination in non-locomotor movements requires the execution of precise and synchronized movements, often involving balance and body positioning.

Yoga is a practical example of coordination with non-locomotor movements. In yoga, the performer moves through a series of postures and positions while maintaining a sense of proprioception and balance. Yoga requires coordination between different elements of kinesthetic fitness, including balance, flexibility, and strength.

In yoga, the performer moves through various postures, such as the downward-facing dog, the tree pose, and the headstand. Each posture requires precise movements and balance to maintain the correct body position. The performer must also exhibit muscular proprioception to control their movements and maintain balance while holding each posture. The coordination required in yoga differs from that in locomotor movements, but it is equally important in maintaining good overall physical health and fitness.

Locomotor movements and coordination

Locomotor coordination involves synchronizing different body parts and movements to move from one location to another. It requires coordination between

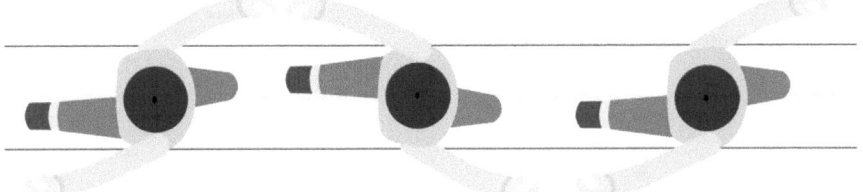

FIGURE 6.4   The limbs, when walking or running (bird's-eye view)

limbs, the left and right sides of the body, and the upper and lower extremities. These movements are essential for daily walking, running, and jumping.

The natural way of walking follows a counterbalanced movement between the left and right hemispheres. As the left foot strides forward, the upper right extremities move in the opposite direction to stabilize the movement. Similarly, the upper left extremities move oppositely as the right foot strides forward. This coordination of movements between the upper and lower extremities is essential for maintaining balance and stability while walking.

When the movement progresses to running (or sprinting), the speed of movement increases, and the force exerted on the lower extremities must be compensated with equal force on the upper extremities to maintain balance and coordination. Coordinating movements between the upper and lower extremities becomes critical in running and sprinting to ensure efficient and effective movement.

Coordination with locomotor movements is essential for daily activities and athletic performance. Athletes in various sports, such as soccer, basketball, and track and field, rely heavily on coordination with locomotor movements to perform at their best. The ability to move efficiently and effectively is critical for success in these sports, and coordination is vital.

Manipulative movements and coordination

Coordination with manipulative movements involves using implements as body extensions to perform tasks. This type of coordination is well known to most people, as it is used in various activities, such as playing sports, handling tools, and performing daily tasks.

Coordination with implements requires the use of sight to determine the location of the implement and proprioception to determine its weight, rigidity, and other physical qualities. Manipulating the implement involves speed control, agility, reaction time, and balance. These elements must be coordinated with the movement of the implement to achieve the desired outcome.

For example, in baseball, the batter must coordinate his or her movements with the bat's swing to contact the ball. This requires coordination between the

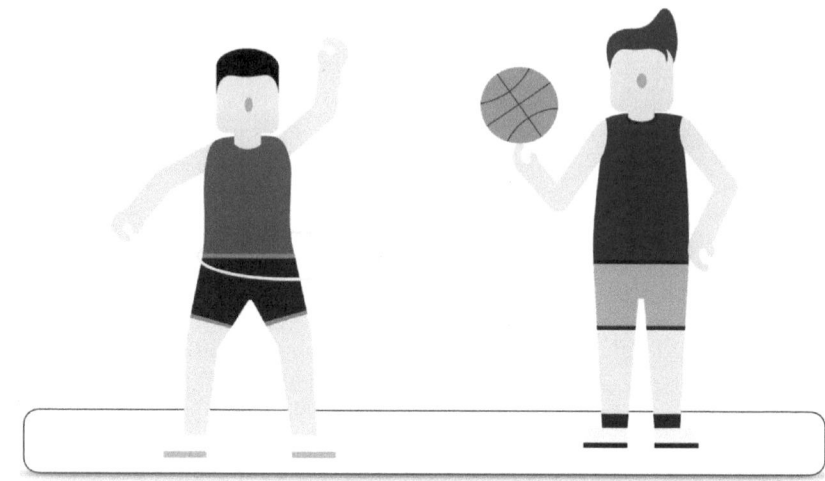

a. keeping an object moving in place

FIGURE 6.5a Manipulative movements

b. sending and receiving objects

FIGURE 6.5b Manipulative movements

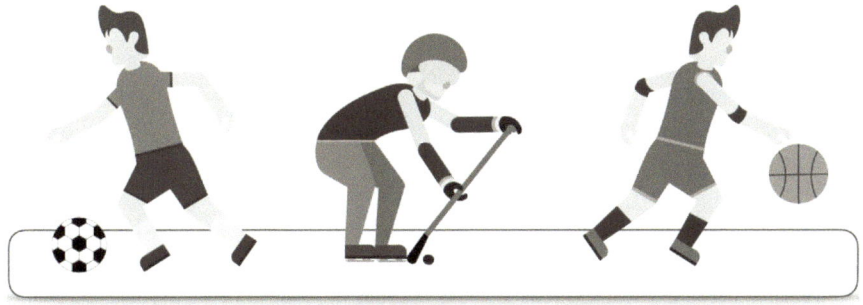

c. travel along with the object

FIGURE 6.5c Manipulative movements

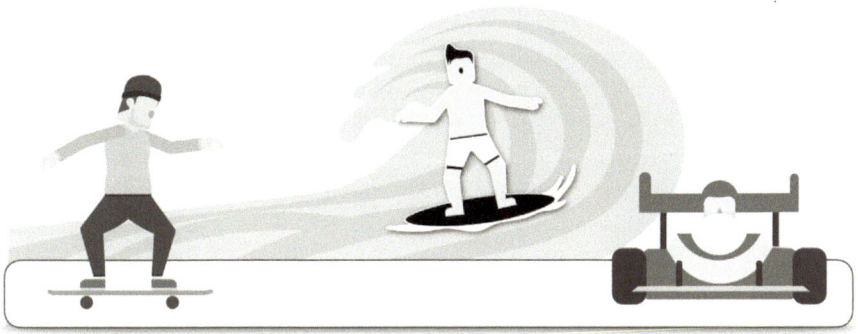

d. operating equipment that transports the body

FIGURE 6.5d Manipulative movements

upper and lower extremities, speed control, agility control, and reaction time. Similarly, in tennis, the player must coordinate his or her movements with the racket's swing to hit the ball accurately. This requires coordination between the upper extremities and the sense of proprioception to determine the weight and rigidity of the racket.

Moving with implements can also be executed in different situations. For example, equipment such as bars, beams, and rings require coordination with manipulative movements in gymnastics. The gymnast must coordinate movements with the equipment to perform flips, spins, and other maneuvers.

Factors that affect coordination

Brain circuits are responsible for coordinating, motor control, and decision-making. Disruptions to these circuits cause abnormal motor behavior in diseases like Parkinson's and Huntington's (Arber & Costa, 2018). The ability of the peripheral nervous system to regulate muscles is affected by neurodegenerative diseases like Alzheimer's disease (AD) and Parkinson's disease (PD), which can lead to noticeable changes in handwriting performance (Impedovo & Pirlo, 2019). Spinocerebellar ataxias (SCAs) are disorders characterized by dysfunction in the cerebellar Purkinje neurons and other neurological components, which can lead to difficulties with balance and coordination (Klockgether et al., 2019).

Information from different parts of the nervous system needs to be put together to control the body's motor units. One of the main signs of motor control disorders like Parkinson's disease and spasticity is the inability to stabilize important variables and use changes in reference coordinates (Latash & Yamagata, 2022). Neurotransmitter activity needs to be balanced to keep coordination. This is shown by the fact that long-term exercise improves motor control and the expression of brain-derived neurotrophic factors in the motor-related cortex (Inoue et al., 2018).

The nervous system's job is to initiate brain–body coordination, which is crucial for moving and staying balanced. Any disruption can significantly impact normal operations, making it difficult to complete tasks and putting physical fitness in a new light.

Summary

This chapter explores the importance of coordination in physical fitness and daily life. It explains how coordination involves harmonizing sensory inputs, body parts, and motor control components to achieve precise and efficient movements. The nervous system orchestrates this synchronization, and the brain plays a crucial role in regulating these elements. Impaired coordination can lead to neurological disorders like dementia, cerebellar issues, or stroke, highlighting the connection between coordination and brain function.

Coordination is not limited to sports but also daily life and work. The brain's ability to gather sensory input, process it, and regulate fitness components like speed, agility, and balance results in precise and effective movement. The chapter comprehensively explains the multifaceted nature of coordination through real-world examples.

Coordination is essential across different movement types, such as non-locomotor, locomotor, and manipulative. Non-locomotor coordination emphasizes balance, flexibility, and strength in static positions, while locomotor coordination synchronizes limbs and extremities. In manipulative movements, coordination with implements reveals how sight, proprioception, and motor skills work together to achieve precise tasks.

Central nervous system disorders and sensory impairments like ataxia can affect coordination. Diagnosis and treatment are essential to enhancing the quality of life for individuals with coordination-related challenges.

Review questions

1. Why is coordination a key component of physical fitness, and what does it mean in that context?
2. What is the primary function of the nervous system in the coordination of movements?
3. What are some typical coordination issues, and how might they impact a person's day-to-day activities?
4. Using examples from the chapter, describe how coordination and brain activity are related.
5. What are the leading fitness metrics that coordination affects, and how do they affect sports performance?
6. Describe the importance that sight, proprioception, and balance play in coordination as sensory inputs.
7. Give instances of tasks requiring non-locomotor coordination and describe their importance.
8. Why is locomotor coordination necessary for walking and running, and how does it differ from non-locomotor coordination?
9. Examine the idea of manipulative coordination and give instances of how it is used in sports and everyday activities.
10. Why must coordination-related issues be addressed for a higher quality of life, and what elements can affect coordination?

Discussion questions

1. Describe how coordination in exercises like yoga and tai chi is aided by integrating sensory inputs, body parts, and motor control elements. Give examples from your experience or observations to demonstrate these components' significance in non-locomotor movements.
2. Examine the connection between coordination and proprioception. How does a person's awareness of their body position improve their capacity to coordinate movements successfully? Give instances of activities where proprioception is essential.
3. Talk about the role vestibular sensation plays in coordination and balance. Examine events that can challenge a person's vestibular sense and how they might respond to them.

4. Utilizing real-world examples, explore the idea of synchronization in manipu-lating movements. How do athletes or specialists in professions like dancing or woodworking use coordination when using implements or tools? Highlight the crucial components that make these actions successful.
5. Consider how neurological conditions like ataxia or cerebellar abnormalities affect coordination. Talk about instances in which people with these diseases experience difficulties with their coordination and the methods or treatments that may be able to help them.

References

Albán, W. E. M., Ruperti, M. J. B., Tumbaco, D. E. S., & Martínez, M. E. M. (2019). Brain and emotions on learning process. *International Journal of Health and Medical Sciences*, *3*(1), 17–20. https://dx.doi.org/10.31295/ijhms.v3n1.108

Andrews, B. S. (2014). *Sprinting kinematics of athletes with selected disabilities* [Doctoral dissertation, Stellenbosch University]. http://bit.ly/3PxoUHx

Arber, S., & Costa, R. (2018). Connecting neuronal circuits for movement. *Science*, *360*, 1403–1404. https://doi.org/10.1126/science.aat5994

Impedovo, D., & Pirlo, G. (2019). Dynamic handwriting analysis for the assessment of neurodegenerative diseases: A pattern recognition perspective. *IEEE Reviews in Biomedical Engineering*, *12*, 209–220. https://doi.org/10.1109/RBME.2018.2840679

Inoue, T., Ninuma, S., Hayashi, M., Okuda, A., Asaka, T., & Maejima, H. (2018). Effects of long-term exercise and low-level inhibition of GABAergic synapses on motor control and the expression of BDNF in the motor related cortex. *Neurological Research*, *40*, 18–25. https://doi.org/10.1080/01616412.2017.1382801

Klockgether, T., Mariotti, C., & Paulson, H. (2019). Spinocerebellar ataxia. *Nature Reviews Disease Primers*, *5*, 1–21. https://doi.org/10.1038/s41572-019-0074-3

Latash, M., & Yamagata, M. (2022). Recent advances in the neural control of movements: Lessons for functional recovery. *Physical Therapy Research*, *25*(1), 1–11. https://doi.org/10.1298/ptr.r0018

McShane, D. (2023). Using personalised music to enhance the well-being of people with dementia. *Mental Health Practice*, *26*(1). http://doi.org/10.7748/mhp.2023.e1637

Moore, A., Goss-Hill, B., & Dening, K. H. (2023). Recognition and assessment of dementia in a primary care setting. *Primary Health Care*, *33*(2). http://doi.org/10.7748/phc.2023.e1794

Musaeus, C. S., Frederiksen, K. S., Andersen, B. B., Høgh, P., Kidmose, P., Fabricius, M., Hribljan, M. C., Hemmsen, M. C., Rank, M. L., Waldemar, G., & Kjær, T. W. (2023). Detection of subclinical epileptiform discharges in Alzheimer's disease using long-term outpatient EEG monitoring. *Neurobiology of Disease*, *183*, 106149. https://doi.org/10.1016/j.nbd.2023.106149

Rodrigues, P. (2020). Sports vision: Influence on athlete's performance. *Acta Sci Ophthalmol*, *3*, 61–68.

Szabo, D. A., Neagu, N., Teodorescu, S., & Sopa, I. S. (2020). Eye-hand relationship of proprioceptive motor control and coordination in children 10–11 years old. *Health, Sports & Rehabilitation Medicine*, *21*(3), 185–191. https://doi.org/10.26659/pm3.2020.21.3.185

Wilson, P. H., Ruddock, S., Smits-Engelsman, B., Polatajko, H., & Blank, R. (2013). Understanding performance deficits in developmental coordination disorder: A meta-analysis of recent research. *Developmental Medicine & Child Neurology, 55*(3), 217–228. https://doi.org/10.1111/j.1469-8749.2012.04436.x

Wong, T. K., Ma, A. W., Liu, K. P., Chung, L. M., Bae, Y. H., Fong, S. S., Ganesan, B., & Wang, H. K. (2019). Balance control, agility, eye–hand coordination, and sport performance of amateur badminton players: A cross-sectional study. *Medicine, 98*(2). https://doi.org/10.1097%2FMD.0000000000014134

Yulianti, M. (2017). Contribution of leg muscle explosive power and eye-hand coordination to the accuracy smash of athletes in volleyball club of Universitas Islam Riau. *Journal of Physical Education Health and Sport, 4*(2), 70–74. https://doi.org/10.15294/jpehs.v4i2.10571

7

ESSENTIALS OF THE UNIFIED SYSTEM FITNESS DESIGN

A synthesis

Nguyen Tra Giang and Oliver Napila Gomez

The Unified System Fitness Design (USFD) has successfully placed physical fitness within various interconnected human organism body systems, enabling it to be seen from a transformative perspective. Specifically, the model identifies four grouped system functions: movement, energy regulation, physiological health, and homeostasis as physical fitness representations. The USFD approach provides an inclusive and holistic view of what constitutes physical fitness. The movement function closely corresponds to skill-related fitness components, including motor control, energy production and utilization, and aerobic control. Energy regulation fills the gap between energy production and utilization and body composition while maintaining physiological health as a critical function. Regarding the overall goodness of a healthy environment towards engagement in physical activities for increased quality service provision nowadays, homeostasis should be identified as a one-way exercise that benefits students physically. All these are combined into one by coordination and control mechanisms within the nervous system, which comprise the core of all other bodily functions constituting physical body exercises and their essentialness for life sustainability among humans or animals.

Outcomes

By the end of this chapter, you will be able to

* examine the development and evolution of the physical fitness components across time

DOI: 10.4324/9781003502937-8

- critically analyze arguments for the traditional classification of physical fitness components connected to health and explore their relevance in various health and fitness scenarios
- discuss grouped system functions and how they relate to physical fitness
- describe the significance of considering the nervous system functions, such as coordination and control, to achieve a healthy level of physical fitness
- explore understandable vocabularies for fair fitness evaluations and practices

The unknown development of physical fitness components

Exploring the development of physical fitness provides valuable insight into its components' evolution over time. We must comprehend the roots and growth of a concept with such relevance in the modern world. Despite its importance, the developmental history of physical fitness has been largely neglected, leaving us famished to discover information that may help us make sense of this essential concept.

We see how fitness components were grouped with body composition to form the health-related suite of physical fitness (cardiorespiratory fitness and endurance, muscular strength, muscular endurance, and flexibility). These grouped components are "health-related" because of their association with health. For instance, cardiorespiratory fitness is associated with an increased risk of coronary heart disease, and several other research studies have been conducted to link health concepts to energy regulation components.

However, this grouping needs to make sense and justify the health context of fitness. Furthermore, we believe this concept only emerged from the need to promote exercise and physical activity engagement for health. Of course, operationalization in the health context is all right, but it should be well established and supported by science.

The HRF–SRF model's substantial emphasis on peak performance is also commendable since it is consistent with the initiative to encourage fitness, physical activities, and sports. As advocates, we are ecstatic about this attention. However, physical fitness should not focus only on sports and performance. It is a concept that covers all people, regardless of their participation in sports. Everyone should be able to benefit from physical fitness. While it is permissible to operationalize it within the framework of sports and performance, we stress the necessity for an extensive understanding that transcends this context. By assuring a broad and thorough approach, we may appreciate the holistic character of physical fitness.

Development of USFD

With the USFD, we look at physical fitness as a multifaceted construct. First, we let go of the performance and health contexts and set it to the *"human as an organism with inter-connected body systems"* context, as in the systems theory. We began with four primary building block systems – nervous, musculoskeletal, cardiorespiratory, and endocrine systems – establishing the first four primary functions necessary for survival: coordination and control, body structure, energy, and body functions.

The four primary systems we identified form a unified structure and function related to physical fitness. This is consistent with the authors' objectives to conceptualize a unified approach for fitness construct and its components presented by the HRF–SRF model. At this point, we successfully unite the HRF–SRF components in the USFD under the *movement component* of fitness. However, our attempt to unify the HRF–SRF components has led us to open a Pandora's box, which can be considered a breakthrough. As a result, we were able to expound the construct, which provided a comprehensive concept that covers not only the movement components but also energy regulation, physiological health, and homeostasis components.

We paired each system from the four primary systems with its corresponding function, which formed six paired systems and six functions using a matrix. We discerned six functions: motor control, aerobic control, body function regulation, energy production and utilization, body composition, and metabolism. We called these the paired system functions.

Then, the primary systems were grouped into three, yielding four group combinations. We discerned the primary function of each group of three, which caused us movement, energy regulation, physiological health, and homeostasis.

Our take on physical fitness is based on these four grouped system functions. The *movement function* is a group of well-known physical fitness components in the HRF–SRF model, heavily concentrated in the context of sports performance and emphasizing optimum levels. Nevertheless, under USFD, these formerly known as fitness components were shared by the movement and energy regulation grouped system functions, which may be related to sports performance. Body composition was odd in the HRF–SRF model as this is the only component not heavily emphasized in the performance context.

The *movement function* has three paired system functions: motor control, energy production and utilization, and aerobic control. The HRF–SRF model has extensively emphasized motor control (balance, coordination, speed, agility, reaction time, and flexibility) and energy production and utilization (muscular strength, muscular endurance). We can draw some similarities to the HRF–SRF model. Motor control can be seen as a skill-related fitness component. In the same way, energy production and utilization may be seen as the muscular fitness components, including strength, endurance, and power. Aerobic control may be viewed as cardiorespiratory fitness in the HRF–SRF model. In other words, we have almost covered the entire HRF–SRF model with just one USFD grouped system function, i.e., movement. Hence, we unified all HRF–SRF fitness components under the movement function.

It is crucial to emphasize enhancing movement function through exercise and physical activity to achieve optimum levels. However, we must emphasize the criteria of task requirement and success to be explicit, inclusive, and universal, ensuring that physical fitness is accessible to people from all walks of life instead of being dominated by a restricted sports and performance environment. We recognize the value of individuality and the diversity of people's fitness goals.

Considering this, we shift our emphasis from pursuing optimum performance to fundamental nervous system functions such as coordination, control, and regulation. Not all real-world tasks demand maximal performance levels; they often require regulated and adjustable ones. Every activity has an ideal combination of speed, agility, balance, reaction time, flexibility, and strength, which, when adequately coordinated, results in exceptional movement and performance quality. It is crucial to recognize that excessively high or low levels of movement and performance may not provide the intended results for a specific task.

Additionally, we coined kinesthetic fitness to highlight motor control and kinetic fitness to emphasize the energy-regulating nature of the indicators (as in kinetic energy). Moreover, we added flexibility to the suite as it is more of a motor control indicator for posture and range of motion than a product of energy regulation.

Energy regulation is another well-known physical fitness component in the HRF–SRF model. It includes energy production (muscular fitness, strength, endurance, and power), utilization, and body composition. Energy regulation is unique because metabolism is an additional indicator.

In this book, we will discuss several energy systems pathways, such as the anaerobic lactic energy system for muscular strength, aerobic energy system for muscular endurance, and phosphocreatine energy system for muscular power, to shed light on the relationship between energy production and utilization through movements and metabolic processes. This is essential knowledge not only in exercise and athletic contexts but also in general. Understanding how energy is produced through the energy system pathways and how they are utilized through metabolism and kinetic fitness to exercise and engage in physical activities will affect the growth and development of healthy body composition.

Moreover, maintaining *physiological health* is an essential function of fitness. This involves motor control, body composition, and body function regulation. This component is unique in USFD, which values the regulation of physiological health by engaging in exercise and physical activities with motor control, maintaining healthy body composition through proper diet, and monitoring physiological conditions and hormone levels to ensure proper body functioning.

Additionally, our perspective on health-related fitness is different from the HRF–SRF model. Cardiorespiratory fitness, muscular strength, endurance, and flexibility are essential to health due to their relatedness with other indicators. However, it makes much more sense to classify them under the movement function. These are performance-based operationalizations of physical fitness, after all. Besides, only the body composition can be considered a health component. Our take on health-related fitness is the exercise–diet–hormone formula, which describes physiological health components.

We also added homeostasis as a fitness function, which pertains to the balanced state of the internal environment. Internal balance is an essential precursor to health. Many medical tests emphasize "normal levels," such as average sugar, cholesterol, or hormone levels. The temperature should be 37 degrees Celsius. The water levels should not go down below a well-hydrated level. Otherwise, people will get dehydrated.

Homeostasis is a precursor to physiological health and a requirement for physical activity engagement. For example, exercising while the body is dehydrated will harm it and increase the risk of injury. Another example is when an athlete has a fever and continues training, it may worsen the underlying sickness, increase the risk of injury, and spread the disease if it is contagious.

Moreover, we described the role of the brain in coordinating all these fitness components. We used neurological disorders as examples to support that the absence of brain control over the voluntary and involuntary functions of the organs and muscles can seriously affect a person's physical fitness, particularly in completing tasks. For this, we consider coordination and control as the core of physical fitness. These mechanisms bind the components together, which occur voluntarily or involuntarily inside the body. It is important to note that the involuntary functions of the nervous system are a part of a person's overall fitness.

The system functions for health and skill

It is essential to stress that our framework recognizes the HRF–SRF model, which we consider a good model. We have extended and reinforced the model by critically analyzing it to understand physical fitness better. With this book, we have effectively envisioned reforming the model by integrating grouped and paired system functions and comprehending them holistically through the lens of systems theory. We are now comfortable characterizing the *system functions for health* (physiological health and homeostasis) and *system functions for skills* (movement and energy control) rather than labeling them merely as health-related or skill-related. In addition, we have convincingly highlighted the interconnectedness of these elements through coordination, emphasizing their holistic and interdependent linkages. This positive approach has enabled us to extend and modify the current model, resulting in a thorough knowledge of physical fitness.

Now, there is a balance between system functions for health and skill. We removed the term "related," which only indicated an association with health or skill context. We refrained from using the term components because of the

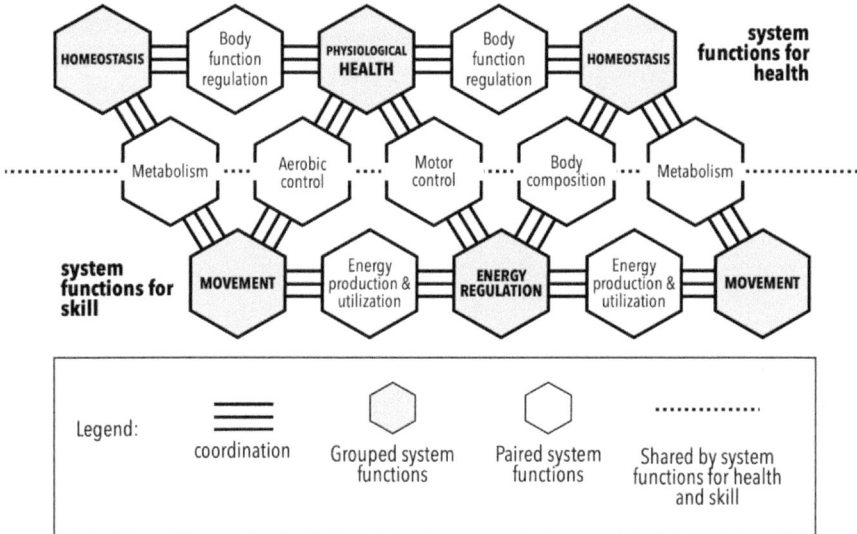

FIGURE 7.1   The system functions for health and skill in the USFD

complexity of the functions we presented. Instead, we are confident that physiological health and homeostasis comprise the system functions for health, while motor control and energy regulation are the system functions for skill. In Figure 7.1, we further illustrate that metabolism, aerobic control, motor control, and body composition share the attributes of system functions for health and skill.

Perpetual complementation

Physical fitness is a shared construct for all, regardless of their contexts. It is a multifaceted construct for everyone. With this, we are introducing the USFD as a holistic fitness framework that unifies the system functions for skill and adds system functions for health based on the four primary body systems. This holistic approach to physical fitness promotes a healthy and active lifestyle for all.

We also observed that the two functions are interrelated in our practice. We discussed how HRF components were unknowingly perceived as prerequisites to SRF components by professors we know. This idea could either be wrong, or something must be fixed with our understanding. However, instead of using the term "prerequisite," we prefer calling it a *"perpetual complementation,"* i.e., enhancing the system functions for health boosts the system functions for skill and vice versa in a cyclical perpetuity. Figure 7.2 shows this cyclical complementation between the two components.

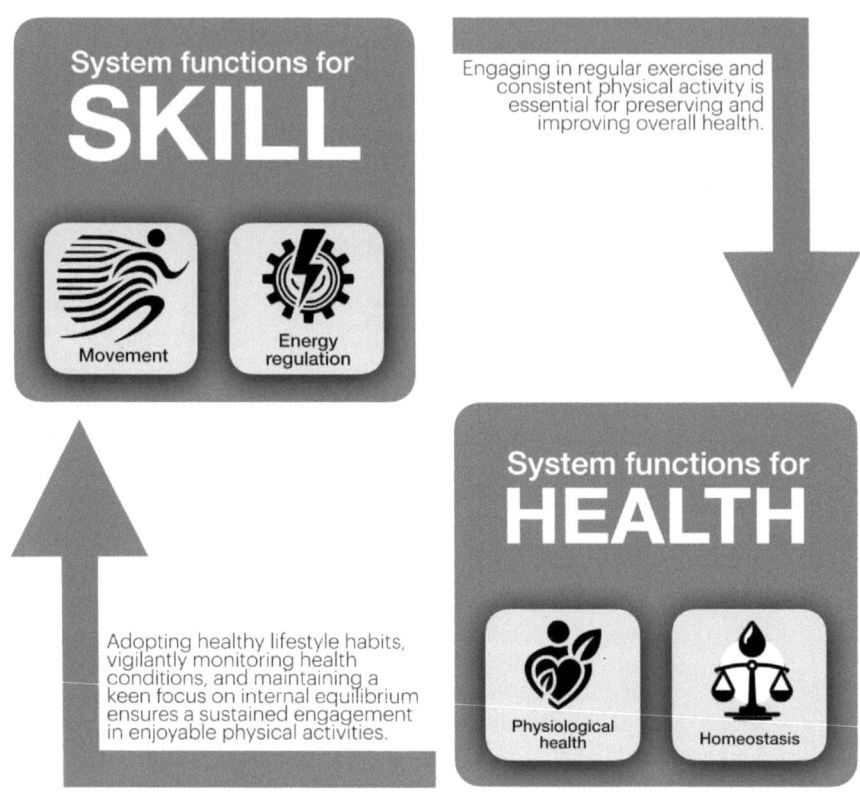

FIGURE 7.2 Perpetual complementation of system functions for health and skill

Enhancing skill components through regular exercise and physical activity participation boosts physiological health and homeostasis. Ensuring the body is in optimum physiological health and internal balance reduces the risk of falls and injury. It ensures that tasks are effectively and efficiently performed through movements and energy.

By using this design, fitness professionals can identify the specific system function of physical fitness that needs to be targeted for improvement. Individuals seeking to improve their fitness can better understand the different aspects of their physical fitness that need attention. Utilizing attribute-based language that is easy for everyone to understand and use, the USFD furthers social justice and inclusion in fitness practices and evaluations. The USFD offers an all-encompassing and multifaceted method of describing and evaluating the fitness construct, which aligns with our theoretical viewpoints and assumptions. This is crucial for discussions regarding physical fitness in the future and its promising advancements.

Summary

By bringing together the many interdependent systems of the human body, the Unified System Fitness Design (USFD) offers a new way of looking at physical fitness. As a representation of physical fitness, the model classifies four grouped system functions: homeostasis, physiological health, energy regulation, and movement. Motor control and energy production are part of the movement function, a fitness component related to skills. Energy regulation connects production, utilization, and body composition. Maintaining homeostasis and good physiological health are critical to general health. The nervous system's control and coordination mechanisms support these fundamental bodily functions, highlighting their vital role in human existence.

The chapter examines conventional categorizations and offers a holistic view. It delves into the evolution of physical fitness components throughout history. The USFD model provides a comprehensive perspective on physical fitness, emphasizing the interdependence of its components by classifying system functions according to health and skill. Personal fitness objectives go beyond just athletic performance, underscoring the importance of integrating movement with energy regulation. Homeostasis further emphasizes the importance of internal balance for general health.

The USFD Framework stresses the importance of continuous complementarity between health and skill system functions to promote a well-rounded strategy for improving fitness. It gives fitness experts and people who want to get in better shape a clear picture of which parts of physical fitness need work. The US Fitness Foundation (USFD) promotes social justice and inclusion by using attribute-based language accessible to everyone. In sum, the USFD provides a solid framework for characterizing and assessing the fitness construct, which aligns with theoretical viewpoints and sets the stage for further developments in physical fitness discourse.

Review questions

1. What is the significance of the developmental history of physical fitness?
2. Why did the authors see that the usual grouping of fitness components in the health-related suite of physical fitness was inadequate?
3. What is the relationship between cardiorespiratory fitness and health, and why is it crucial to understand?
4. What are the authors' take on the HRF–SRF model's emphasis on optimum performance in physical fitness?
5. What is the chapter's case for physical fitness being a term that should apply to all people, not just athletes or sports enthusiasts?
6. How do the authors' understanding of physical fitness benefit from the systems theory approach?

7. What are four basic building block systems, and how do they relate to physical fitness?
8. Describe the concept of "perpetual complementation" between system functions for health and skill.
9. What does the USFD Framework mean for fitness professionals and individuals looking to enhance their physical fitness?
10. In what ways does the chapter argue that the USFD offers a complete and multifaceted approach to defining and measuring fitness?

Discussion questions

1. How can the USFD Framework's holistic approach to physical fitness be utilized in fitness evaluations and training programs for individuals with various goals and backgrounds?
2. How can the concept of "perpetual complementation" between health and skill components of physical fitness be used to aid fitness professionals in designing exercise and wellness programs for their clients?
3. Discuss the practical consequences of emphasizing physical fitness programs from optimum performance to fundamental coordination and control. How may this help people in their daily lives?
4. Investigate practical approaches to improving social justice and inclusiveness in physical fitness practices and evaluations, as the USFD Framework proposes. How can fitness professionals ensure that all people have access to fitness opportunities?
5. Given the chapter's emphasis on the interconnection of multiple fitness functions, how can individuals and fitness professionals apply this knowledge to create well-rounded and effective training routines that address health and skills functions?

PART II

The system functions of fitness

Exploring the interconnected system functions of physiological health, homeostasis, motor control, and energy regulation

8

BODY FUNCTION REGULATION

Oliver Napila Gomez and Nguyen Tra Giang

Physiological well-being and homeostasis rely on the function of body function regulation. Hormones secreted by the endocrine and nervous systems, which work in tandem, modulate metabolic rate, growth rate, and reproductive success. Genetic and behavioral variables, including food, exercise, illness, and natural factors, all impact the body's functions. Vital signs such as blood pressure, heart rate, breathing rate, and body temperature must be within normal ranges to evaluate physiological health. The vestibular, cardiovascular, and neurological systems do not work well when feeling lightheaded or vertigo. A healthy mind is crucial to being healthy, and interoception helps control our feelings and actions. Additional factors contributing to physiological health include being at a healthy weight, having strong muscles and joints, an efficient digestive system, a robust immune system, and getting enough sleep. A balanced body and mind that can handle the stresses of everyday life are crucial functions of fitness and task performance. Overall, health and task performance are impacted by many factors, but one thing necessary for maintaining homeostasis is the regulation of bodily functions. People can improve their physiological health and overall well-being by monitoring their vital signs, encouraging healthy lifestyle habits, and dealing with discrepancies or problems.

Outcomes

By the end of the chapter, you will be able to

- explain how hormones play a crucial role in regulating many physiological activities and how hormonal abnormalities might affect overall health

DOI: 10.4324/9781003502937-10

- reflect on the various elements influencing body functions, such as heredity, lifestyle choices, and natural developmental changes
- recognize the significance of vital indicators such as blood pressure, heart rate, breathing rate, and body temperature in assessing physiological health and sustaining homeostasis
- explore the relationship between digestive health, gut microbiota, and general physiological health, focusing on the importance of food choices, lifestyle variables, and the gut–brain connection in promoting and maintaining optimal health
- discuss the complex relationship between mental health and interoception, including how disruptions in this system can contribute to mental health problems

What is body function regulation?

In the USFD Framework, body function regulation, a crucial component shared by physiological health and homeostasis, relies on the paired function of the nervous and endocrine systems. The two grouped system functions are both for health. In other words, this intricate coordination ensures that the organs in the body function optimally and in equilibrium for optimum health.

The endocrine system, comprising various glands distributed throughout the body, plays a pivotal role in maintaining this balance (Lee & Tsai, 2017). These glands, such as the pituitary gland, thyroid gland, adrenal gland, pancreas, and gonads, secrete hormones that control many physiological functions (Walling & Rosol, 2019). Hormones released by these endocrine glands serve multiple purposes (Belfiore & Leroith, 2018). They regulate emotions and stress levels, stimulate tissue growth and development, impact the functions of various organs, support metabolic processes, and govern the intricate processes of the reproductive system (Ahsan et al., 2020). It is important to note that a range of factors, including hormones, natural factors, genetic factors, lifestyle behaviors, and overall health, can influence the functions of the body's organs (Bigzad, 2022). These influences can induce temporary and permanent changes in an individual's physiological health. In essence, hormones are indispensable regulators of the body's internal metabolic processes and profoundly influence an individual's overall bodily functions (Stucker et al., 2021).

Hormones influence physiological health by impacting body functions (Cicatiello et al., 2018). For example, insulin, produced by the pancreas, regulates the body's metabolism of carbohydrates and fat (Venditti et al., 2019). Insulin helps to move glucose from the bloodstream into the cells, where it can be used for energy or stored as glycogen (Jayanthi & Srinivasan, 2019). When insulin levels are consistently high, as in the case of individuals with insulin resistance or type 2 diabetes, the body may be likely to store excess glucose as fat, leading to weight gain, visible through the changes in body composition (Sharma et al., 2015).

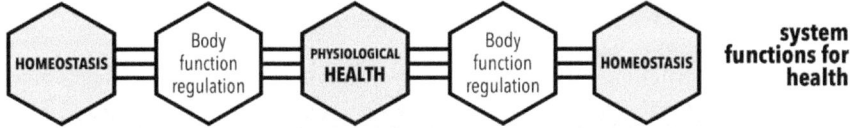

FIGURE 8.1   Body function regulation – shared by physiological health and homeostasis

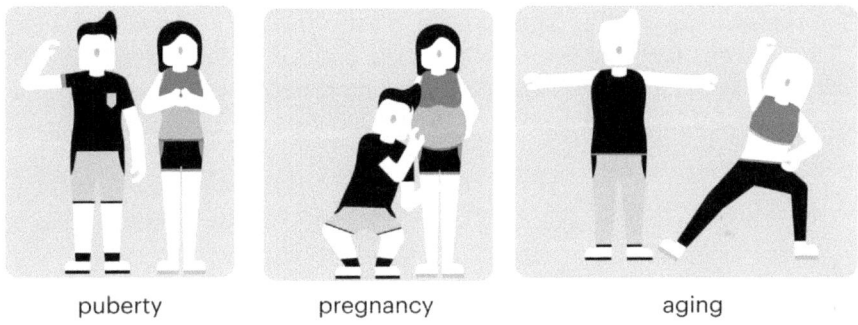

FIGURE 8.2   Natural factors

Similarly, thyroid hormones, produced by the thyroid gland, play a crucial role in regulating metabolism and energy expenditure (Eliasson, 2017). When the thyroid gland produces too little thyroid hormone, as in individuals with hypothyroidism, the body's metabolism may slow down, leading to weight gain, fatigue, and changes in body functions (Chaker et al., 2017). Conversely, when the thyroid gland produces too much thyroid hormone, as in individuals with hyperthyroidism, the body's metabolism may increase, leading to weight loss and changes in body composition (Bobryk, 2015).

Other hormones also affect body functions. For example, testosterone, produced by the testes in males and smaller amounts by the ovaries in females, is essential for developing and maintaining muscle mass and bone density. Insulin-like growth factor 1 (IGF-1), produced by the liver in response to growth hormone, also plays a critical role in muscle growth and development (Ahmed et al., 2020).

Moreover, throughout people's lifespans, puberty, pregnancy among women, and aging are three of the most common causes of *natural developmental changes* in the structural fitness of the body (Connelly et al., 2015). When boys and girls reach sexual maturity, testosterone (male sex hormone) and estrogen (female sex hormone) stimulate the secondary sex characteristics (Vlot et al., 2017). Boys will develop broader shoulders and increase muscle mass, while girls will notice changes around the structure of their breasts, hips, and waist (Gharahdaghi et al., 2021).

Among women, pregnancy is another major factor in body function changes. During pregnancy, women experience increases in maternal fat, fat-free mass, total body water content, and intrauterine growth caused by the development of the fetus (Subhan et al., 2019). The increased weight from conception to birth is called *gestational weight gain* (GWG). After giving birth, GWG affects the postpartum accumulation of visceral fat mass in the adipose tissues (Subhan et al., 2019; Vesco et al., 2022).

In continuation with the chronological events throughout people's lifespans, aging is only natural. The body is biologically programmed to increase fat mass and decrease lean mass, which is caused by a decreased metabolic rate as people age (Conte et al., 2019; Ponti et al., 2020).

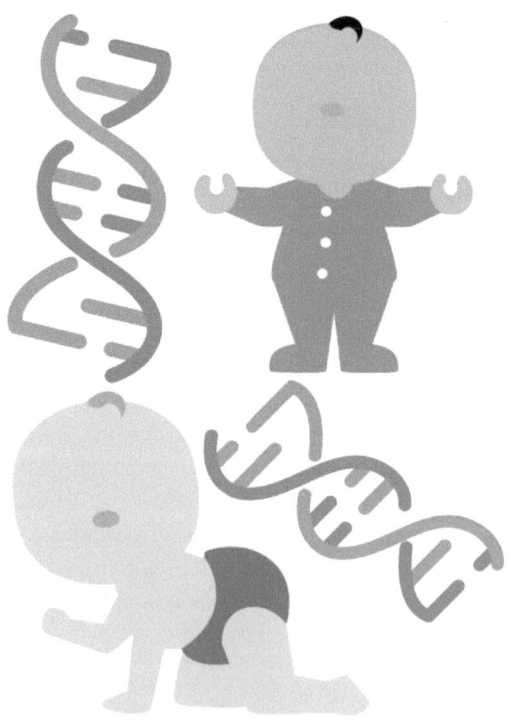

FIGURE 8.3 Genes regulate traits, appearance, and body functions

Moreover, children are born with genes they inherited from their parents. DNA containing genetic codes is like a program instructing how the body functions and shapes physical appearance, including primary (before puberty) and secondary sex characteristics during adolescence (Boyle et al., 2017). Body function is influenced by natural factors such as a person's unique genetic makeup. This factor explains children's apparent differences in body structure (Locke et al., 2015). Genes control the development and growth of the body, including hereditary conditions affecting body functions, appearance, and composition (El-Hattab & Scaglia, 2016).

Aside from natural factors, *behavioral factors* such as lifestyle (diet and physical activity) and health conditions (diseases and medication) also affect body functions (Ling & Rönn, 2019). Lifestyle involves metabolic processes, including balancing food intake and energy expenditure (Landrier et al., 2019). A person's behavioral lifestyle will determine gains in body mass if the metabolic process works perfectly. Some diseases, such as hypothyroidism and insulin resistance, may slow metabolism, resulting in weight gain (Cicatiello et al., 2018). Some conditions, such as hyperthyroidism and type 2 diabetes, may increase metabolism, causing extreme weight loss (Taylor et al., 2018). Medications can help to stabilize these medical conditions. However, some medicines, such as antibiotics, may disrupt the body's natural immunity (Stangierski et al., 2015). In addition, *supplementation* may alter body functions and composition. For example, protein supplements may increase muscle mass and weight training among bodybuilders (Rabbani et al., 2021).

In a nutshell, body function regulation influences physiological health while maintaining homeostasis. The status of a person's body functions is an essential indicator of physiological health regulation and homeostasis. Normal body functions, indicated by vital signs (blood pressure, heart rate, breathing rate), steadiness, healthy weight, good musculoskeletal condition, good digestive health, restfulness, and mental health, may be checked on a daily, weekly, monthly, biyearly, or yearly basis depending on the task requirement. These indicators can also determine the readiness of a person to engage in rigorous physical activity for overall wellness and safety.

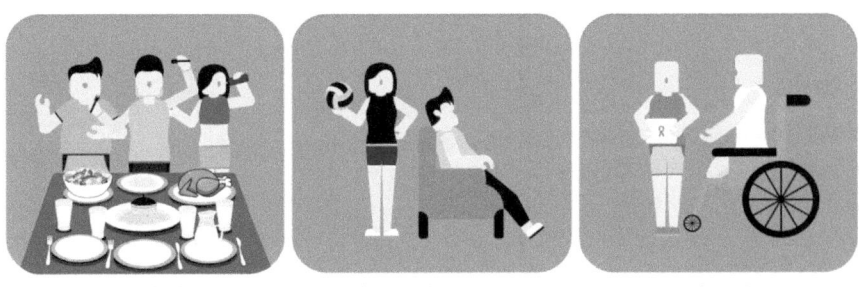

dietary habits   physical activity   medication

FIGURE 8.4   Behavioral and health factors

The body function regulation for homeostasis

The body's homeostatic regulation includes several critical factors that ensure our well-being – maintaining average vital indicators that provide insights into the body's healthy functioning and can aid in the early detection of potential health issues. Furthermore, steadiness, or the lack of dizziness and related symptoms, emphasizes the need to address any dizziness-related concerns. Finally, mental health is critical to total functioning, regulating emotions, perceptions, and physiological health. Let us explore the regulation of body functions for homeostasis deeply.

Normal vital signs

Vital signs are observable indicators that can be used to determine whether the body is functioning correctly. Maintaining normal blood pressure is a primary requirement for good health and crucial to living a healthy life (Chen et al., 2015). Additionally, a continual shift in blood pressure can result in significant health issues like hypertension, fatal cardiovascular illnesses, and kidney failure (Gupta et al., 2022).

Also, one of the most fundamental indicators of life and health is a normal heart rate, which shows blood flowing freely (Hutchon, 2016). When at rest, the heart rate should be between 60 and 100 beats per minute (BPM), but when running, the heart rate will rise with the intensity of the exercise (Ichwana et al., 2018).

The number of breaths a typical person or individual takes in a minute is their normal breathing rate (Qadir & Saleem, 2019). According to Qadir and Hassan (2019), an underlying sickness may cause an individual's breathing rate, typically monitored by a respirometer when the person is at rest, to increase.

Moreover, body temperature indicates human physiological activity and health, particularly in pediatrics, surgery, and general emergency departments (Kumar & Kumar, 2022). A high or low body temperature suggests the individual is afflicted with an illness. Hypothermia is indicated by a low body temperature (Karn, 2020), but an increased body temperature may suggest a bacterial illness (Sahagun & Pineda, 2018).

Steadiness

Dizziness is an experience of disrupted or impaired spatial orientation with a misleading sense of motion (Lin et al., 2014). (Malak et al., 2021). It characterizes symptoms such as haziness, nausea, wooziness, or unsteadiness (Wells, 2022), which may be caused by a range of illnesses, such as vestibular, cardiac, neurological, and psychosomatic entities (Van der Zaag-Loonen & van Leeuwen, 2015). It may also indicate diabetes and anemia (low blood levels) (Asare &

Danquah, 2017) or that medication or therapy has begun to take action (Wilhelm et al., 2018).

On the other hand, steadiness is a sign of physiological health since it indicates the absence of dizziness and its symptoms. Steadiness indicates steady spatial alignment and a distinct perception of motion (Lin et al., 2014). This absence of lightheadedness indicates a healthy vestibular system, cardiovascular system, neurological system, and general physiological health (Malak et al., 2021). Balance and steadiness are requirements for proper functioning, indicating good body functions.

Furthermore, monitoring and addressing dizziness symptoms is essential to reach and maintain optimum stability and general physiological health (Wells, 2022; Van der Zaag-Loonen & van Leeuwen, 2015). Identifying the underlying reasons for dizziness, such as diabetes, anemia, or drug side effects, is essential for establishing equilibrium and sustaining good physiological health (Asare & Danquah, 2017; Wilhelm et al., 2018).

Mental health

Mental health is essential to an individual's general functioning and capacity to deal with life's challenges (Colizzi et al., 2020). Meanwhile, interoception, which includes the signaling, encoding, integration, and psychological expression of internal body status information, impacts perceptions, cognitions, actions, and emotions and contributes to physiological health by coordinating homeostatic reflexes and allostatic responses (Quadt et al., 2018). The dysfunction of interoception has been identified as a significant factor in several mental health conditions, including anxiety disorders, mood disorders, eating disorders, addictive disorders, and somatic symptom disorders, highlighting its role in mapping the body's internal landscape across conscious and unconscious levels (Khalsa et al., 2018). Interoception reveals the underlying processes of mental health disorders and implies that disturbances in this system may lead to the development of anxiety, depression, and psychosis (Nord & Garfinkel, 2022).

The body function regulation for physiological health

Some aspects of body function regulation support physiological health, contributing to overall well-being. Let us look at significant body function regulation functions for physiological health. These functions include maintaining a healthy weight, maintaining good musculoskeletal function, cultivating good digestive health, boosting immunity, and enjoying restfulness when sleeping. These factors substantially impact numerous physiological systems and can significantly impact a person's overall health and quality of life.

Healthy weight

A healthy weight is another sign of physiological health. A body mass index of at least 19 and less than 25 is healthy for people under 20 years old (Usman et al., 2022). While an unhealthy weight is considered a major global health risk (Vaquera et al., 2018), maintaining a healthy weight entails ensuring the diet has enough calories to sustain growth and exercise (Meyer et al., 2013).

Maintaining a healthy weight is also crucial for health, particularly as people age, and for managing obesity in young adults (Atukunda, 2019; Hill, 2022). Exercise is crucial to achieving and maintaining a healthy weight since carrying pounds puts the spine under unneeded strain (Cooper, 2015). A healthy weight is crucial to lowering cancer risk and other chronic diseases like heart disease, diabetes, and chronic cardiometabolic diseases (Asuncion, 2014; Kang & Kong, 2021).

Good musculoskeletal function

The musculoskeletal system is profoundly impacted by aging, with loss of muscle mass and bone density beginning in midlife, leading to increased physical weakness, falls, fractures, and loss of independence. However, good musculoskeletal function is essential for healthy and active old age (Whittaker et al., 2018).

Additionally, elevating serum vitamin D levels may decrease the prevalence of gastrointestinal and general cancer, as Kokturk and colleagues (2018) found that vitamin D insufficiency is connected to cancer and muscle weakness. Healthy organ function is a physiological and biomechanical prerequisite for good musculoskeletal function (Sorenson & Wallden, 2016).

Therefore, regular monitoring of joint range of motion, muscle volume and strength, gait, and adequate and effective exercise performance all contribute to safe sports participation to prevent weight gain and preserve good musculoskeletal function and fitness (Chen et al., 2016).

Good digestive health

Maintaining good gut health is vital for overall physiological health, necessitating a holistic strategy that involves attentive dietary selections, lifestyle decisions, and physical activity (Nawab, 2023). Dietary fibers, with their varying physical and chemical properties, have been found to exhibit various physiological effects beyond enhanced laxation, such as benefits on cardiovascular health, weight maintenance, immune function, and colonic health. This highlights the importance of consuming fiber from various sources for health promotion and disease prevention (Slavin, 2013).

In addition, the gastrointestinal tract acts as a vital interface for nutritional absorption while maintaining a protective barrier against dangerous chemicals since alterations in intestinal barrier function have been linked to various illnesses and disorders (Konig et al., 2016). The gut microbiota, which is influenced by genetics, diet, and metabolism, plays a significant role in human health and disease, necessitating additional research to understand its complexities and develop interventions for gastrointestinal and neurological conditions, with a focus on addressing gut dysbiosis (Olvera-Rosales et al., 2021).

Furthermore, recent developments in gut microbiome research have shown its wide-ranging effects on host physiology and health. It is essential to appreciate the link between the gut microbiota and the aging process to devise treatments that promote healthy aging (Wilmanski et al., 2022). Thus, the strong relationship between digestive health, gut microbiota, and overall physiological health highlights the importance of food choices and lifestyle variables in sustaining optimum health (Guinane & Cotter, 2013; Makki et al., 2018).

Immunity

The immune system comprises many organs, cellular structures, and signaling molecules. It is vital for protecting against infections, but its ability to eradicate infections while preventing immune-related harm is limited in its precision. An enhanced immune system is essential for many physiological processes; maintaining a healthy immune system requires a well-rounded diet high in antioxidant-rich vitamins, minerals, and other nutrients (Calder, 2021).

When the immune system is weak, as in the case of acquired immunodeficiency syndrome (AIDS), the number and function of T cells decrease, and the remaining T cells eventually become functionally exhausted. The clearance of infected and activated cells can be hindered, and inflammation markers that damage tissue can be elevated, leading to severe inflammatory responses (Diao et al., 2020). Regarding coronavirus disease (COVID-19), the mucosal immune system is crucial, as it guards the primary sites of infection and sheds light on asymptomatic and mild cases (Russell et al., 2020).

The immune system protects the body's physiological health from harmful pathogens. Keeping the immune function healthy is highlighted because it can cause serious health problems when impaired. A weak or overactive immune response can cause severe outcomes in cases of COVID-19, while a robust immune system is associated with milder disease. Considering this, it is crucial to learn about and take care of the immune system, especially in times of global health crises like the COVID-19 pandemic (Manna et al., 2022)

Restfulness

Restfulness during sleep indicates excellent physiological health since it reflects the restorative aspect of sleep and is strongly correlated with sleep quality

(Hernandez, 2023; Kohyama, 2021). Sleep quality, which includes duration, timing, absence of sleep disorders, and restfulness, plays a crucial role in overall health, with insufficient sleep linked to a variety of health issues, such as obesity, type 2 diabetes, hypertension, cardiovascular disease, depression, and increased mortality (Chaput et al., 2018). In addition, sleep quality affects cortisol stress reactivity because cortisol, the stress hormone, is controlled by sleep patterns and plays critical roles in several physiological processes (Bassett et al., 2015). Short sleep duration, poor sleep quality, and late bedtimes are all connected with excessive food consumption, a poor diet, and obesity in teenagers (Chaput & Dutil, 2016). Poor sleep quality has also been associated with adverse health outcomes such as osteoporosis (Sasaki et al., 2016), increased arterial stiffness (Osonoi et al., 2015), insulin resistance (Kline et al., 2018), weight gain, and depressive symptoms (Hawes et al., 2019), highlighting the importance of restful sleep in maintaining good physiological health.

Body function regulation and task performance

Keeping the body and mind in a state of homeostasis allows for optimal performance on tasks (Serrador, 2019). For example, the cardiovascular system's capacity to maintain constant blood pressure and blood flow to the brain is crucial for activities that demand sustained physical exertion and mental concentration. Cognitive functions required for complex tasks are also supported by glucose metabolism that is adequately controlled. Regulating bodily functions is critical for task completion and success.

Physiological changes, such as fluctuations in blood pressure or heart rate variability, can majorly impact an individual's ability to work. For example, dizziness caused by uncontrolled blood pressure can impair a person's ability to focus and maintain their balance – two factors that are particularly problematic when requiring fine motor skills or making rapid decisions (Wuehr et al., 2017). Furthermore, it can be challenging to perform lightheaded tasks, particularly those requiring physical stability or careful movement (Dieterich & Staab, 2017).

It might be challenging to complete tasks when dealing with mental health issues such as anxiety, depression, or chronic stress (Hopstaken et al., 2015). Additionally, fatigue, uneasiness, inactivity, weight gain, impaired alertness, and difficulty completing tasks are all symptoms of insomnia or lack of sleep, which necessitates rest for the brain (Rodrigues et al., 2021).

In addition, metabolic syndrome, insulin resistance, and chronic low-grade inflammation are all associated with obesity, which in turn makes it harder to perform physical and mental activities. It becomes challenging to complete tasks due to this impact on immunity and pathogen defense (Andersen et al., 2016). Infections and chronic diseases are common in people with compromised immune systems, which compromises lymphoid tissue integrity and alters leukocyte activity, making it difficult to carry out daily tasks effectively (Andersen et al., 2016).

D'Onghia and colleagues (2021) found that fibromyalgia is common in obese individuals, which has repercussions for their quality of life, pain tolerance, activity level, and overall musculoskeletal health. As a result, these factors may influence their ability to perform tasks effectively. Because pain influences thinking, feeling, and physical abilities, arthritis also impacts the ability to perform tasks (Connolly et al., 2015).

Finally, while there may be a lack of research directly examining the correlation between gastrointestinal issues and task performance, the consensus holds that the latter can impede the former. Discomforts related to the digestive system, such as gas, queasy stomach, and indigestion, can distract a person from their tasks.

Summary

In order to keep the body in a state of homeostasis, it is essential to regulate its functions. Ensuring optimal functioning of organs and metabolic processes involves coordinating various systems, including the nervous and endocrine systems. Hormones influence metabolism, development, growth, and reproduction, among other bodily functions. Along with genetic factors, natural factors like puberty, pregnancy, and aging impact the regulation of bodily functions.

Body functions can be influenced by behavioral factors such as food, exercise, and health conditions, which in turn can cause changes in weight, muscle mass, and general health. In order to evaluate the regulation and homeostasis of bodily functions, it is crucial to monitor vital signs, steadiness, and mental health.

Keeping mental and physical health in check is essential for homeostasis. The physiological systems operate as they should when vital signs like temperature, pulse, and respiration rate are within normal ranges. Mental health is essential for overall well-being and homeostasis, while steadiness indicates the absence of dizziness.

Being physically fit includes being at a healthy weight, having strong muscles and joints, a healthy digestive system, a robust immune system, and getting enough sleep. These elements enhance a person's health and happiness.

Keeping physiological parameters under control is crucial for optimal task performance because changes in these parameters can affect physical and mental capacities. Task performance can be impacted by factors like mental health, obesity, chronic diseases, and gastrointestinal issues, which impact energy levels, pain tolerance, and overall well-being.

Review questions

1. What are the primary systems regulating physiological health and homeostasis, and how do they interact?
2. Explain the role of the endocrine system in maintaining body balance. What glands are essential in this process?

3. How do hormones affect our physiology, such as emotions, stress levels, and reproductive processes?
4. Describe how hormones affect metabolic processes and body composition.
5. What are the long-term effects of elevated insulin levels in the body? What does this have to do with insulin resistance and type 2 diabetes?
6. Discuss the role of thyroid hormones in metabolic regulation. How do hypothyroidism and hyperthyroidism affect a person's physiological health?
7. How do natural processes like puberty, pregnancy, and aging influence changes in the structural fitness of the body? Give concrete examples for each stage of life.
8. Discuss how genetics influences features, appearance, and body functions. What variables can cause inherited diseases that impact physiology?
9. Investigate the effect of behavioral factors on physiological processes, such as lifestyle choices (diet and physical activity) and health conditions (diseases and medication). Give instances of how these variables can affect physiology.
10. Why is it essential to monitor and maintain typical vital signs, steadiness, healthy weight, good musculoskeletal function, digestive health, restfulness, and mental health for overall physiological health? What are the potential consequences of neglecting these aspects of physiological health regulation?

Discussion questions

1. How can an understanding of physiological health and homeostasis be practically utilized to assist those suffering from nonconventional health issues such as insomnia or substance abuse in improving their overall well-being? What approaches might be practical?
2. How do changes in physiological health regulation affect treatment outcomes and overall quality of life in the context of HIV and cancer? What actions or changes in lifestyle can be suggested to lessen these effects?
3. Discuss the obstacles and potential for fostering physical fitness in people living with HIV. How can individualized workout routines be created to meet their unique demands and limitations?
4. Cancer survivors may encounter physiological health difficulties as a result of treatments such as chemotherapy and radiation. How can exercise and diet assist them in regaining and maintaining their physiological health? What are some practical considerations when creating exercise plans for cancer survivors?
5. Investigate the role of physiological health control in mental illnesses such as depression and anxiety. To improve overall outcomes, how might physical fitness and lifestyle changes be integrated into mental health treatment plans?

References

Ahmed, T., Alattar, M., Pantalone, K., & Haque, R. (2020). Is testosterone replacement safe in men with cardiovascular disease? *Cureus*, *12*. https://doi.org/10.7759/cureus.7324

Ahsan, A., Khan, A., Farooq, M., Naveed, M., Baig, M., & Tian, W. (2020). Physiology of endocrine system and related metabolic disorders. *Endocrine Disrupting Chemicals-induced Metabolic Disorders and Treatment Strategies*, 3–41. https://doi.org/10.1007/978-3-030-45923-9_1

Andersen, C., Murphy, K., & Fernández, M. (2016). Impact of obesity and metabolic syndrome on immunity. *Advances in Nutrition*, *7*(1), 66–75. https://doi.org/10.3945/an.115.010207

Asare, M., & Danquah, S. A. (2017). The need for clearance in relaxation therapy: Development of the relaxation clearance tool for practitioners. *Journal of General Practice (Los Angeles)*, *5*(324), 2. https://doi.org/10.4172/2329-9126.1000324

Asuncion, A. (2014). *Diet and physical activity: What's the cancer connection? Control your weight*. Philippine Cancer Society. https://policycommons.net/artifacts/1614243/diet-and-physical-activity/2304170/

Atukunda, C. (2019). *Barriers and facilitators to weight loss among young adults aged 18–25 years undertaking weight loss programs in Makerere University* [Doctoral dissertation, Makerere University]. https://bit.ly/3PAFBCe

Bassett, S. M., Lupis, S. B., Gianferante, D., Rohleder, N., & Wolf, J. M. (2015). Sleep quality but not sleep quantity effects on cortisol responses to acute psychosocial stress. *Stress*, *18*(6), 638–644. https://doi.org/10.3109/10253890.2015.1087503

Belfiore, A., & Leroith, D. (2018). *Principles of endocrinology and hormone action*. Springer. https://doi.org/10.1007/978-3-319-44675-2

Bigzad, A. (2022). An observation on endocrine glands with low secretions but high effects. *International Journal for Research in Applied Sciences and Biotechnology*, *9*(1), 191–195. https://doi.org/10.31033/ijrasb.9.1.24

Bobryk, M. (2015). Mutual influence of thyroid and carbohydrate metabolism: Paradigms and paradoxes. *International Journal of Endocrinology*, *3*(67)127–132. https://doi.org/10.22141/2224-0721.3.67.2015.75284

Boyle, F., Li, Y., & Pritchard, J. (2017). An expanded view of complex traits: From polygenic to omnigenic. *Cell*, *169*, 1177–1186. https://doi.org/10.1016/j.cell.2017.05.038

Calder, P. (2021). Nutrition and immunity: Lessons for COVID-19. *European Journal of Clinical Nutrition*, *75*, 1309–1318. https://doi.org/10.1038/s41430-021-00949-8

Chaker, L., Bianco, A., Jonklaas, J., & Peeters, R. (2017). Hypothyroidism. *The Lancet*, *390*, 1550–1562. https://doi.org/10.1016/S0140-6736(17)30703-1

Chaput, J. P., & Dutil, C. (2016). Lack of sleep as a contributor to obesity in adolescents: Impacts on eating and activity behaviors. *International Journal of Behavioral Nutrition and Physical Activity*, *13*, 1–9. https://doi.org/10.1186/s12966-016-0428-0

Chaput, J. P., Dutil, C., & Sampasa-Kanyinga, H. (2018). Sleeping hours: What is the ideal number and how does age impact this? *Nature and Science of Sleep*, 421–430. http://doi.org/10.2147/NSS.S163071

Chen, C. M., Yang, Y. H., Chang, C. H., Chen, C. C., & Chen, P. C. (2016). The utilization of rehabilitation in patients with hemophilia A in Taiwan: A nationwide population-based study. *PLoS One*, *11*(9). https://doi.org/10.1371/journal.pone.0164009

Chen, S., Cao, P., Dong, N., Peng, J., Zhang, C., Wang, H., Zhou, T., Yang, J., Zhang, Y., Martelli, E. E., Naga Prasad, S. V., & Wu, Q. (2015). PCSK6-mediated corin activation is essential for normal blood pressure. *Nature Medicine*, *21*(9), 1048–1053. https://doi.org/10.1038/nm.3920

Cicatiello, A., Girolamo, D., & Dentice, M. (2018). Metabolic effects of the intracellular regulation of thyroid hormone: Old players, new concepts. *Frontiers in Endocrinology*, *9*. https://doi.org/10.3389/fendo.2018.00474

Colizzi, M., Lasalvia, A., & Ruggeri, M. (2020). Prevention and early intervention in youth mental health: Is it time for a multidisciplinary and trans-diagnostic model for care? *International Journal of Mental Health Systems*, *14*(1), 1–14. https://doi.org/10.1186/s13033-020-00356-9

Connelly, K., Larson, E., Marks, D., & Klein, R. (2015). Neonatal estrogen exposure results in biphasic age-dependent effects on the skeletal development of male mice. *Endocrinology*, *156*(1), 193–202. https://doi.org/10.1210/en.2014-1324

Connolly, D., Fitzpatrick, C., O'Toole, L., Doran, M., & O'Shea, F. (2015). Impact of fatigue in rheumatic diseases in the work environment: A qualitative study. *International Journal of Environmental Research and Public Health*, *12*, 13807–13822. https://doi.org/10.3390/ijerph121113807

Conte, M., Martucci, M., Sandri, M., Franceschi, C., & Salvioli, S. (2019). The dual role of the pervasive "fattish" tissue remodeling with age. *Frontiers in Endocrinology*, *10*. https://doi.org/10.3389/fendo.2019.00114

Cooper, G. (2015). Exercises for lower back pain. *Non-Operative Treatment of the Lumbar Spine*, 85–87. https://doi.org/10.1007/978-3-319-21443-6_16

D'Onghia, M., Ciaffi, J., Lisi, L., Mancarella, L., Ricci, S., Stefanelli, N., Meliconi, R., & Ursini, F. (2021, April). Fibromyalgia and obesity: A comprehensive systematic review and meta-analysis. In *Seminars in arthritis and rheumatism* (Vol. 51, No. 2, pp. 409–424). WB Saunders. https://doi.org/10.1016/j.semarthrit.2021.02.007

Diao, B., Wang, C., Tan, Y., Chen, X., Liu, Y., Ning, L., Chen, L., Li, M., Liu, Y., Wang, G., & Yuan, Z. (2020). Reduction and functional exhaustion of t cells in patients with coronavirus disease 2019 (COVID-19). *Frontiers in Immunology*, *11*. https://doi.org/10.3389/fimmu.2020.00827

Dieterich, M., & Staab, J. (2017). Functional dizziness: From phobic postural vertigo and chronic subjective dizziness to persistent postural-perceptual dizziness. *Current Opinion in Neurology*, *30*(1), 107–113. https://doi.org/10.1097/WCO.0000000000000417

El-Hattab, A., & Scaglia, F. (2016). Mitochondrial cytopathies. *Cell Calcium*, *60*(3), 199–206. https://doi.org/10.1016/j.ceca.2016.03.003

Eliasson, L. (2017). Reduced blood glucose through thyroid hormone degradation product. *Acta Physiologica*, *220*. https://doi.org/10.1111/apha.12847

Gharahdaghi, N., Phillips, B., Szewczyk, N., Smith, K., Wilkinson, D., & Atherton, P. (2021). Links between testosterone, oestrogen, and the growth hormone/insulin-like growth factor axis and resistance exercise muscle adaptations. *Frontiers in Physiology*, *11*. https://doi.org/10.3389/fphys.2020.621226

Guinane, C. M., & Cotter, P. D. (2013). Role of the gut microbiota in health and chronic gastrointestinal disease: Understanding a hidden metabolic organ. *Therapeutic Advances in Gastroenterology*, *6*(4), 295–308. http://doi.org/10.1177/1756283X13482996

Gupta, K., Jiwani, N., & Afreen, N. (2022, April). Blood pressure detection using CNN-LSTM model. In *2022 IEEE 11th international conference on communication systems and network technologies (CSNT)* (pp. 262–366). IEEE. https://doi.org/10.1109/CSNT54456.2022.9787648

Hawes, N. J., Wiggins, A. T., Reed, D. B., & Hardin-Fanning, F. (2019). Poor sleep quality is associated with obesity and depression in farmers. *Public Health Nursing*, *36*(3), 270–275. https://doi.org/10.1111/phn.12587

Hernandez, M. (2023). The benefits of sleep. In *General surgery residency survival guide* (pp. 165–172). Springer International Publishing. http://doi.org/10.1007/978-3-031-25617-2_39

Hill, S. (2022). *Healthy habits to lose weight more quickly*. Lifespan Extension Advocacy Foundation. https://www.lifespan.io/topic/healthy-habits-to-lose-weight-more-quickly/

Hopstaken, J., Linden, D., Bakker, A., & Kompier, M. (2015). The window of my eyes: Task disengagement and mental fatigue covary with pupil dynamics. *Biological Psychology*, *110*, 100–106. https://doi.org/10.1016/j.biopsycho.2015.06.013

Hutchon, D. J. (2016). The normal range of heart rate at birth in a healthy term neonate: A critical review of the evidence. *Current Pediatric Research*, *20*(1–2), 7–10. https://www.currentpediatrics.com/articles/the-normal-range-of-heart-rate-at-birth-in-a-healthy-term-neonate-a-critical-review-of-the-evidence.html

Ichwana, D., Ikhlas, R. Z., & Ekariani, S. (2018, October). Heart rate monitoring system during physical exercise for fatigue warning using non-invasive wearable sensor. In *2018 international conference on information technology systems and innovation (ICITSI)* (pp. 497–502). IEEE.

Jayanthi, R., & Srinivasan, A. (2019). Biochemical isthmus [nexus] between type 2 diabetes mellitus and thyroid status-an update. *Diabetes & Metabolic Syndrome*, *13*(2), 1173–1177. https://doi.org/10.1016/J.DSX.2019.01.037

Kang, I. S., & Kong, K. A. (2021). Body mass index and severity/fatality from coronavirus disease 2019: A nationwide epidemiological study in Korea. *PloS One*, *16*(6). https://doi.org/10.1371/journal.pone.0253640

Karn, K. K. L. (2020). Study of health care diagnostic system in human patient by fuzzy logic implication. *World Journal of Pharmaceutical Research*, *9*(6), 466–471. http://doi.org/10.20959/wjpr20206-17531

Khalsa, S. S., Adolphs, R., Cameron, O. G., Critchley, H. D., Davenport, P. W., Feinstein, J. S., Garfinkel, S. N., Lane, R. D., Mehling, W. E., & Meuret, A. E., & Zucker, N. (2018). Interoception and mental health: A roadmap. *Biological Psychiatry: Cognitive Neuroscience and Neuroimaging*, *3*(6), 501–513. https://doi.org/10.1016/j.bpsc.2017.12.004

Kline, C. E., Hall, M. H., Buysse, D. J., Earnest, C. P., & Church, T. S. (2018). Poor sleep quality is associated with insulin resistance in postmenopausal women with and without metabolic syndrome. *Metabolic Syndrome and Related Disorders*, *16*(4), 183–189. https://doi.org/10.1089/met.2018.0013

Kohyama, J. (2021). Which is more important for health: Sleep quantity or sleep quality? *Children*, *8*(7), 542. http://dx.doi.org/10.3390/children8070542

Kokturk, N., Baha, A., Oh, Y. M., Young Ju, J., & Jones, P. W. (2018). Vitamin D deficiency: What does it mean for chronic obstructive pulmonary disease (COPD)? A comprehensive review for pulmonologists. *The Clinical Respiratory Journal*, *12*(2), 382–397. https://doi.org/10.1111/crj.12588

König, J., Wells, J., Cani, P. D., García-Ródenas, C. L., MacDonald, T., Mercenier, A., Whyte, J., Troost, F., & Brummer, R. J. (2016). Human intestinal barrier function in health and disease. *Clinical and Translational Gastroenterology*, *7*(10), e196. https://doi.org/10.1038%2Fctg.2016.54

Kumar, A., & Kumar, A. (2022). Contactless temperature and distance measuring device: A low-cost, novel infrared-based—Badgel-shaped structural model for measuring physical distance and body temperature. *AIMS Electronics and Electrical Engineering*, *6*(1), 43–60. http://doi.org/10.3934/electreng.2022004

Landrier, J., Derghal, A., & Mounien, L. (2019). MicroRNAs in obesity and related metabolic disorders. *Cells*, *8*. https://doi.org/10.3390/cells8080859

Lee, H., & Tsai, S. (2017). Endocrine targets of hypoxia-inducible factors. *The Journal of Endocrinology*, *234*(1), R53–R65. https://doi.org/10.1530/JOE-16-0653

Lin, J. G., Chen, K. B., & Lee, Y. C. (2014). Dizziness. *Acupuncture for Pain Management*, 265–266. https://doi.org/10.1007/978-1-4614-5275-1_46

Ling, C., & Rönn, T. (2019). Epigenetics in human obesity and type 2 diabetes. *Cell Metabolism*, *29*, 1028–1044. https://doi.org/10.1016/j.cmet.2019.03.009

Locke, A., Kahali, B., Berndt, S. I., Justice, A. E., Pers, T. H., Day, F. R., Powell, C., Vedantam, S., Buchkovich, M. L., Yang, J., & Croteau-Chonka, D. C. (2015). Genetic studies of body mass index yield new insights for obesity biology. *Nature, 518*, 197–206. https://doi.org/10.1038/nature14177

Makki, K., Deehan, E. C., Walter, J., & Bäckhed, F. (2018). The impact of dietary fiber on gut microbiota in host health and disease. *Cell Host & Microbe, 23*(6), 705–715. https://doi.org/10.1016/j.chom.2018.05.012

Malak, W., Hagiwara, M., & Nguyen, V. (2021). Neuroimaging of dizziness and vertigo. *Otolaryngologic Clinics of North America, 54*(5), 893–911. https://doi.org/10.1016/j.otc.2021.06.001

Manna, P., Gray, Z., & Reddy, P. (2022). Healthy immunity on preventive medicine for combating COVID-19. *Nutrients, 14*. https://doi.org/10.3390/nu14051004

Meyer, S., Shelnutt, K. P., & Kauwell, G. (2013). Raising healthy children: Health risks of obesity: FCS80023/FY1356, 4/2013. *EDIS, 2013*(4). https://journals.flvc.org/edis/article/download/120894/119438

Nawab, A. (2023). The best foods for digestive health: A comprehensive guide. In *Vedicalhealth*. https://vedicalhealth.com/articles/best-foods-for-digestive-health/

Nord, C. L., & Garfinkel, S. N. (2022). Interoceptive pathways to understand and treat mental health conditions. *Trends in Cognitive Sciences, 26*(6), 499–513. https://doi.org/10.1016/j.tics.2022.03.004

Olvera-Rosales, L. B., Cruz-Guerrero, A. E., Ramírez-Moreno, E., Quintero-Lira, A., Contreras-López, E., Jaimez-Ordaz, J., Castañeda-Ovando, A., Añorve-Morga, J., Calderón-Ramos, Z. G., Arias-Rico, J., & González-Olivares, L. G. (2021). Impact of the gut microbiota balance on the health-disease relationship: The importance of consuming probiotics and prebiotics. *Foods, 10*(6), 1261. http://doi.org/10.3390/foods10061261

Osonoi, Y., Mita, T., Osonoi, T., Saito, M., Tamasawa, A., Nakayama, S., Someya, Y., Ishida, H., Kanazawa, A., Gosho, M., Fujitani, Y., & Watada, H. (2015). Poor sleep quality is associated with increased arterial stiffness in Japanese patients with type 2 diabetes mellitus. *BMC Endocrine Disorders, 15*(1), 1–7. https://doi.org/10.1186/s12902-015-0026-1

Ponti, F., Santoro, A., Mercatelli, D., Gasperini, C., Conte, M., Martucci, M., Sangiorgi, L., Franceschi, C., & Bazzocchi, A. (2020). Aging and imaging assessment of body composition: from fat to facts. *Frontiers in Endocrinology, 10*, 488049. https://doi.org/10.3389/fendo.2019.00861

Qadir, M. I., & Hassan, A. (2019). Does normal breathing rate effects interest of people in cricket? *Online Journal of Cardiovascular Research, 1*(4), 517. http://doi.org/10.33552/OJCR.2019.01.000517

Qadir, M. I., & Saleem, Z. (2019). Is there any relation between normal breathing rate and falooda ice cream loving? *ARC Journal of Immunology and Vaccines, 4*(1), 28–30. https://www.arcjournals.org/pdfs/ajiv/v4-i1/5.pdf

Quadt, L., Critchley, H. D., & Garfinkel, S. N. (2018). The neurobiology of interoception in health and disease. *Annals of the New York Academy of Sciences, 1428*(1), 112–128. https://doi.org/10.1111/nyas.13915

Rabbani, E., Golgiri, F., Janani, L., Moradi, N., Fallah, S., Abiri, B., & Vafa, M. (2021). Randomized study of the effects of zinc, vitamin A, and magnesium co-supplementation on thyroid function, oxidative stress, and hs-CRP in patients with hypothyroidism. *Biological Trace Element Research, 199*, 4074–4083. https://doi.org/10.1007/s12011-020-02548-3

Rodrigues, G., Fiorelli, E., Furlan, L., Montano, N., & Tobaldini, E. (2021). Obesity and sleep disturbances: The "chicken or the egg" question. *European Journal of Internal Medicine, 92*, 11–16. https://doi.org/10.1016/j.ejim.2021.04.017

Russell, M., Moldoveanu, Z., Ogra, P., & Mestecky, J. (2020). Mucosal immunity in COVID-19: A neglected but critical aspect of SARS-CoV-2 infection. *Frontiers in Immunology, 11*. https://doi.org/10.3389/fimmu.2020.611337

Subhan, F. B., Shulman, L., Yuan, Y., McCargar, L. J., Kong, L., & Bell, R. C. (2019). Association of pre-pregnancy BMI and gestational weight gain with fat mass distribution and accretion during pregnancy and early postpartum: a prospective study of Albertan women. *BMJ Open, 9*(7). https://doi.org/10.1136/bmjopen-2018-026908

Sahagun, M. A. M., & Pineda, C. N. (2018, November). A telemonitoring system for remote pediatric application using cloud computing. In *2018 IEEE 10th international conference on humanoid, nanotechnology, information technology, communication and control, environment and management (HNICEM)* (pp. 1–6). IEEE. https://doi.org/10.1109/HNICEM.2018.8666284

Sasaki, N., Fujiwara, S., Yamashita, H., Ozono, R., Teramen, K., & Kihara, Y. (2016). Impact of sleep on osteoporosis: Sleep quality is associated with bone stiffness index. *Sleep Medicine, 25*, 73–77. https://doi.org/10.1016/j.sleep.2016.06.029

Serrador, J. (2019). The cardiovascular dizziness connection: Role of vestibular autonomic interactions in aging and dizziness. In B. W. Kesser & A. T. Gleason (Eds.), *Dizziness and vertigo across the lifespan* (pp. 175–190). Elsevier Health Sciences. https://doi.org/10.1016/B978-0-323-55136-6.00015-0

Sharma, P., Tripathi, G., Kumar, P., Sharma, R., Kishore, K., & Saran, M. (2015). Thyroid disorders in type-II diabetes mellitus. *Indian Journal of Public Health Research and Development, 6*, 26–28. https://doi.org/10.5958/0976-5506.2015.00192.8

Slavin, J. (2013). Fiber and prebiotics: Mechanisms and health benefits. *Nutrients, 5*(4), 1417–1435. https://doi.org/10.3390/nu5041417

Sorenson, M., & Wallden, M. (2016). Visceral factors in rehabilitation & health. *Journal of Bodywork and Movement Therapies, 20*(4), 920–925. https://doi.org/10.1016/j.jbmt.2016.09.007

Stangierski, A., Ruchała, M., Krauze, T., Moczko, J., & Guzik, P. (2015). Treatment of severe thyroid function disorders and changes in body composition. *Endokrynologia Polska, 67*(4), 359–366. https://doi.org/10.5603/EP.a2016.0025

Stucker, S., Angelis, J., & Kusumbe, A. (2021). Heterogeneity and dynamics of vasculature in the endocrine system during aging and disease. *Frontiers in Physiology, 12*. https://doi.org/10.3389/fphys.2021.624928

Taylor, P., Albrecht, D., Scholz, A., Gutierrez-Buey, G., Lazarus, J., Dayan, C., & Okosieme, O. (2018). Global epidemiology of hyperthyroidism and hypothyroidism. *Nature Reviews Endocrinology, 14*, 301–316. https://doi.org/10.1038/nrendo.2018.18

Usman, Y. B., Shittu, O. I., Aloysius, M. T., Aliyu, A. O., & Igho, V. G. (2022). Performance criteria of modified multihalver technique for detecting outlying values of body mass index (BMI): A higher risk factor and prognosis of COVID-19 infections. *International Journal of Statistics and Applied Mathematics, 7*(2), 99–104. https://doi.org/10.22271/maths.2022.v7.i2b.800

Van der Zaag-Loonen, H. J., & van Leeuwen, R. B. (2015). Dizziness causes absence from work. *Acta Neurologica Belgica, 115*, 345–349. https://doi.org/10.47494/cajmns.v1i1.36

Vaquera, E., Jones, R., Marí-Klose, P., Marí-Klose, M., & Cunningham, S. A. (2018). Unhealthy weight among children in Spain and the role of the home environment. *BMC Research Notes, 11*, 1–8. https://doi.org/10.1186/s13104-018-3665-2

Venditti, P., Reed, T., Víctor, V., & Meo, S. (2019). Insulin resistance and diabetes in hyperthyroidism: A possible role for oxygen and nitrogen reactive species. *Free Radical Research, 53*, 248–268. https://doi.org/10.1080/10715762.2019.1590567

Vesco, K. K., Marshall, N. E., Baetscher, E., Leo, M. C., Rooney, W., Francisco, M., Baker, E., King, J. C., Catalano, P., Frias, A. E., & Purnell, J. Q. (2022). Changes in visceral and ectopic adipose tissue stores across pregnancy and their relationship to gestational weight gain. *The Journal of Nutrition, 152*(4), 1130–1137. https://doi.org/10.1093/jn/nxac010

Vlot, M., Klink, D., Heijer, M., Blankenstein, M., Rotteveel, J., & Heijboer, A. (2017). Effect of pubertal suppression and cross-sex hormone therapy on bone turnover markers and bone mineral apparent density (BMAD) in transgender adolescents. *Bone*, *95*, 11–19. https://doi.org/10.1016/j.bone.2016.11.008

Walling, B., & Rosol, T. (2019). Pathology of the endocrine system. *Toxicologic Pathology for Non-Pathologists*, 537–569. https://doi.org/10.1007/978-1-4939-9777-0_13

Wells, L. (2022). Dizziness and vertigo. *Quick References*, *2022*. https://doi.org/10.1542/aap.ppcqr.396061

Whittaker, A. C., Delledonne, M., Finni, T., Garagnani, P., Greig, C., Kallen, V., Kokko, K., Lord, J., Maier, A. B., Meskers, C. G., Santos, N. C., & van Riel, N. (2018). Physical activity and nutrition influences in ageing (PANINI): Consortium mission statement. *Aging Clinical and Experimental Research*, *30*(6), 685–692. https://doi.org/10.1007/s40520-017-0823-7

Wilhelm, M., Rief, W., & Doering, B. K. (2018). Decreasing the burden of side effects through positive message framing: An experimental proof-of-concept study. *International Journal of Behavioral Medicine*, *25*, 381–389. https://doi.org/10.1007/s12529-018-9726-z

Wilmanski, T., Gibbons, S. M., & Price, N. D. (2022). Healthy aging and the human gut microbiome: Why we cannot just turn back the clock. *Nature Aging*, *2*(10), 869–871. https://doi.org/10.1038/s43587-022-00294-w

Wuehr, M., Brandt, T., & Schniepp, R. (2017). Distracting attention in phobic postural vertigo normalizes leg muscle activity and balance. *Neurology*, *88*, 284–288. https://doi.org/10.1212/WNL.0000000000003516

9

METABOLISM

Nguyen Tra Giang and Oliver Napila Gomez

This chapter explores the complex interplay of metabolism, movement, and homeostasis. Essential for development, reproduction, and reactions to the environment, metabolism is a web of cellular processes that generate life energy necessary for healthy physiological functioning. Homeostasis maintains internal condition stability in the face of external perturbations. Learning new skills and being able to adapt are aided by movement, including structured and unstructured physical activities. There are two primary types of metabolic energy expenditure: homeostasis and movement. The resting metabolic rate (BMR) and the thermal effect of food (TEF) are part of homeostasis. In contrast, exercise energy expenditure (EEE) and non-exercise activity thermogenesis (NEAT) are part of movement. Insight into these factors allows for personalizing exercise and food plans for peak health. Substrate utilization, hormonal regulation, body composition, and metabolic disorders are integral to operationalizing metabolic fitness. Energy expenditure during exercise is affected by metabolic efficiency, especially in athletes. Metabolic diseases have far-reaching effects on health, while hormones and body type influence metabolic function. BMR, TEF, EEE, and NEAT affect task performance. Metabolic health and task performance are both enhanced by regular physical activity, but there may be adverse side effects from exercising too much. A balance between exercise volume and intensity is encouraged to maximize metabolic health and performance.

DOI: 10.4324/9781003502937-11

Outcomes

By the end of this chapter, you will be able to

- explore and explain how metabolism serves as a shared system function between homeostasis and movement
- reflect on the practical implications of the integrated perspective on metabolism for their health
- apply knowledge of metabolism, energy expenditure, and metabolic fitness to create tailored strategies for maintaining or improving health and well-being
- assess the importance of metabolic fitness in the context of overall health and physical performance
- analyze the impact of metabolic disorders on individuals' lives and health, exploring the role of genetics and lifestyle in the development of these disorders

Movement and homeostasis

Metabolism is necessary for sustaining overall health and optimal physiological function. The interaction between movement and homeostasis ensures that the organism has a steady energy source, maintains stable internal conditions, and reacts appropriately to external stimuli.

Metabolism is a complex network of metabolic events inside cells to provide the energy required for the body's proper functioning (Sánchez López de Nava & Raja, 2019). These processes are vital for life because they enable growth, reproduction, structural maintenance, and environmental responses (Kuuva, 2016). Although metabolism comprises all metabolic activities in an organism, it is frequently used to define the particular reactions involved in obtaining energy

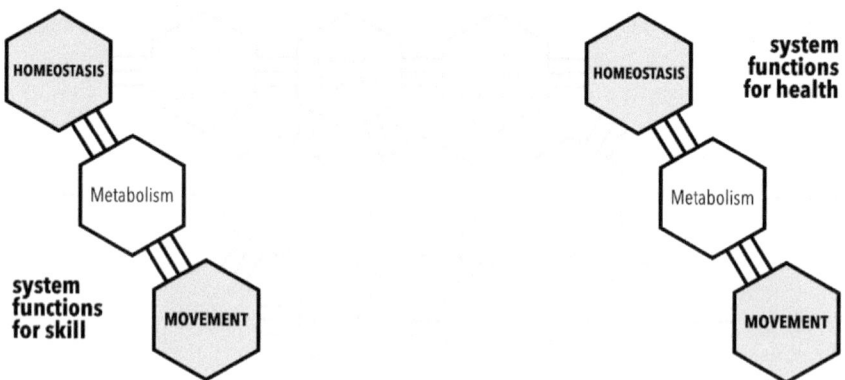

FIGURE 9.1   Metabolism – shared by homeostasis and movement

from food (Wotring, 2012). Hence, the breakdown of nutrients via metabolism is essential for maintaining life and supporting various physiological processes.

Meanwhile, maintaining homeostasis is essential for general health because it helps the body control its internal environment in reaction to external changes, consequently avoiding the onset of illness by guaranteeing stability and correct physiological functioning (Vithalani et al., 2017). Homeostasis is the capacity of organisms and cells to maintain a steady internal environment despite a fluctuating external environment (Tveit & Thorsen, 2017). This automatic tendency of the body to maintain a relatively constant internal environment, including factors such as temperature, cardiac output, ion concentrations, blood pH, hydration, and blood glucose concentration, is essential for maintaining the body's physiological processes despite the constant entry and exit of energy and molecules (Caon, 2020).

Metabolism is an important indicator to determine the right amount of food and water needed to support movement and homeostasis. Additionally, metabolic rate refers to the pace at which metabolism processes occur, such as the conversion rate of food into energy, measured by the number of calories burned per unit of time (hour or day) (Lawler et al., 2019).

Energy metabolism

When talking about metabolism, it is essential to understand total daily energy expenditure (TDEE). In the USFD Framework, the total daily energy expenditure is the sum of all energy expenditures from homeostasis and movement.

Energy spent for homeostasis includes resting metabolic rate (energy required for maintenance and repair) and the thermic impact of eating (energy required to digest, absorb, and store food). Energy spent for homeostasis comprises around 60–75% of resting energy expenditure and 10% of food thermogenesis (Fonseca et al., 2018).

On the other hand, the energy spent on movement includes organized and spontaneous physical activity (Ravussin & Peterson, 2015). Around 15–30% of energy expenditure during physical activity (Fonseca et al., 2018).

Energy expenditure through homeostasis

Energy expenditure via homeostasis is critical to understanding how the human body controls and consumes energy for essential physiological activities. We delve into the various processes that underpin this aspect of metabolism in this part, offering light on essential components such as basal metabolic rate (BMR) and the thermal effect of food (TEF). BMR represents the lowest energy required to maintain vital biological functions at rest, providing crucial insights into individual energy requirements and metabolic health. Meanwhile, TEF emphasizes the energy expended during nutrition digestion, absorption, and utilization, providing critical information for balancing energy intake and expenditure. We learn better how our bodies maintain homeostasis and support general health by investigating these aspects of energy consumption.

Basal metabolic rate (BMR)

The basal metabolic rate (BMR) measures the body's energy metabolism rate at rest, independent of muscular activity, external temperature fluctuations, food consumption, and mental stress (Xiao, 2022; Yu, 2021; Zhao, 2014). It is the least energy required to maintain fundamental physiological activities in a calm and awake state at ambient temperature. However, it is essential to note that BMR is relative from person to person because it is influenced by factors such as age, sex, physical activity, body composition, and body function control (hormone levels).

Knowing the BMR is essential because it gives crucial information on the minimal amount of energy the body requires at rest to sustain fundamental physiological activities. For visualization purposes, we will use the US Department of Agriculture (USDA) guidelines for the recommended daily calorie consumption of 2,000 calories for adults (VanEpps et al., 2016; Pang & Hammond, 2013; Heller & Keoleian, 2015) as the recommended daily caloric intake. Everyone has a relative daily dietary caloric intake regarding individuality and many other factors. Hence, 2,000 calories are only used here for discussion.

According to Fonseca and colleagues (2018), around 60–75% of calories are utilized for resting energy expenditure or BMR. With this, we can predict that around 1,200–1,500 calories is the energy required to support and maintain essential functions while at rest, including breathing, maintaining average temperature, sustaining brain functions, and maintaining continuous heartbeat, among others.

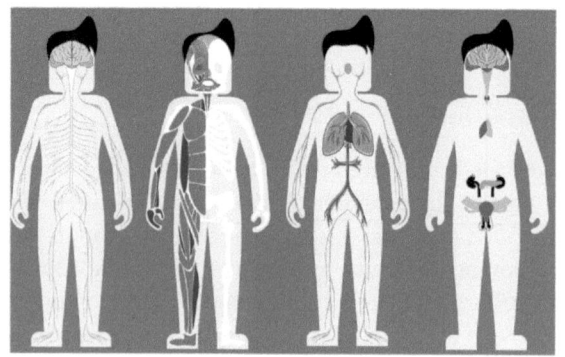

BMR reflects the energy required to maintain essential functions at rest, such as breathing, maintaining normal temperature, sustaining brain functions, and maintaining a continuous heartbeat.

FIGURE 9.2   The basal metabolic rate

Hence, knowing an individual's BMR makes it possible to predict daily calorie requirements correctly. This information is precious for establishing tailored nutrition and activity regimens since it helps identify the optimum calorie intake for weight control, regardless of whether the objective is weight reduction, maintenance, or gain. In addition, knowing individual BMR may aid in monitoring general metabolic health and spotting any abnormalities that may need further assessment and treatment.

Thermal effect of food (TEF)

In addition, the body expends energy on the thermal effect of feeding, the energy spent on food digestion. The thermal effect of food refers to the energy expenditure generated by digestion, absorption, transport, processing, assimilation, and storage of nutrients, which varies depending on the substrate ingested and accounts for 5–15% of the TEE (Sanches et al., 2016). It is believed that the thermal impact of a typical mixed meal (including lipids, carbs, and proteins) accounts for around 5–7% of its energy content (Sanches et al., 2016). However, Fonseca and colleagues (2018) have claimed that 10% of energy is used for food thermogenesis.

Understanding TEF is crucial because it reflects the energy expenditure involved with the digestion, absorption, transport, and storage of nutrients derived from food. This information is significant since it adds to calculating the total energy balance and caloric needs. For example, if a typical mixed meal delivers 2,000 calories based on USDA recommendations (VanEpps et al., 2016; Pang & Hammond, 2013; Heller & Keoleian, 2015), the TEF allotment of 10% would equate to around 200 calories. Understanding TEF helps fine-tune dietary recommendations and ensure that energy intake aligns with energy expenditure for weight management and overall metabolic health.

Energy expenditure through movement

Movement-based energy expenditure is a dynamic and multidimensional part of our metabolic physiology, covering numerous physical activity characteristics and their impact on overall energy balance. This section explores the complexities of energy expenditure during movement, focusing on two critical components: exercise energy expenditure (EEE) and non-exercise activity thermogenesis (NEAT). As a pillar of scientific growth, EEE throws light on the energy expended during structured physical exercise, providing essential insights towards enhancing fitness regimens and reaching health goals. Meanwhile, NEAT sheds light on the often overlooked area of energy used during spontaneous, nonconscious physical activity, emphasizing its importance in sustaining metabolic health and assisting with weight management. We fully understand how our bodies adapt to various forms of physical activity and their critical role in our general well-being as we delve into these elements of energy expenditure through movement.

Exercise energy expenditure (EEE)

Gong and He (2020) said that measuring human exercise energy expenditure (EEE) is the cornerstone of scientific progress. It is a highly regarded variable component of TEE (Hannon et al., 2021) that contributes 15–30% of energy expenditure during physical exercise (Fonseca et al., 2018). However, Hannon and colleagues (2021) reported that the contributions of EEE to TEE in healthy, physically active individuals varied from 20–60% This estimate of EEE in the work of Hannon and colleagues (2021) is modified for athletes, especially endurance athletes, based on variables such as exercise type, duration, intensity, and individual characteristics.

Effective monitoring of exercise energy expenditure is essential for active persons to modify their physical activity to attain their fitness objectives (Yan & Chen, 2022). This enables people to make educated choices about their exercise routines, optimizing the efficacy and efficiency of their exercises while reducing the danger of overtraining or undertraining. By measuring exercise energy expenditure, people may measure their progress, establish realistic goals, and modify their training regimens, improving their overall health and fitness.

Non-exercise activity thermogenesis (NEAT)

Non-exercise activity thermogenesis (NEAT) is the energy used during spontaneous physical movements such as sitting, standing, walking, and fidgeting that are not consciously motivated by exercise. Work, leisure, genetics, and the diet's

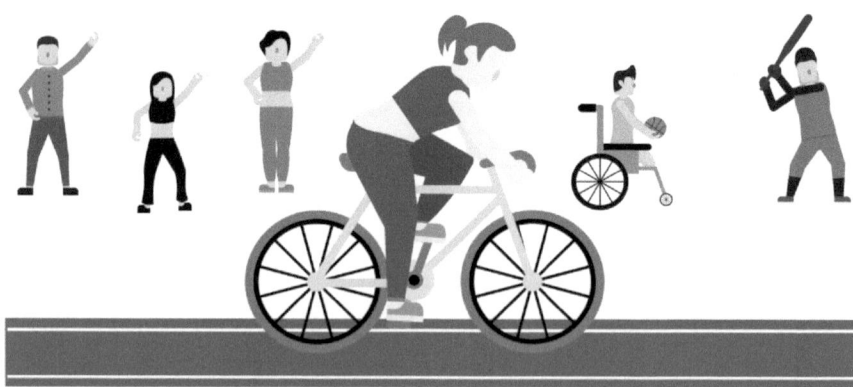

FIGURE 9.3 Exercise energy expenditure (EEE) – the energy utilized during physical activity (Brooks, 2021)

impact on physical activity may explain the wide variability in NEAT, contributing to the varied susceptibility of people to weight gain, emphasizing the need to understand energy balance and weight control (von Loeffelholz & Birkenfeld, 2018; Malaeb et al., 2019).

NEAT was not in Fonseca and colleagues' (2018) components of TDEE. NEAT was previously ignored in metabolic definitions until recently when NEAT became a highly variable component of daily TEE and a low level of NEAT associated with obesity (Chung et al., 2018). As a metabolism component, NEAT helps explain the complex relationship between energy intake, expenditure, and body weight management, emphasizing the need for planned and spontaneous physical activity for metabolic health. Since then, Malaeb and colleagues (2019) mentioned that NEAT may range from approximately 15–50% or above of TDEE. Based on this information, NEAT can range from approximately 300–1,000 calories out of a 2,000-calorie daily intake.

Understanding NEAT, its causes, fluctuations, and effects on energy expenditure is essential for understanding energy balance and weight management. By understanding NEAT's significance in daily energy expenditure, people may maximize their spontaneous physical activities by adding movement to their

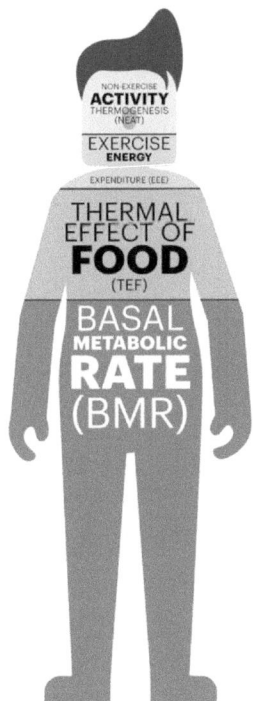

FIGURE 9.4   The total daily energy expenditure (TDEE) – how the body expends energy

daily routines, adopting active work and leisure habits, and encouraging a physically active atmosphere. Understanding energy intake and expenditure helps people control their weight and metabolic health. NEAT may also maintain a healthy weight beyond food and exercise.

Implications for homeostasis and movement

The new perspective on metabolism provided by the USFD Framework, particularly its integration with homeostasis and movement, has substantial implications for our knowledge of energy expenditure and its role in maintaining general health and physiological function. This viewpoint emphasizes the complex interplay between metabolism, homeostasis (the system function for health), and movement (the system function for skill), emphasizing metabolism's critical role in maintaining these fundamental features of human biology.

Metabolism, commonly regarded as the body's energy currency, is central to this framework. It powers growth, reproduction, structural upkeep, and environmental adaption. Importantly, metabolism involves an extensive network of cellular activities, allowing the body to respond to its surroundings rather than only producing energy. This extensive view of metabolism lays the groundwork for understanding how energy is directed toward basic survival and complicated processes, such as skill development and adaptability to external stimuli.

The concept of homeostasis is critical to sustaining internal equilibrium in the face of a constantly changing external environment. It includes a variety of physiological mechanisms that maintain stability in variables like temperature, ion concentrations, blood pH, and hydration. Homeostasis, mediated by metabolism, enables the organism to adjust quickly and respond to external changes. The new viewpoint stresses metabolism as a significant participant in the background, ensuring that the body can sustain these consistent internal circumstances. This acknowledgment of metabolism's function in homeostasis emphasizes its significance in overall health maintenance.

Meanwhile, movement is more than just a physical act; it is a competence the body must acquire, adapt to, and excel at. Movement includes planned acts, such as exercise, and unplanned acts, such as fidgeting or walking. It is fascinating to contemplate how these seemingly unconnected actions are linked through metabolism. The energy consumed during organized and unplanned physical activities has an everyday metabolic basis. This realization emphasizes the importance of metabolism in supporting our physical capabilities and facilitating skill development.

Moreover, TDEE is defined in the USFD Framework as the total energy expended on homeostasis and movement. This holistic view of energy expenditure recognizes that sustaining health and acquiring skills necessitate balancing these two factors. The total calories an individual can burn daily are represented by TDEE, which includes BMR, TEF, EEE, and NEAT. It is a comprehensive measure of how the body uses energy.

The interdependence of metabolism, homeostasis, and movement has practical ramifications. Knowing BMR, for example, can provide valuable insights into daily calorie requirements, allowing for individualized nutrition and activity planning. Recognizing the importance of the TEF aids in fine-tuning dietary recommendations to balance energy intake and expenditure. Meanwhile, EEE and NEAT provide information on how to improve fitness regimens and encourage spontaneous physical activity.

Finally, the USFD Framework's perspective on metabolism as a shared system function between homeostasis and movement provides a comprehensive understanding of how our bodies manage energy. It emphasizes the importance of metabolism in sustaining internal stability and skill development and ensuring our general health. This new perspective enables us to investigate the complicated web of energy expenditure, allowing us to better understand how our bodies adapt and prosper in a changing world.

Operationalizing metabolic fitness

Since 1994, the word metabolic fitness has been used to refer to glucose tolerance, insulin sensitivity, lipid profile, and the ratio of lipid to carbohydrate oxidized during steady-state exercise (Bouchard & Shephard, 1994; Nwimo & Orji, 2015). Thus, a metabolically fit individual often has regulated blood glucose levels, efficient energy intake, proper nutrient utilization, and healthy lipid and hormone profiles. Good metabolic fitness is associated with a lower risk of chronic metabolic illnesses, such as obesity, type 2 diabetes, cardiovascular disease, and metabolic syndrome. Typically, attaining and maintaining metabolic fitness requires regular physical activity, a healthy diet, enough rest, and other lifestyle factors that support optimal metabolic function.

Metabolic efficiency

In athletic performance, metabolic efficiency refers to an athlete's capacity to use available energy sources efficiently during activity. It is affected by several variables, including core temperature, muscle fiber type, and substrate consumption (Dolci et al., 2018). Athletes with high metabolic efficiency can maximize their energy usage, enabling them to endure extended physical activity while limiting energy expenditure and conserving necessary energy storage (Bellofiore & Chesler, 2013).

From this, we can deduce that metabolic efficiency refers to the body's capacity to consume and digest energy from dietary sources in a manner that promotes overall health and well-being. It entails the effective metabolism of macronutrients, such as carbs, lipids, and proteins, to fulfill the body's energy requirements and maintain optimum physiological function.

Substrate utilization

The synthesis of acetyl-CoA inside the mitochondrial matrix and its entrance into the tricarboxylic acid (TCA) cycle is a crucial step in the production of energy through substrate usage, which includes the oxidation of ingested carbohydrates and lipids as well as protein metabolism (DiMauro et al., 2014). The body's ability to properly convert and use available nutrients to fulfill energy needs indicates metabolic fitness, as it can optimally utilize these substrates for energy generation (Frankenfield, 2001).

For example, the body needs energy to fuel muscle contractions and maintain performance during physical exercise. During this process, muscle cells break down and oxidize substrates such as carbs and lipids to produce ATP, the body's principal energy currency. The body's capacity to use these substrates effectively is critical for maximum performance during exercise. A well-trained endurance athlete who has built metabolic fitness via constant training may display increased substrate utilization, utilizing carbohydrates and lipids effectively to maintain extended activity. In contrast, an unskilled person may need help efficiently using these substrates, resulting in tiredness and diminished physical performance.

Hormonal regulation

Various metabolic functions, including glucose absorption, energy generation, and the body's reaction to stress, depend on hormone levels. Assessing hormone levels such as insulin, glucagon, thyroid hormones, and cortisol may offer helpful information on the regulation and function of the body's metabolism. Understanding these hormone levels may aid in evaluating metabolic health and creating treatments, such as fitness training, to enhance hormonal balance and promote general health (Sellami et al., 2019).

Body composition

The composition of the human body, which refers to the quantity and distribution of lean tissue, adipose tissue, and bone (Hemke et al., 2020), plays a vital role in metabolism. Variations in body fat distribution and the expandability of subcutaneous fat tissue might result in varying metabolic and cardiovascular risks in people with comparable BMI (Piché et al., 2018). Understanding these variations in body fat distribution is essential for appreciating the many metabolic consequences of obesity and its influence on cardiovascular health.

In addition, body fatness has a significant impact on blood parameters linked to glucose and lipid metabolism (Matsushita et al., 2014). Due to the metabolic repercussions of diminished muscle mass, the steady rise in body fat mass and loss of lean body mass that occur with biological aging might lead to metabolic illnesses. Dietary adjustments, increased physical activity, and exercise are essential for preventing and treating obesity and boosting metabolic health. For instance, resistance exercise may have a role in strengthening metabolic regulation by increasing muscle mass and changing body fat distribution (Strasser, 2013).

Metabolic disorders

Metabolic disorders relate to several medical issues that impact the body's metabolic processes to obtain or produce energy, resulting in metabolic diseases (Boia et al., 2015; Ferrante, 2013). However, certain metabolic illnesses are inherited, complicated genetic abnormalities that disrupt a person's metabolism. Several metabolic diseases result in a range of prevalent disease states, such as obesity, diabetes, hypercholesterolemia, and hypertriglyceridemia. Obesity is perhaps the most frequent of these diseases (Bell, 2012). We consider metabolic disorders indicators of metabolic fitness due to their impact on the body's metabolic processes and energy regulation.

Metabolism and task performance

All the biochemical reactions in an organism to keep it alive are included in metabolism. The conversion of food into energy is an essential process that powers many bodily functions and tasks. A person's capacity to carry out routine tasks and strenuous physical and mental tests is directly related to how well their metabolic processes work.

The body's energy while at rest in a temperature-neutral environment is called the basal metabolic rate (BMR) (Kumar et al., 2019). Age, sex, body composition, and genetic predisposition are the factors that cause basal metabolic rate (BMR) to differ among individuals (Olejníčková et al., 2019). With an extensive energy reservoir, an individual with a higher basal metabolic rate (BMR) may be better able to maintain energy-intensive tasks, improving performance in various settings (Heer et al., 2015).

Due to the energy required for digestion, absorption, and distribution of nutrients, there is an increase in energy expenditure above the basal metabolic rate after eating. This phenomenon is known as the thermal effect of food (TEF). The timing of calorie intake has been found to affect thermogenesis and metabolic patterns, which in turn affects task performance. Consuming food first thing in the morning, instead of later in the day, may increase resting metabolic rates, giving energy to get things done after breakfast (Bo et al., 2015).

A person's ability to perform, particularly when faced with physically demanding tasks, directly correlates to their exercise energy expenditure (Sanchez-Delgado et al., 2015). A person's ability to carry out activities is enhanced through optimizing energy utilization brought about by adaptive responses to exercise, including improvements in cardiovascular health and muscle efficiency (Sepa-Kishi & Ceddia, 2016). In addition, the effects of exercise on both brown and white adipose tissue can affect thermogenesis and overall energy metabolism, which could lead to better performance by making energy available and efficient (Aldiss et al., 2018).

Energy expenditure during non-exercise activity thermogenesis (NEAT) does not involve physical activity such as sleeping, eating, or performing sports. Regarding profession and lifestyle choices, NEAT varies among individuals (Chung et al., 2018). An individual's total energy expenditure – the amount of energy used for non-exercise movements like walking and standing – affects their ability to perform tasks, and increasing NEAT can impact this (Horswill et al., 2017). Task performance can be enhanced by increasing total energy expenditure and metabolic health through lifestyle modifications that enhance NEAT (Rizzato et al., 2022).

On the one hand, the increased risk of diseases like type 2 diabetes and coronary heart disease caused by metabolic syndrome – a condition defined by obesity, insulin resistance, hypertension, and hyperlipidemia – influences global health (Saklayen, 2018). Regular aerobic and resistance training exercises can improve metabolic syndrome symptoms, increase cardiorespiratory fitness, and positively impact aging people's muscle mass, strength, and metabolic health. This can potentially delay or reduce metabolic syndrome severity (Distéfano & Goodpaster, 2018). People who suffer from metabolic syndrome have impaired cognitive function, which becomes even more pronounced when they do not move around much. Physical activity affects metabolic syndrome patients, including enhanced cognitive function and increased cerebral oxygenation (Guicciardi et al., 2019). Managing and reducing metabolic syndrome requires regular physical exercise and improved fitness levels, which generally affect the disease's components and health outcomes (Myers et al., 2019). By alleviating metabolic diseases, exercise-induced myokines mediate the positive effects of physical activity on health. Adipose tissue is one of the many tissues with which myokines interact to enhance the immune-metabolic factor interface and the health benefits of exercise (Leal et al., 2018).

Conversely, the effects of a metabolically active lifestyle on physical fitness and task performance bring to light several critical factors, emphasizing how exercise and physical training affect metabolic health. Resistance training and high-intensity interval training (HIIT) can improve glucose control and metabolic health in various people, including those with type 2 diabetes. These exercises increase insulin sensitivity and muscle mitochondrial capacity (Little et al.,

2011). Aerobic interval training, strength training, or a mix of the two can improve endothelial function and decrease waist circumference – two of the metabolic syndrome-related physiological abnormalities – without affecting body weight, fasting plasma glucose, or HDL levels (Stensvold et al., 2010). Myokines are peptides muscle fibers release during exercise with local and systemic effects. These effects include improvements in glucose and lipid metabolism and anti-inflammatory activities. The myokines IL-6, IL-10, and IL-1ra mediate the communication between muscle and adipose tissue, which is essential for the health benefits of exercise (Leal et al., 2018).

Maintaining energy homeostasis during exercise is crucial, and an exceptionally active metabolism, marked by improved metabolic flexibility, enables efficient adaptation to changes in energy demand and nutrient availability. Consistent exercise improves this metabolic flexibility, which occurs when the body switches between burning carbohydrates and fat, depending on the intensity and length of the exercise (Pedersen & Saltin, 2006). Excessive exercise training has been found to impair mitochondrial function and decrease glucose tolerance in otherwise healthy people, suggesting that there is a limit to how much exercise can improve metabolic health (Flockhart et al., 2021).

Lastly, a slow metabolism dramatically affects a person's capacity to carry out duties and keep themselves physically fit. However, by improving metabolic health, cognitive function, general physical fitness, and task performance, regular physical activity – including aerobic and resistance exercises – can mitigate the adverse effects of poor metabolism. Meanwhile, it is crucial to balance exercise volume and intensity to prevent the potential adverse effects of overtraining.

Summary

Metabolism is crucial to maintaining overall health and physiological function, as it powers growth, reproduction, structural maintenance, and environmental responsiveness. The chapter emphasizes the interconnectedness of metabolism, homeostasis, and movement. Homeostasis is the body's ability to maintain a stable internal environment, while metabolism provides the energy necessary for the body to respond rapidly to external changes.

TDEE is the sum of energy expenditures for both homeostasis and movement. RMR represents the minimum energy required to sustain essential physiological activities at rest, while TEF accounts for energy expended during food digestion, absorption, and utilization. Understanding these components helps determine daily calorie requirements and tailor nutrition and activity regimens to individual needs.

BMR, a measure of the body's energy metabolism rate at rest, is influenced by age, sex, physical activity, body composition, and hormonal levels. Knowledge about BMR empowers individuals to make informed choices regarding calorie intake and monitor overall metabolic health.

Movement-based energy expenditure includes EEE and NEAT, essential for metabolic health. Achieving and maintaining metabolic fitness requires regular physical activity, a balanced diet, adequate rest, and lifestyle factors supporting optimal metabolic function.

A better understanding of these factors allows for customizing exercise and food plans, optimizing energy balance, and promoting metabolic health. Metabolic fitness is highlighted in the text as an essential factor that includes hormone regulation, body composition, substrate utilization, and metabolic disorders. The effects of exercise on metabolic efficiency, task performance, and general fitness are covered. While regular exercise can improve metabolic health, it is essential to avoid overexertion to avoid adverse effects on energy homeostasis.

Review questions

1. Why is the relationship between metabolism, homeostasis, and movement crucial for overall health?
2. How do the components of TDEE relate to homeostasis and movement?
3. Why is BMR important to consider when planning tailored nutrition and exercise?
4. Explain the implications of TEF for energy expenditure and dietary recommendations.
5. What factors determine EEE, and how does it contribute to TDEE?
6. Define NEAT and its significance in TDEE. How can we improve NEAT in our daily lives?
7. How does metabolism contribute to the body's ability to maintain internal stability, as stated in terms of homeostasis?
8. What is the significance of comprehending the metabolic efficiency of energy utilization during physical activity?
9. Explain substrate use and its importance in metabolic fitness, particularly during exercise.
10. What role does understanding hormone control, body composition, and metabolic disorders play in enhancing metabolic health and overall well-being?

Discussion questions

1. How can knowing your BMR and TDEE help you make better decisions about your daily calorie intake and effectively control your weight?
2. How can NEAT knowledge be used in everyday routines to promote better metabolic health and reduce sedentary behaviors?
3. Discuss how EEE can be used to create tailored exercise programs. How can people maximize their workout programs based on how much energy they lose during physical activity?

4. What is the TEF, and how does it influence meal planning and dietary choices? What tactics can we use daily to make energy-efficient food choices?
5. Consider the following scenario: someone is attempting to enhance their metabolic fitness. How can knowledge of substrate use, hormone regulation, and body composition be incorporated into a holistic approach to attain their objectives?

References

Aldiss, P., Betts, J., Sale, C., Pope, M., Budge, H., & Symonds, M. (2018). Exercise-induced "browning" of adipose tissues. *Metabolism, 81*, 63–70. https://doi.org/10.1016/j.metabol.2017.11.009

Bell, C. (2012). Regulation of metabolism. In *Primer on the autonomic nervous system* (pp. 253–255). Academic Press.

Bellofiore, A., & Chesler, N. C. (2013). Methods for measuring right ventricular function and hemodynamic coupling with the pulmonary vasculature. *Annals of Biomedical Engineering, 41*, 1384–1398. https://doi.org/10.1007/s10439-013-0752-3

Bo, S., Fadda, M., Castiglione, A., Ciccone, G., Francesco, A., Fedele, D., Guggino, A., Caprino, M., Ferrara, S., Boggio, M., Mengozzi, G., Ghigo, E., Maccario, M., & Broglio, F. (2015). Is the timing of caloric intake associated with variation in diet-induced thermogenesis and in the metabolic pattern? A randomized cross-over study. *International Journal of Obesity, 39*, 1689–1695. https://doi.org/10.1038/ijo.2015.138

Boia, M., Manea, A., & Bilav, O. (2015). Features of the endocrine-metabolic plurimal formative syndrome. *Revista Societății Române de Chirurgie Pediatrică, 68*. http://www.jurnalulpediatrului.ro/archive/71-72/71-72-15.pdf

Bouchard, C., & Shephard, R. (1994). Physical activity, fitness and health: The model and key concepts. In C. Bouchard, R. Shephard, & T. Stephens (Eds.), *Physical activity, fitness and health* (pp. 77–88). Human Kinetics.

Brooks, S. (2021). *Nutrient intake, body composition, and performance measures of wildland firefighters: A longitudinal analysis*. University of Idaho.

Caon, M. (2020). Homeostasis. *Examination Questions and Answers in Basic Anatomy and Physiology: 2900 Multiple Choice Questions and 64 Essay Topics*, 173–183. https://doi.org/10.1007/978-3-030-47314-3_6

Chung, N., Park, M. Y., Kim, J., Park, H. Y., Hwang, H., Lee, C. H., Han, J. S., So, J., Park, J., & Lim, K. (2018). Non-exercise activity thermogenesis (NEAT): A component of total daily energy expenditure. *Journal of Exercise Nutrition & Biochemistry, 22*(2), 23–30. https://doi.org/10.20463/jenb.2018.0013

DiMauro, S., Nishino, I., & Hirano, M. (2014). Mitochondrial myopathies. *Neuromuscular Disorders in Clinical Practice*, 1335–1353. https://doi.org/10.1007/978-1-4614-6567-6_64

Distéfano, G., & Goodpaster, B. (2018). Effects of exercise and aging on skeletal muscle. *Cold Spring Harbor Perspectives in Medicine, 8*(3). https://doi.org/10.1101/cshperspect.a029785

Dolci, F., Hart, N. H., Kilding, A., Chivers, P., Piggott, B., & Spiteri, T. (2018). Movement economy in soccer: Current data and limitations. *Sports, 6*(4), 124. https://doi.org/10.3390/sports6040124

Ferrante, C. (2013). Management of inborn errors of metabolism and metabolic disorders, on march 7–8, 2013 in association with international union of biochemistry and molecular biology (IUBMB). The meeting was successful with the participation of renowned. *Indian Journal of Biochemistry and Biophysics, 50*, 335–336. https://niscpr.res.in/jinfo/IJBB/IJBB%2050(5)%20(Preface).pdf

Flockhart, M., Nilsson, L., Tais, S., Ekblom, B., Apró, W., & Larsen, F. (2021). Excessive exercise training causes mitochondrial functional impairment and decreases glucose tolerance in healthy volunteers. *Cell Metabolism, 33*(5), 957–970. https://doi.org/10.1016/j.cmet.2021.02.017

Fonseca, D. C., Sala, P., Ferreira, B. D. A. M., Reis, J., Torrinhas, R. S., Bendavid, I., & Waitzberg, D. L. (2018). Body weight control and energy expenditure. *Clinical Nutrition Experimental, 20*, 55–59. https://doi.org/10.1016/j.yclnex.2018.04.001

Frakenfield, D. (2001). Energy and macrosubstrate requirements. *The Science and Practice of Nutrition Support: A Case-Based Core Curriculum*, 31–52.

Gong, X., & He, H. (2020). Signal extraction and monitoring of motion loads based on wearable online device. *Computer Communications, 154*, 138–147. https://doi.org/10.1016/j.comcom.2020.02.072

Guicciardi, M., Crisafulli, A., Doneddu, A., Fadda, D., & Lecis, R. (2019). Effects of metabolic syndrome on cognitive performance of adults during exercise. *Frontiers in Psychology, 10*. https://doi.org/10.3389/fpsyg.2019.01845

Hannon, M. P., Flueck, J. L., Gremeaux, V., Place, N., Kayser, B., & Donnelly, C. (2021). Key nutritional considerations for youth winter sports athletes to optimize growth, maturation and sporting development. *Frontiers in Sports and Active Living, 2*. https://doi.org/10.3389/fspor.2021.599118

Heer, M., Titze, J., Smith, S., & Baecker, N. (2015). Energy, macronutrient supply, and effects of spaceflight. *Nutrition Physiology and Metabolism in Spaceflight and Analog Studies*, 11–19. https://doi.org/10.1007/978-3-319-18521-7_3

Heller, M. C., & Keoleian, G. A. (2015). Greenhouse gas emission estimates of US dietary choices and food loss. *Journal of Industrial Ecology, 19*(3), 391–401. https://doi.org/10.1111/jiec.12174

Hemke, R., Buckless, C., & Torriani, M. (2020, August). Quantitative imaging of body composition. In *Seminars in musculoskeletal radiology* (Vol. 24, No. 4, pp. 375–385). Thieme Medical Publishers. https://doi.org/10.1055/s-0040-1708824

Horswill, C., Scott, H., & Voorhees, D. (2017). Effect of a novel workstation device on promoting non-exercise activity thermogenesis (NEAT). *Work, 58*(4), 447–454. https://doi.org/10.3233/WOR-172640

Kumar, A. S., Maiya, G., Shastry, B., Vaishali, K., Maiya, S., & Umakanth, S. (2019). Correlation between basal metabolic rate, visceral fat and insulin resistance among type 2 diabetes mellitus with peripheral neuropathy. *Diabetes & Metabolic Syndrome, 13*(1), 344–348. https://doi.org/10.1016/j.dsx.2018.10.005

Kuuva, S. (2016). Metabolism of visual symbols: Case Madonna. *International Journal of the Image, 7*(2).

Lawler, K., Bell, I., Bryant, C., Pickering, S. H., Gillding, E. R., Rapley, S., & Rolfe, M. (2019). Jump distance of Monistria concinna in relation to metabolic rate and femur length: Mass ratio. *Field Studies in Ecology, 2*(1). https://studentjournals.anu.edu.au/index.php/fse/article/view/224

Leal, L., Lopes, M., & Batista, M. (2018). Physical exercise-induced myokines and muscle-adipose tissue crosstalk: A review of current knowledge and the implications for health and metabolic diseases. *Frontiers in Physiology, 9*. https://doi.org/10.3389/fphys.2018.01307

Little, J., Gillen, J., Percival, M., Safdar, A., Tarnopolsky, M., Punthakee, Z., Jung, M., & Gibala, M. (2011). Low-volume high-intensity interval training reduces hyperglycemia and increases muscle mitochondrial capacity in patients with type 2 diabetes. *Journal of Applied Physiology, 111*(6), 1554–1560. https://doi.org/10.1152/japplphysiol.00921.2011

Malaeb, S., Perez-Leighton, C. E., Noble, E. E., & Billington, C. (2019). A "NEAT" approach to obesity prevention in the modern work environment. *Workplace Health & Safety, 67*(3), 102–110. https://doi.org/10.1177/2165079918790980

Matsushita, M., Yoneshiro, T., Aita, S., Kameya, T., Sugie, H., & Saito, M. (2014). Impact of brown adipose tissue on body fatness and glucose metabolism in healthy humans. *International Journal of Obesity*, *38*(6), 812–817. https://doi.org/10.1038/ijo. 2013.206

Myers, J., Kokkinos, P., & Nyelin, E. (2019). Physical activity, cardiorespiratory fitness, and the metabolic syndrome. *Nutrients*, *11*. https://doi.org/10.3390/nu11071652

Nwimo, I. O., & Orji, S. A. (2015). Physical fitness among school children: Review of empirical studies and implications for physical and health education. *Journal of Tourism, Hospitality and Sports*, *10*, 2312–5179.

Olejníčková, J., Forejt, M., Čermáková, E., & Hudcová, L. (2019). Factors influencing basal metabolism of Czechs of working age from South Moravia. *Central European Journal of Public Health*, *27*(2), 135–140. https://doi.org/10.21101/cejph.a5103

Pang, J., & Hammond, D. (2013). Efficacy and consumer preferences for different approaches to calorie labeling on menus. *Journal of Nutrition Education and Behavior*, *45*(6), 669–675. https://doi.org/10.1016/j.jneb.2013.06.005

Pedersen, B., & Saltin, B. (2006). Evidence for prescribing exercise as therapy in chronic disease. *Scandinavian Journal of Medicine & Science in Sports*, *16*. https://doi. org/10.1111/J.1600-0838.2006.00520.X

Piché, M. E., Poirier, P., Lemieux, I., & Després, J. P. (2018). Overview of epidemiology and contribution of obesity and body fat distribution to cardiovascular disease: An update. *Progress in Cardiovascular Diseases*, *61*(2), 103–113. https://doi. org/10.1016/j.pcad.2018.06.004

Ravussin, E., & Peterson, C. M. (2015). Physical activity and the missing calories. *Exercise and Sport Sciences Reviews*, *43*(3), 107–108. https://doi.org/10.1249/ JES.0000000000000052

Rizzato, A., Marcolin, G., & Paoli, A. (2022). Non-exercise activity thermogenesis in the workplace: The office is on fire. *Frontiers in Public Health*, *10*. https://doi.org/ 10.3389/fpubh.2022.1024856

Saklayen, M. (2018). The global epidemic of the metabolic syndrome. *Current Hypertension Reports*, *20*. https://doi.org/10.1007/s11906-018-0812-z

Sanches, A. C. S., Góes, C. R. D., Bufarah, M. N. B., Balbi, A. L., & Ponce, D. (2016). Resting energy expenditure in critically ill patients: Evaluation methods and clinical applications. *Revista da Associação Médica Brasileira*, *62*, 672–679. https://doi. org/10.1590/1806-9282.62.07.672

Sanchez-Delgado, G., Martinez-Tellez, B., Olza, J., Aguilera, C. M., Labayen, I., Ortega, F. B., Chillon, P., Fernandez-Reguera, C., Alcantara, J. M., Martinez-Avila, W. D., & Munoz-Hernandez, V. (2015). Activating brown adipose tissue through exercise (ACTIBATE) in young adults: Rationale, design and methodology. *Contemporary Clinical Trials*, *45*(Pt B), 416–425. https://doi.org/10.1016/j.cct.2015.11.004

Sánchez López de Nava, A., & Raja, A. (2019). Physiology, metabolism. In *StatPearls*. StatPearls Publishing. https://europepmc.org/article/nbk/nbk546690

Sellami, M., Bragazzi, N. L., Slimani, M., Hayes, L., Jabbour, G., De Giorgio, A., & Dugué, B. (2019). The effect of exercise on glucoregulatory hormones: A countermeasure to human aging: Insights from a comprehensive review of the literature. *International Journal of Environmental Research and Public Health*, *16*(10), 1709. https://doi.org/10.3390/ijerph16101709

Sepa-Kishi, D. M., & Ceddia, R. B. (2016). Exercise-mediated effects on white and brown adipose tissue plasticity and metabolism. *Exercise and Sport Sciences Reviews*, *44*(1), 37–44. https://doi.org/10.1249/JES.0000000000000068

Stensvold, D., Tjønna, A., Skaug, E., Aspenes, S., Stølen, T., Wisløff, U., & Slørdahl, S. (2010). Strength training versus aerobic interval training to modify risk factors of metabolic syndrome. *Journal of Applied Physiology*, *108*(4), 804–810. https://doi.org/ 10.1152/japplphysiol.00996.2009

Strasser, B. (2013). Physical activity in obesity and metabolic syndrome. *Annals of the New York Academy of Sciences, 1281*(1), 141–159. https://doi.org/10.1111/j.1749-6632.2012.06785.x

Tveit, D. M., & Thorsen, K. (2017). Passivity-based analysis of biochemical networks displaying homeostasis. In *Proceedings of the 58th conference on simulation and modelling, Reykjavik, Iceland, September 25–27, 2017* (pp. 108–113). Linköping Electronic Conference Proceedings 138:14. http://dx.doi.org/10.3384/ecp17138108

VanEpps, E. M., Downs, J. S., & Loewenstein, G. (2016). Calorie label formats: Using numeric and traffic light calorie labels to reduce lunch calories. *Journal of Public Policy & Marketing, 35*(1), 26–36. https://doi.org/10.1509/jppm.14.112

Vithalani, L. V., Sakharkar, B. V., & Dalvi, S. A. (2017). Shatkriyakala with special reference to homeostasis and pathogenesis- a brief review. *An International Journal of Research in AYUSH and Allied Systems, 4*(6), 1467–1473. https://core.ac.uk/download/pdf/333809984.pdf

von Loeffelholz, C., & Birkenfeld, A. (2018). *The role of non-exercise activity thermogenesis in human obesity.* Endotext [Internet]. https://www.ncbi.nlm.nih.gov/sites/books/NBK279077/

Wotring, V. E. (2012). Metabolism and excretion. *Space Pharmacology,* 27–32. https://doi.org/10.1007/978-1-4614-3396-5_4

Xiao, P. (2022). Cardiopulmonary resistance in obese individuals during different aerobic exercises. *Revista Brasileira de Medicina do Esporte, 28,* 486–488. https://doi.org/10.1590/1517-8692202228052022_0056

Yan, Y., & Chen, Q. (2022). Energy expenditure estimation of tabata by combining acceleration and heart rate. *Frontiers in Public Health, 9,* 2098. https://doi.org/10.3389/fpubh.2021.804471

Yu, S. (2021). Application of blockchain-based sports health data collection system in the development of sports industry. *Mobile Information Systems, 2021,* 1–6. https://doi.org/10.1155/2021/4663147

Zhao, B. (2014). Analysis on the differences of body composition and maximal oxygen uptake between sports and non-sports male students. In *Advanced materials research* (Vol. 934, pp. 38–43). Trans Tech Publications Ltd. https://doi.org/10.4028/www.scientific.net/AMR.934.38

10

AEROBIC CONTROL

Oliver Napila Gomez and Nguyen Tra Giang

The fitness of the cardiorespiratory and nervous systems is essential for general health and task performance, and this chapter explores the complex relationship between aerobic control, movement, and physiological health. It emphasizes the significance of breathing and blood flow efficiency for optimal health, especially in predicting health outcomes like hypertension, lung function changes, and death. Efforts to enhance cardiorespiratory fitness are currently being investigated. One promising intervention is high-intensity aerobic interval training, which aims to increase aerobic capacity and endurance. The capacity to regulate breathing, heart rate, and exercise intensity while engaging in physical activity is introduced in this chapter as the notion of aerobic control. The Karvonen formula and other heart rate monitoring methods are covered, as well as the importance of aerobic endurance for maintaining physical exertion for long periods. The effects of diseases like COVID-19 on aerobic capacity and task performance are discussed, along with factors influencing aerobic control, such as obesity and risk factors for cardiovascular disease. Despite the difficulties brought on by long-term health conditions and other variables, the chapter stresses the significance of aerobic control and cardiorespiratory health for optimum physiological function and movement competency.

Outcomes

By the end of this chapter, you will be able to

- explain aerobic efficiency and how the cardiovascular and respiratory systems help the body transport and use oxygen efficiently

DOI: 10.4324/9781003502937-12

- explore the substantial effects of aerobic fitness on physiological health
- discuss the switch from VO_2 max and endurance to aerobic control in the USFD Framework, emphasizing the control of cardiorespiratory capacity and endurance to match work needs
- elaborate aerobic control, including heart rate and breathing, altering aerobic capacity and endurance for safe and efficient workouts
- reflect on how lifestyle choices, regular aerobic exercise, and risk factors like smoking and obesity affect aerobic control

Physiological health and movement

Breathing and blood flow are two ways the cardiorespiratory system shows its efficiency. Achieving and sustaining general health and wellness depends on the respiratory and cardiovascular systems' capacity to cooperate efficiently and effectively during physical activity (Cheifetz, 2014; Stensvold et al., 2017).

Similar to the current understanding of cardiorespiratory fitness, it was previously a factor in predicting both high blood pressure and alterations in lung function with aging (Dogra et al., 2017). Cardiorespiratory fitness predicts clinical issues, length of hospital stay, and mortality in older COVID-19 survivors (Antunes et al., 2022), and increases cancer risk (Grote et al., 2020). Cardiovascular events occur daily in men and women with low cardiorespiratory fitness (Ferentinos et al., 2022). To put it differently, cardiorespiratory fitness is associated with health because it is a predictor of death and the prevalence of chronic diseases (Zisman-Ilani et al., 2020; Arcila et al., 2022; Barbagelata et al., 2022; Leija, 2019).

Current cardiorespiratory fitness research focuses on improving aerobic capacity and endurance; for example, in patients with stable coronary artery

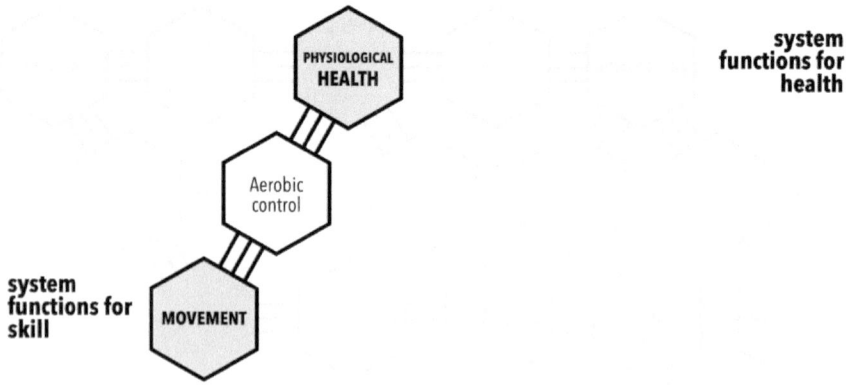

FIGURE 10.1   Aerobic control – shared by physiological health and movement

disease, increasing VO$_2$ max through high-intensity aerobic interval training is more effective than moderate-intensity exercise (Rognmo et al., 2004). The capacity of the cardiorespiratory system to supply oxygen to working muscles is directly related to aerobic capacity, also known as VO$_2$ max, and hence to physical performance (Karpoor et al., 2011). Improved exercise capacity and health outcomes result from aerobic endurance, which is essential for maintaining moderate-intensity activities through efficient oxygen utilization by muscles (Haykowsky et al., 2012). Performance success is contingent upon several variables, including aerobic capacity, endurance, neuromuscular function, and movement economy. Cardiorespiratory fitness can be improved by combining strength training with aerobic exercise, increasing neuromuscular economy and muscle oxidative capacity (Cadore et al., 2011).

Optimal aerobic performance, in the context of modern sports, is the driving force behind the current obsession with aerobic fitness. People have been led to believe that being fit means having a higher VO$_2$ max and sustaining intense exercises for long periods. When compared, optimal levels can get things done efficiently. However, peak VO$_2$ max and endurance levels are optional for some tasks.

Aerobic control is a critical function in the USFD Framework. It refers to the ability of a person to be aware of their cardiorespiratory capacity and endurance, manage their breathing, monitor their heart rate, and match the aerobic capacity and endurance required by the task at hand. When a person has reasonable aerobic control, they should be able to closely monitor their breathing and heart rate to ensure they exercise at the right intensity.

Aerobic control

We are now releasing a new fitness system function representing an individual's capacity to control their breathing and heart rate during strenuous exercise. This function shows that managing aerobic capacity and endurance with the intensity of aerobic exercise means a person can work out longer without getting sick.

Studies showing the powerful and opposing effects of vagal sensory neurons in the vagus nerve demonstrate the precision needed for breathing regulation (Chang et al., 2018; Kupari et al., 2019). The brain's GPR4 receptor is essential for CO_2-stimulated breathing, highlighting CO_2 detection's role in respiratory control (Kumar & Kumar, 2015; Hosford et al., 2018). Diaphragmatic breathing improves sustained attention, reduces negative affect, and lowers cortisol, suggesting mental health and stress management benefits (Ma et al., 2017). However, obesity significantly affects lung volumes, respiratory mechanics, and breathing efficiency, emphasizing the importance of weight management in respiratory health (Steier et al., 2014).

Today, people rely on monitoring methods for accuracy when exercising (Stahl et al., 2016) since heart rate monitoring has become passive.

Photoplethysmography (PPG) and other newly developed HR monitoring methods work effectively even during vigorous exercise (Zhang, 2015). However, the USFD Framework sees breathing and heart rate monitoring as an active fitness skill under aerobic control. It can be used to proactively adjust the intensity of workouts and make sure that everyone is exercising safely.

One can measure resting heart rate (RHR) by getting up first thing in the morning and then sitting or lying down for ten minutes (Venkat et al., 2022). Even when someone is not moving around or sleeping, the heart constantly pumps blood (Dong et al., 2015). A person's pulse is a simple way to track their heart rate and activity (Venkat et al., 2022). An adult's typical RHR is between 60 and 100 beats per minute (BPM). While RHRs can vary from person to person, a lower RHR might indicate aerobic fitness (Russell et al., 2019). In contrast, if the heart rate is consistently over 100 BPM, it could be a sign of an irregular heart rhythm, weak cardiac muscles due to a virus, or any number of other conditions that cause an increase in heart rate, such as hyperthyroidism, fever, anemia, or caffeine consumption (Sarganas et al., 2017; Harvard Health Publishing, 2021).

When someone moves around and exerts energy, their heart rate goes up. Conventional cardiorespiratory fitness tests allow nonathletes to achieve sub-maximal heart rates (Berglund et al., 2019). Nevertheless, measuring resting heart rate is more straightforward than measuring maximum heart rate (MHR), and using age-based formulas might need to be more accurate, which could cause exercise intensity prescription errors or the early termination of fitness tests (Matabuena et al., 2019). Exercise testing can assess cardiovascular capacity and fitness by gauging the effort required to achieve and sustain maximum heart rate (MHR) (Arena et al., 2016). Thorough monitoring and expert supervision is necessary to avoid complications such as chest pain, muscle fatigue, and oxygen debt from obtaining 100% MHR (Faizan-ul-Haq et al., 2018). The physical stress of MHR clinical testing might harm those not trained to handle it (Nikolaidis, 2015). Predicting or reaching MHR consistently is challenging because of the variability caused by factors such as fitness level, age, body composition, and sex (Gelbart et al., 2017).

The Karvonen method (She et al., 2015) is a famous formula many sports scientists use to estimate age-based MHR instead of this "practical" method. Nevertheless, its validity remains debatable. The formula might give an inflated estimate of the MHR for young adults and a lowered estimate for the old population. One source claims that the formula was initially developed to help people with heart conditions determine appropriate exercise (Kolata, 2001). The need to estimate MHR gradually led to its widespread adoption by the general public worldwide, particularly in the medical sector. To diagnose cardiac problems, doctors employ the formula. A user's target heart rate (THR) zone can be determined on the gym treadmill by subtracting their age from 220. Despite its poor validity, the Karvonen formula is now well known among fitness experts and PE instructors for estimating MHR measurements.

The Karvonen Formula: MHR = 220 − age

TABLE 10.1 Alternative formulas to the Karvonen method for estimating maximum heart rate (Tanaka et al., 2001; Gulati et al., 2010; Porcari et al., 2015)

Method	Formula	Intended for
Tanaka	MHR = 208 − (0.7 × age)	Healthy men and women
Gelish	MHR = 207 − (0.7 × age)	A broad range of fitness levels (male or female)
Gulati	MHR = 206 − (0.88 × age)	Middle-aged women

There might be a need for accuracy in the estimates given by the equations in Table 10.1. A precise measurement of an individual's maximum heart rate is fraught with difficulty and danger, but these alternatives offer a practical means of approximating this number.

Even when at rest or asleep, the RHR must be maintained to keep vital biological processes going. Under highly strenuous physical activity, the maximum heart rate (MHR) is the maximum rate at which the heart pumps blood to meet the body's circulatory demands. Heart rate reserve (HRR) is the difference between the maximum and resting heart rates. To show the degree of physical exertion based on heart rate count, the HRR can be divided into ten levels.

Theoretically, engaging in certain lifestyle activities can raise the heart rate from resting to 50% of HRR. Walking, cleaning, and watering plants are examples of lifestyle activities. People also do these things at home, at work, and school.

Light-intensity activities done at 51% to 60% HRR are warm-ups. They get the muscles and cardiovascular system ready for strenuous exercise. Exercising at a moderate to light intensity, between 61% and 70% of HRR, can help keep the weight off. To keep muscles supplied with oxygen and glucose at this intensity level, the aerobic energy system uses Krebs's cycle and the mitochondria's electron transport chain to generate ATP. Physical activities that are moderate in intensity and done at a heart rate range of 71% to 80% of HRR are great for building aerobic endurance.

Aerobic endurance is more typical than anaerobic endurance in cardiorespiratory fitness tests (Begum et al., 2022). The capacity to maintain aerobic activity for a long time is known as aerobic endurance (Hiremath et al., 2021). In contrast, the ability to maintain anaerobic intensity for a long time is known as anaerobic endurance (Juric et al., 2019). The aerobic energy system requires oxygen for aerobic processes but does not for anaerobic ones (Lee & Stone, 2019). Anaerobic intensity levels are theoretically between 81% and 90% of

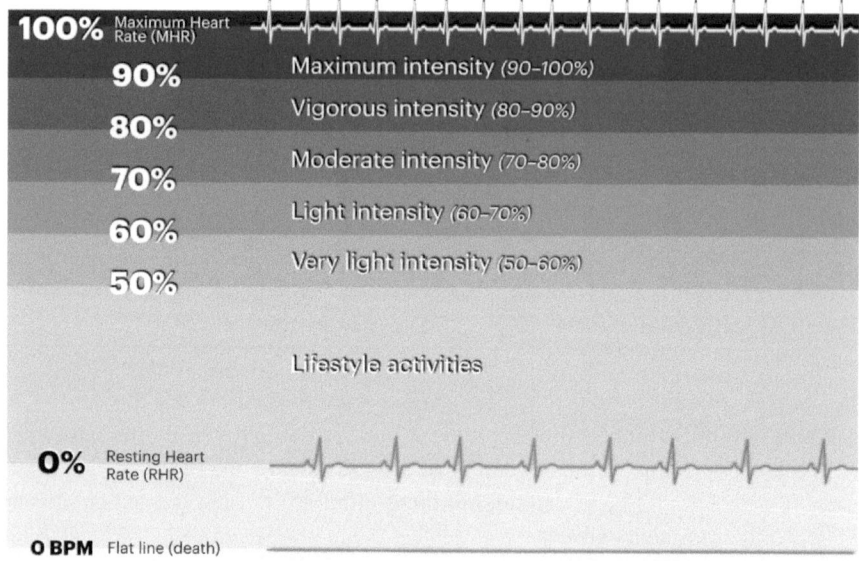

FIGURE 10.2   The concept of heart rate and aerobic intensity system

HRR (Albesa-Albiol et al., 2019). Hydrogen ions are produced in the working muscles as the body taps into the anaerobic lactic energy system (Poole et al., 2020; Brooks, 2020). Acidosis, brought on by an accumulation of hydrogen ions, causes a painful muscle-burning sensation (Miesse & Slaughter, 2020). Muscles can maintain activity for two minutes or beyond because lactate (hydrogen ions that bind with pyruvate) reduces acidosis (Bangsbo, 2019). The burning sensation in the muscles is caused by lactate, which is carried away from the working muscles to neutralize the acidity (Zhao et al., 2019).

Finally, due to the risks involved, untrained populations should not perform maximum-intensity exercises ranging from 91% of HRR to 100% of the MHR. It is feasible to reach this level; however, groups of trained individuals may make it up to two minutes, while untrained individuals may only last 10 to 60 seconds. Trained people have the potential to reach this level. However, this intensity level may need to use the phosphocreatine energy system to meet the rapid and high energy demands, but only briefly.

The target heart rate is 71% and 80% of the HRR to improve aerobic endurance. At this intensity level, exercise is just below the aerobic threshold before feeling the buildup of hydrogen ions, indicating the start of anaerobic intensity (Hansen et al., 2019). The efficiency of the cardiorespiratory system in absorbing, transporting, and utilizing oxygen for aerobic respiration to sustain the working muscles varies from person to person (Rogers & Gronwald, 2022), so this only works in theory.

Aerobic control functions for physiological health and movement

Two essential aspects of aerobic control in the USFD model are aerobic capacity and endurance. The ability to efficiently transport and use oxygen during aerobic activities is known as aerobic capacity, which is vital for physiological health. It measures cardiovascular health and affects aerobic exercise performance. Aerobic endurance, in contrast, refers to a person's capacity to maintain moderate to high levels of aerobic activity for long periods. Skillful movement tasks, such as swimming and long-distance running, require it. In the context of the USFD paradigm, both tasks stress the significance of aerobic control for attaining and sustaining physiological wellness and movement competence.

Aerobic capacity and physiological health

Aerobic capacity is one of the most critical aspects of aerobic control in preserving physiological health in the USFD Framework. This view is based on an in-depth understanding of aerobic capacity's role in a person's general fitness and health.

A vital indicator of the cardiorespiratory system's capacity to transport and utilize oxygen during aerobic physical activity is aerobic capacity, which is also called VO_2 max or maximal oxygen uptake (Kumar & Kumar, 2015; Maurer, 2022; Oluwadare & Olufemi, 2018). It makes it harder to do aerobic activities like swimming, cycling, and running. Aerobic capacity is an essential cardiovascular health indicator and critical for exercise performance.

Aerobic capacity should be treated as a function of aerobic management within the USFD Framework due to the complex interplay between oxygen supply and energy generation during aerobic exercise. In order to sustain energy production through aerobic respiration, individuals who participate in aerobic activities necessitate a steady and sufficient supply of oxygen. The cardiorespiratory system pumps oxygen-rich blood to working muscles, removing waste products like carbon dioxide through the lungs and blood arteries. An individual's aerobic capacity is directly related to the rate at which their functional muscles transport and use oxygen.

To measure and evaluate this crucial physiological parameter, people often take part in maximal exercise tests, which can be done on a treadmill or stationary bike. As the subject works up a sweat, these tests keep close tabs on vitals like heart rate, breathing rate, and oxygen consumption. When one reaches their maximal effort, they can determine their VO_2 max by measuring their oxygen consumption rate at its peak.

Managing and regulating physiological responses during aerobic activities is built upon aerobic capacity, so aerobic control is considered an essential function within the USFD Framework. An impressive capacity to supply working muscles with oxygen, enabling them to function efficiently for extended durations, is indicated by a robust aerobic capacity. Enhanced aerobic control results in better health outcomes, endurance, and a decreased risk of developing a host of chronic disorders – including cardiovascular diseases.

As it may, building aerobic capacity is possible through consistent aerobic exercise, but it must be done within the bounds of legality. The importance of engaging in regular, health-promoting physical activity to maintain an adequate level of aerobic capacity is emphasized by the USFD Framework. Natural heart and lung strengthening, better oxygen utilization by muscles, and enhanced blood circulation are the tenets of this approach. Ultimately, we want people to be able to use aerobic control to get in shape and stay in shape.

Additionally, blood doping and other unlawful methods of increasing aerobic capacity are strongly discouraged by the USFD Framework (Sieljacks et al., 2016). Blood doping, which involves artificially increasing the blood's capacity to carry oxygen, is illegal (Mussack et al., 2021). As far as medical treatments go, this is a lousy way to boost muscle oxygen flow artificially (Nacerbey & Makhlouf, 2022). In order to achieve physiological health, the paradigm stresses the significance of legal and natural ways of increasing aerobic capacity while simultaneously highlighting the ethical concerns and possible health risks connected with such practices.

In the USFD Framework, aerobic capacity is the most critical factor in maintaining physiological health through aerobic management. Improving endurance, health outcomes, and reducing the risk of chronic diseases are all outcomes of effectively monitoring and regulating physiological responses during aerobic exercises, which is where its significance lies. It opposes unlawful activities that endanger health and integrity while promoting aerobic capacity ethically and health-promotingly.

Aerobic endurance and movement

One of the main goals of aerobic regulation of movement in the USFD Framework is aerobic endurance. This perspective is based on a solid understanding of the vital role that aerobic endurance plays in an individual's ability to engage in sustained, skilled movement.

One important aspect of aerobic management in the USFD Framework is aerobic endurance, which is the capacity of the body to transport and use oxygen continuously throughout all of its systems (Ahmad et al., 2014; Smith, 2016; Zhang, 2022). Consistently engaging in aerobic activity at a moderate to high intensity for long durations without experiencing fatigue or weariness is what it means. The ability to engage in deft motions that call for consistent effort over an extended period rests on this foundation of endurance.

Aerobic endurance is the foundation of aerobic regulation of movement because of the close relationship between the cardiorespiratory system and the muscles used during exercise. A highly efficient delivery of oxygen to the working muscles is what the cardiorespiratory system needs to achieve a high degree of aerobic endurance. For this intricate process to work, the heart must pump blood rich in oxygen, the lungs must be able to process large amounts of oxygen, and the circulatory system must effectively transfer this blood to the muscles to generate energy.

Sports like long-distance running, cycling, and swimming demand constant effort for extended periods, making aerobic endurance a must-have. Oxygen availability is crucial to the aerobic energy system, which produces ATP (adenosine triphosphate), the cellular energy currency, to power the working muscles during these activities. The aerobic energy system is crucial for endurance sports because, unlike anaerobic energy systems, it provides sustained energy over long periods rather than rapid but brief bursts.

Within the context of the USFD Framework, aerobic endurance is significant because of the role it plays in enabling skill and duration-defined movement. It paves the way for people to participate in pursuits that call for physical competence and the capacity to maintain it over time. For instance, to complete a marathon without tiring, a long-distance runner needs both the technical running abilities and the aerobic endurance to keep going.

Aerobic exercise is an intricate process that, over time, can improve aerobic endurance. Activities that demand moderate to high intensity, like running, cycling, swimming, and rowing, are great ways to build aerobic endurance. Aerobic exercise, when done consistently over time and with increasing intensity, trains the heart and lungs to deliver oxygen to working muscles better. Aerobic endurance is enhanced as a result of this adaptation.

The USFD Framework celebrates aerobic endurance as the apex of aerobic control for movement. It allows people to perform movement tasks that call for precision and stamina. Because the framework emphasizes building aerobic endurance, which improves overall physical performance and increases movement competence, it enables people to excel in activities that demand sustained, skilled movement.

Aerobic endurance is highly regarded as the foundation of aerobic control for movement within the USFD Framework. It seamlessly integrates with the framework's focus on knowledge, competence, performance, and decision-making in pursuing movement proficiency.

Factors that affect aerobic control

The muscle cells need oxygen to carry out aerobic activities efficiently. Therefore, aerobic fitness is determined mainly by the body's capacity to maximize oxygen uptake. Maintaining an aerobic workout for longer, improving aerobic threshold, and reducing hydrogen ion buildup are all benefits of a good VO_2 max.

Aerobic exercise and other regular physical activity can also raise the aerobic threshold and improve fitness. On the flip side, cardiovascular disease risks and cardiorespiratory fitness can both be worsened by an inactive lifestyle.

Other issues also impact heart and lung function. Impending influences on cardiorespiratory fitness come from heart and pulmonary disease risk factors such as smoking, pollution exposure, high cholesterol, and diabetes (Niemann et al., 2017; Rajagopalan et al., 2018).

Additionally, cardiorespiratory fitness can be impacted by obesity, which is a risk factor for numerous cardiovascular diseases (Oktay et al., 2017). When a person is overweight, their heart has to work harder to pump enough oxygen to their muscles so they can perform aerobic respiration and produce ATP. The detrimental effects of excess body fat on cardiorespiratory functions and the ability of working muscles to absorb oxygen are demonstrated by the fact that functional impairment is directly proportional to the body mass index (BMI) (Setty et al., 2013). As the level of exertion rises during exercise, the blood pressure rises to meet the increased demand for blood distribution by the cardiovascular system. For people who are overweight, this could mean a higher chance of heart attack.

Aerobic control and task performance

The importance of a strong heart in lowering the risk of major cardiovascular events and enhancing performance is highlighted by the fact that individuals with high levels of cardiorespiratory fitness have a lower risk of severe ventricular arrhythmias (Laukkanen et al., 2019). Nonetheless, in line with the HATS Framework, when the health of the cardiorespiratory and nervous systems are impaired, aerobic control diminishes, impacting the capacity to execute tasks efficiently and effectively.

Take the recent COVID-19 pandemic as an example. The disease affected the heart and lungs and left many patients with long-term effects like fatigue and shortness of breath even after they were discharged from the hospital. These symptoms affect the capacity to carry out routine activities, along with a decline in exercise tolerance, cognitive performance, and quality of life (Raman et al., 2020).

Chronic obstructive pulmonary disease (COPD) and heart diseases, such as pulmonary hypertension, are characterized by fatigue and dyspnea, which significantly restrict daily activities for patients. Reduced quality of life and inefficiency in managing daily tasks are associated with exercise intolerance and poor exercise capacity, which are frequently caused by these conditions (Manders et al., 2015; Raman et al., 2020).

Moreover, there is a correlation between cardiovascular diseases, such as heart failure, and an increase in mortality and morbidity rates. These diseases impact various organ systems. Exercise capacity and the ability to perform daily tasks are diminished due to these diseases' effects on ventilatory control and efficiency, cardiac output, systemic and pulmonary vascular resistance, and abnormalities (Verbrugge et al., 2020).

In conclusion, healthy and functional cardiorespiratory and nervous systems are crucial, improving overall performance and lowering the risk of serious cardiovascular events. Nevertheless, diseases like COVID-19 can drastically reduce aerobic control, which in turn causes long-term effects like weariness and decreased exercise tolerance. These difficulties are already tricky enough without adding the limitations imposed by chronic diseases like heart disease and chronic obstructive pulmonary disease (COPD). Furthermore, heart failure and other cardiovascular diseases are associated with higher mortality and morbidity rates; these conditions impact various organ systems and further limit an individual's ability to exercise and carry out daily tasks. Improving health outcomes and quality of life for people dealing with these issues requires a thorough understanding of and attention to these complexities.

Summary

The efficiency of the cardiorespiratory system is demonstrated by breathing and blood flow, which are essential for overall health and well-being. When working out, the cardiovascular and respiratory systems work together, which is crucial for health in general.

Once only a predictor of hypertension and age-related declines in lung function, cardiorespiratory fitness is now an essential component in many clinical outcomes, such as the likelihood of surviving COVID-19 and the likelihood of developing cancer. Low cardiorespiratory fitness is associated with worse health outcomes and a higher prevalence of chronic diseases, including cardiovascular events, which are common in this population.

Most studies aim to increase aerobic capacity and endurance to achieve peak physiological health and performance. When increasing VO_2 max in individuals with coronary artery disease, high-intensity aerobic interval training works better than moderate-intensity exercise. Aerobic endurance affects health outcomes and overall performance because it is necessary to maintain moderate- to high-intensity activities.

An essential part of the USFD Framework, aerobic control involves keeping the breathing, heart rate, and aerobic capacity under control while exercising. Reaching a reasonable level of aerobic control allows people to keep a close eye on their body's reactions during exercise, which leads to effective and safe sessions.

Muscle cell oxygen uptake, individual lifestyle factors, and disease risk factors like obesity and cardiovascular disease all impact aerobic control. Reduced aerobic control affects task efficiency and general health when cardiorespiratory and nervous system health is impaired.

In order to enhance health outcomes and quality of life, it is crucial to comprehend the complexities of aerobic control and how it affects physiological health and movement. People can improve their aerobic control and general health by focusing on aerobic fitness, regular physical activity, and addressing underlying health issues.

Review questions

1. Why is an efficient cardiorespiratory system important for overall health and well-being?
2. Discuss the health consequences of cardiorespiratory fitness, such as its link to age-related lung function loss and high blood pressure.
3. How does aerobic fitness affect clinical outcomes in older COVID-19 survivors, and what does this mean?
4. Using relevant literature, explain the association between aerobic fitness and cancer mortality.
5. Contrast the usual emphasis on VO_2 max and endurance with the USFD Framework's concept of "aerobic control."
6. What is aerobic control, and how does it help with good workout management?
7. Describe the difficulties and hazards involved in establishing maximum heart rate and other approaches for measuring it.
8. What exactly is heart rate reserve (HRR), and how is it used to determine the level of physical exertion or intensity during exercise?
9. What effects do lifestyle factors such as frequent aerobic exercise, smoking, and obesity have on aerobic control and cardiorespiratory fitness?
10. What practical methods and lifestyle changes may people make to improve their aerobic control and general well-being?

Discussion questions

1. Assume you are dealing with a client who wants to improve cardiovascular health by participating in aerobic exercise. What strategies would you offer to assist them in improving their aerobic control? How would you assess their present aerobic capacity and endurance?
2. How can aerobic control be implemented into schools' physical education curriculum to encourage lifetime fitness habits among students? What specific activities or approaches do you recommend to achieve this goal?
3. Many people need help to stick to a regular aerobic exercise plan. How can fitness trackers and mobile apps be used to assist people to monitor and control their heart rate and breathing during workouts? What are the benefits and drawbacks of adopting technology in this situation?

4. Discuss the significance of customizing aerobic control measures to specific populations, such as older adults, those with chronic health issues, and athletes. How might the strategy for aerobic control differ for each group, and what factors should be considered?
5. Workplace wellness programs are frequently designed to promote employee health while lowering healthcare expenditures. How can these programs combine an awareness of aerobic control and efficiency to encourage physical exercise and overall well-being among employees? What kinds of incentives or efforts might work in this situation?

References

Ahmad, H., Ishak, N. A., & Ishak, A. (2014). Optimizing physiological and performance outcomes using recovery strategies among junior cyclists. *Jurnal Sains Sukan & Pendidikan Jasmani*, *3*(1), 1–10. https://ojs.upsi.edu.my/index.php/JSSPJ/article/view/630

Albesa-Albiol, L., Serra-Payá, N., Garnacho-Castaño, M., Cano, L., Cobo, E., Maté-Muñoz, J., & Garnacho-Castaño, M. (2019). Ventilatory efficiency during constant-load test at lactate threshold intensity: Endurance versus resistance exercises. *PLoS One*, *14*. https://doi.org/10.1371/journal.pone.0216824

Antunes, E. L., Costa, B. M., Sochodolak, R. C., Vargas, L. M., & Okuno, N. M. (2022). The influence of physical activity level on the length of stay in hospital in older men survivors of COVID-19. *Sport Sciences for Health*, *18*(4), 1483–1490. https://doi.org/10.1007/s11332-022-00948-7

Arcila, E., Restrepo, C., Valbuena, L., Quintero, M. A., Marino, F., Osorio, J. A., Gallo-Villegas, J., & Saldarriaga Franco, J. F. (2022). Validity and reproducibility of a method to estimate cardiorespiratory fitness in college adults. *Biomédica*, *42*(4), 611–622. https://doi.org/10.7705/biomedica.6404

Arena, R., Myers, J., & Kaminsky, L. (2016). Revisiting age-predicted maximal heart rate: Can it be used as a valid measure of effort? *American Heart Journal*, *173*, 49–56. https://doi.org/10.1016/j.ahj.2015.12.006

Bangsbo, J. (2019). Energy demands in competitive soccer. *Journal of Sports Sciences*, *12*, S5–S12. https://doi.org/10.1080/02640414.1994.12059272

Barbagelata, L., Masson, W., Bluro, I., Lobo, M., Iglesias, D., & Molinero, G. (2022). Prognostic role of cardiopulmonary exercise testing in pulmonary hypertension: A systematic review and meta-analysis. *Advances in Respiratory Medicine*, *90*(2), 109–117. https://doi.org/10.5603/ARM.a2022.0030

Begum, A., Lakshmi, T., & Syed, S. (2022). Assessment of cardiovascular fitness among young sedentary adults using 1600 M walking test. *Medical and Health Science Journal*, *6*(2), 1–6. https://doi.org/10.33086/mhsj.v6i02.3213

Berglund, I., Sørås, S., Relling, B., Lundgren, K., Kiel, I., & Moholdt, T. (2019). The relationship between maximum heart rate in a cardiorespiratory fitness test and in a maximum heart rate test. *Journal of Science and Medicine in Sport*, *22*(5), 607–610. https://doi.org/10.1016/j.jsams.2018.11.018

Brooks, G. (2020). Lactate as a fulcrum of metabolism. *Redox Biology*, *35*. https://doi.org/10.1016/j.redox.2020.101454

Cadore, E., Pinto, R., Alberton, C., Pinto, S., Lhullier, F., Tartaruga, M., Correa, C., Almeida, A., Silva, E., Laitano, O., & Kruel, L. (2011). Neuromuscular economy, strength, and endurance in healthy elderly men. *Journal of Strength and Conditioning Research*, *25*, 997–1003. https://doi.org/10.1519/JSC.0b013e3181d650ba

Chang, R., Strochlic, D., Nonomura, K., Patapoutian, A., & Liberles, S. (2018). Airway mechanoreceptors that control breathing. *The FASEB Journal, 32*, 893.3. https://doi.org/10.1096/fasebj.2018.32.1_supplement.893.3

Cheifetz, I. (2014). Cardiorespiratory interactions: The relationship between mechanical ventilation and hemodynamics. *Respiratory Care, 59*, 1937–1945. https://doi.org/10.4187/respcare.03486

Dogra, S., Froehle, A. W., & Peterson, M. (2017). Novel predictors of age-related changes in lung function. *Medicine and Science in Sports and Exercise, 49*(5S), 788. http://doi.org/10.1249/01.mss.0000519104.70462.6f

Dong, B., Wang, Z., Wang, H., & Ma, J. (2015). The association between resting heart rate and blood pressure among children and adolescents with different waist circumferences. *European Journal of Pediatrics, 174*, 191–197. https://doi.org/10.1007/s00431-014-2377-4

Faizan-ul-Haq, F., Yaqoob, U., & Khan, M. (2018). Our pulse – best in-build fitness monitor. *Indian Heart Journal, 70*, 584–584. https://doi.org/10.1016/j.ihj.2018.02.004

Ferentinos, P., Tsakirides, C., Swainson, M., Davison, A., James, M. S., & Ispoglou, T. (2022). The impact of different forms of exercise on endothelial progenitor cells in healthy populations. *European Journal of Applied Physiology*, 1–37. https://doi.org/10.1007%2Fs00421-022-04921-7

Gelbart, M., Ziv-Baran, T., Williams, C., Yarom, Y., & Dubnov-Raz, G. (2017). Prediction of maximal heart rate in children and adolescents. *Clinical Journal of Sport Medicine, 27*, 139–144. https://doi.org/10.1097/JSM.0000000000000315

Grote, S., Ricci, J. M., Dehom, S., Modeste, N., Sealy, D. A., & Tarleton, H. P. (2020). Heart rate variability and cardiovascular adaptations among cancer-survivors following a 26-week exercise intervention. *Integrative Cancer Therapies, 19*, 1–11. https://doi.org/10.1177/1534735420969816

Gulati, M., Shaw, L. J., Thisted, R. A., Black, H. R., Bairey Merz, C. N., & Arnsdorf, M. F. (2010). Heart rate response to exercise stress testing in asymptomatic women: The St. James women take heart project. *Circulation, 122*(2), 130–137. https://doi.org/10.1161/circulationaha.110.939249

Hansen, D., Bonné, K., Alders, T., Hermans, A., Copermans, K., Swinnen, H., Maris, V., Jansegers, T., Mathijs, W., Haenen, L., Vaes, J., Govaerts, E., Reenaers, V., Frederix, I., & Dendale, P. (2019). Exercise training intensity determination in cardiovascular rehabilitation: Should the guidelines be reconsidered?. *European Journal of Preventive Cardiology, 26*, 1921–1928. https://doi.org/10.1177/2047487319859450

Harvard Health Publishing. (2021, June). *Should I worry about my fast pulse?* [Internet]. https://www.health.harvard.edu/heart-health/should-i-worry-about-my-fast-pulse

Haykowsky, M., Brubaker, P., Stewart, K., Morgan, T., Eggebeen, J., & Kitzman, D. (2012). Effect of endurance training on the determinants of peak exercise oxygen consumption in elderly patients with stable compensated heart failure and preserved ejection fraction. *Journal of the American College of Cardiology, 60*(2), 120–128. https://doi.org/10.1016/j.jacc.2012.02.055

Hiremath, S., Patil, P., & Goudar, S. (2021). Evaluation of basal heart rate and cardio respiratory endurance among wrestlers-a cross-sectional study. *National Journal of Physiology, Pharmacy and Pharmacology, 12*(7), 974–977. https://doi.org/10.5455/njppp.2022.12.11423202116122021

Hosford, P., Mosienko, V., Kishi, K., Jurisic, G., Seuwen, K., Kinzel, B., Ludwig, M., Wells, J., Christie, I., Koolen, L., Abdala, A., Liu, B., Gourine, A., Teschemacher, A., & Kasparov, S. (2018). CNS distribution, signalling properties and central effects of G-protein coupled receptor 4. *Neuropharmacology, 138*, 381–392. https://doi.org/10.1016/j.neuropharm.2018.06.007

Juric, I., Labor, S., Plavec, D., & Labor, M. (2019). Inspiratory muscle strength affects anaerobic endurance in professional athletes. *Archives of Industrial Hygiene and Toxicology, 70*, 42–48. https://doi.org/10.2478/aiht-2019-70-3182

Karpoor, C., Shettar, S., & Dv, D. (2011). Cardiovascular endurance [physical fitness index] and maximal aerobic capacity [Vo2 max] in young male wrestlers. *Indian Journal of Public Health Research and Development, 2*(1).

Kolata, G. (2001, April 24). "Maximum" heart rate theory is challenged. *New York Times*. https://www.nytimes.com/2001/04/24/health/maximum-heart-rate-theory-is-challenged.html

Kumar, A., & Kumar, M. (2015). Effect of body composition and aerobic capacity on blood pressure in young Indian adult males of age group 18–21 years. *International Journal of Science and Research (IJSR), 4*(10), 816–820. http://bit.ly/44iZNfV

Kupari, J., Häring, M., Agirre, E., Castelo-Branco, G., & Ernfors, P. (2019). An atlas of vagal sensory neurons and their molecular specialization. *Cell Reports, 27*(8), 2508–2523. https://doi.org/10.1016/j.celrep.2019.04.096

Laukkanen, J., Lavie, C., Khan, H., Kurl, S., & Kunutsor, S. (2019). Cardiorespiratory fitness and the risk of serious ventricular arrhythmias: A prospective cohort study. *Mayo Clinic Proceedings, 94*, 833–841. https://doi.org/10.1016/j.mayocp.2018.11.027

Lee, J., & Stone, A. (2019). Combined aerobic and resistance training for cardiorespiratory fitness, muscle strength, and walking capacity after stroke: A systematic review and meta-analysis. *Journal of Stroke and Cerebrovascular Diseases: The Official Journal of National Stroke Association, 104498.* https://doi.org/10.1016/j.jstrokecerebrovasdis.2019.104498

Leija, R. G. (2019). *The utilization of verification trials for $\dot{V}O_2MAX$ determination in the heat* [Doctoral dissertation, California State University].

Ma, X., Yue, Z., Gong, Z., Zhang, H., Duan, N., Shi, Y., Wei, G., & Li, Y. (2017). The effect of diaphragmatic breathing on attention, negative affect and stress in healthy adults. *Frontiers in Psychology, 8*. https://doi.org/10.3389/fpsyg.2017.00874

Manders, E., Rain, S., Bogaard, H., Handoko, M., Stienen, G., Vonk-Noordegraaf, A., Ottenheijm, C., & Man, F. (2015). The striated muscles in pulmonary arterial hypertension: Adaptations beyond the right ventricle. *European Respiratory Journal, 46*, 832–842. https://doi.org/10.1183/13993003.02052-2014

Matabuena, M., Vidal, J., Hayes, P., Saavedra-García, M., & Trillo, F. (2019). Application of functional data analysis for the prediction of maximum heart rate. *IEEE Access, 7*, 121841–121852. https://doi.org/10.1109/ACCESS.2019.2938466

Maurer, A. (2022). *Aerobic capacity alters susceptibility to hepatic steatosis via bile acid signaling* [Doctoral dissertation, University of Kansas]. https://www.proquest.com/openview/f555461feb6380693eb56d703ce32f46/1?pq-origsite=gscholar&cbl=18750&diss=y

Miesse, P., & Slaughter, G. (2020). Flexible electrochemical lactate biosensor. In *2020 IEEE 15th international conference on nano/micro engineered and molecular system (NEMS)* (pp. 580–583). IEEE. https://doi.org/10.1109/NEMS50311.2020.9265579

Mussack, V., Wittmann, G., & Pfaffl, M. W. (2021). On the trail of blood doping – microRNA fingerprints to monitor autologous blood transfusions in vivo. *American Journal of Hematology, 96*(3), 338–353. https://doi.org/10.1002/ajh.26078

Nacerbey, K., & Makhlouf, H. (2022). Blood doping in sport. *Laboratory Records Review, 17*(1), 430–447. https://www.asjp.cerist.dz/en/downArticle/483/17/1/191917

Niemann, B., Rohrbach, S., Miller, M. R., Newby, D. E., Fuster, V., & Kovacic, J. C. (2017). Oxidative stress and cardiovascular risk: Obesity, diabetes, smoking, and pollution: Part 3 of a 3-part series. *Journal of the American College of Cardiology, 70*(2), 230–251. https://doi.org/10.1016/j.jacc.2017.05.043

Nikolaidis, P. (2015). Maximal heart rate in soccer players: Measured versus age-predicted. *Biomedical Journal, 38*, 84–89. https://doi.org/10.4103/2319-4170.131397

Oktay, A. A., Lavie, C. J., Kokkinos, P. F., Parto, P., Pandey, A., & Ventura, H. O. (2017). The interaction of cardiorespiratory fitness with obesity and the obesity paradox in cardiovascular disease. *Progress in Cardiovascular Diseases, 60*(1), 30–44. https://doi.org/10.1016/j.pcad.2017.05.005

Oluwadare, O. A., & Olufemi, O. O. (2018). Aerobic fitness levels among undergraduate students of a Nigerian university using Cooper's 12-minute walk test. *International Journal of Advanced Research and Publications*, *2*(4), 6–8. http://bit.ly/3JAAi1T

Poole, D., Rossiter, H., Brooks, G., & Gladden, L. (2020). The anaerobic threshold: 50+ years of controversy. *The Journal of Physiology*, *599*. https://doi.org/10.1113/JP279963

Porcari, J., Bryant, C., & Comana, F. (2015). *Exercise physiology*. FA Davis.

Rajagopalan, S., Al-Kindi, S. G., & Brook, R. D. (2018). Air pollution and cardiovascular disease: JACC state-of-the-art review. *Journal of the American College of Cardiology*, *72*(17), 2054–2070. https://doi.org/10.1016/j.jacc.2018.07.099

Raman, B., Cassar, M. P., Tunnicliffe, E. M., Filippini, N., Griffanti, L., Alfaro-Almagro, F., Okell, T., Sheerin, F., Xie, C., Mahmod, M., & Mózes, F. E. (2020). Medium-term effects of SARS-CoV-2 infection on multiple vital organs, exercise capacity, cognition, quality of life and mental health, post-hospital discharge. *Eclinicalmedicine*, *31*. https://doi.org/10.1016/j.eclinm.2020.100683

Rogers, B., & Gronwald, T. (2022). Fractal correlation properties of heart rate variability as a biomarker for intensity distribution and training prescription in endurance exercise: An update. *Frontiers in Physiology*, *13*. https://doi.org/10.3389/fphys.2022.879071

Rognmo, Ø., Hetland, E., Helgerud, J., Hoff, J., & Slørdahl, S. (2004). High intensity aerobic interval exercise is superior to moderate intensity exercise for increasing aerobic capacity in patients with coronary artery disease. *European Journal of Preventive Cardiology*, *11*, 216–222. https://doi.org/10.1097/01.hjr.0000131677.96762.0c

Russell, A., Heneghan, C., & Venkatraman, S. (2019). Investigation of an estimate of daily resting heart rate using a consumer wearable device. *Medrxiv*, *19008771*. https://doi.org/10.1101/19008771

Sarganas, G., Rosario, A., & Neuhauser, H. (2017). Resting heart rate percentiles and associated factors in children and adolescents. *The Journal of Pediatrics*, *187*, 174–181. https://doi.org/10.1016/j.jpeds.2017.05.021

Setty, P., Padmanabha, B. V., & Doddamani, B. R. (2013). Correlation between obesity and cardio respiratory fitness. *International Journal of Medical Science and Public Health*, *2*(2), 300–304. http://doi.org/10.5455/ijmsph.2013.2.298-302

She, J., Nakamura, H., Makino, K., Ohyama, Y., & Hashimoto, H. (2015). Selection of suitable maximum-heart-rate formulas for use with Karvonen formula to calculate exercise intensity. *International Journal of Automation and Computing*, *12*, 62–69. https://doi.org/10.1007/s11633-014-0824-3

Sieljacks, P., Thams, L., Nellemann, B., Larsen, M. S., Vissing, K., & Christensen, B. (2016). Comparative effects of aerobic training and erythropoietin on oxygen uptake in untrained humans. *Journal of Strength and Conditioning Research*, *30*(8), 2307–2317. https://doi.org/10.1519/JSC.0000000000001314

Smith, T. M. (2016). Physical and psychological effects of a 12-session cancer rehabilitation exercise program. *Number 6/December 2016*, *20*(6), 653–659.

Stahl, S., An, H., Dinkel, D., Noble, J., & Lee, J. (2016). How accurate are the wrist-based heart rate monitors during walking and running activities? Are they accurate enough? *BMJ Open Sport – Exercise Medicine*, *2*. https://doi.org/10.1136/bmjsem-2015-000106

Steier, J., Lunt, A., Hart, N., Polkey, M. I., & Moxham, J. (2014). Observational study of the effect of obesity on lung volumes. *Thorax*, *69*(8), 752–759. https://thorax.bmj.com/content/69/8/752

Stensvold, D., Sandbakk, S. B., Viken, H., Zisko, N., Reitlo, L. S., Nauman, J., Gaustad, S. E., Hassel, E., Moufack, M., Brønstad, E., & Aspvik, N. P. (2017). Cardiorespiratory reference data in older adults: The generation 100 study. *Medicine and Science in Sports and Exercise*, *49*, 2206–2215. https://doi.org/10.1249/MSS.0000000000001343

Tanaka, H., Monahan, K. D., & Seals, D. R. (2001). Age-predicted maximal heart rate revisited. *Journal of the American College of Cardiology*, *37*(1), 153–156. https://doi.org/10.1016/S0735-1097(00)01054-8

Venkat, S., Preejith, S., & Sivaprakasam, M. (2022). Comparative analysis of resting heart rate measurement at multiple instances in a single day. *2022 44th Annual International Conference of the IEEE Engineering in Medicine & Biology Society (EMBC)*, 824–827. https://doi.org/10.1109/EMBC48229.2022.9871825

Verbrugge, F., Guazzi, M., Testani, J., & Borlaug, B. (2020). Altered hemodynamics and end-organ damage in heart failure. *Circulation, 142*, 1012–998. https://doi.org/10.1161/CIRCULATIONAHA.119.045409

Zhang, L. (2022, May). Gamification exploration of military sports training projects based on deep learning. In *International conference on electronic information technology (EIT 2022)* (Vol. 12254, pp. 722–728). SPIE. https://doi.org/10.1117/12.2639426

Zhang, Z. (2015). Photoplethysmography-based heart rate monitoring in physical activities via joint sparse spectrum reconstruction. *IEEE Transactions on Biomedical Engineering, 62*, 1902–1910. https://doi.org/10.1109/TBME.2015.2406332

Zhao, L., Wu, H., Sun, J., Liao, L., Cui, C., Liu, Q., Luo, J., Tang, X., Luo, W., Ma, J., Ye, X., Li, S., & Yang, S. (2019). MicroRNA-124 regulates lactate transportation in the muscle of largemouth bass (Micropterus salmoides) under hypoxia by targeting MCT1. *Aquatic Toxicology, 218*, 105359. https://doi.org/10.1016/j.aquatox.2019.105359

Zisman-Ilani, Y., Fasing, K., Weiner, M., & Rubin, D. J. (2020). Exercise capacity is associated with hospital readmission among patients with diabetes. *BMJ Open Diabetes Research and Care, 8*(1), e001771. https://doi.org/10.1136/bmjdrc-2020-001771

11

MOTOR CONTROL

Nguyen Tra Giang and Oliver Napila Gomez

Through the perspective of kinesthetic fitness, the complex interplay among motor control, physiological well-being, and energy regulation is brought to light in the chapter. It emphasizes the importance of motor control and other kinesthetic functions in health and energy regulation. Balance, aided by proprioceptive feedback and the integration of sensory data for spatial orientation and movement control, is emphasized in the summary as being important in both static and dynamic situations. Moreover, this chapter goes beyond eating right and exercising regularly to improve physiological health. The importance of joint mobility and flexibility in injury prevention and musculoskeletal health is also addressed. Concepts like reaction time, speed control, and agility control are also introduced, which goes on to explore motor control functions for energy regulation. This highlights the importance of controlling speed to complete tasks efficiently rather than just optimum speed, as is the complexity of reaction time in response to environmental stimuli. Sports and everyday life place a premium on agility control, the ability to quickly and precisely change directions while retaining balance and coordination.

Outcomes

By the end of this chapter, you will be able to

- discuss the fundamental principles and mechanisms of motor control, such as the integration of neural, muscular, and sensory systems
- appreciate the importance of motor control in maintaining physiological health, with a particular emphasis on balance and flexibility

DOI: 10.4324/9781003502937-13

- explain how motor control affects energy regulation in physical activities by optimizing energy expenditure through reaction time, speed control, and reactive agility
- apply motor control concepts to sports performance and fitness activities to improve their capacity to excel in a variety of physical undertakings
- consider the everyday significance of motor control, recognizing how increased motor control abilities can positively impact daily activities, safety, and the pursuit of an active lifestyle

Fundamentals of physiological health and energy regulation

Kinesthetics, or motor control, facilitates efficient and effective movement and improves physiological health via physical activity and exercise. As a result, we are introducing the concept of kinesthetic fitness to describe the USFD's motor control functions for health-enhancing performance and movement. The way a person moves is a good indicator of their kinesthetic functions. The musculoskeletal system, responsible for the actual movement, and the nervous system, which includes the visual and vestibular systems and proprioceptive signals, work together (through brain–body coordination) to produce these effects. Furthermore, the regulation of physiological health also depends on motor control. In addition to a balanced diet and regular exercise, a healthy lifestyle that includes regular physical activity also improves health.

Motor control functions for physiological health

Among the motor control tasks linked to physiological health in the USFD Framework is balance, which is necessary for stability in static and dynamic

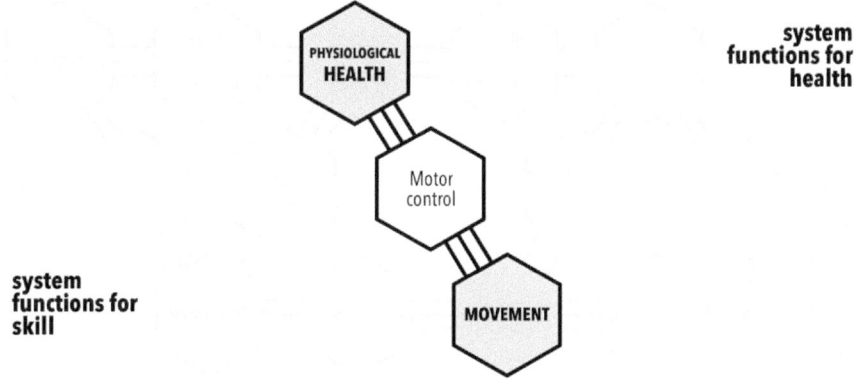

FIGURE 11.1   Motor control – shared by physiological health and energy regulation

conditions. Essential for everyday injury prevention, the vestibular, visual, and proprioceptive systems communicate with the brain to relay information about the body's position and movement. Regular stretching and exercise improve joint health and general physiological wellness, crucial for efficient mobility and musculoskeletal health.

Balance

Maintaining a center of gravity on the ground with the help of one or both feet is a fundamental motor control element in a wide variety of sports (Gong, 2020; Ha et al., 2019). This skill is essential for bringing the body's resistance to external, internal, and gravitational forces down to zero (Tanir, 2018). According to Ha and colleagues (2019), being able to respond to environmental stimuli or move around while maintaining equilibrium is known as dynamic balance. When a person does not move while remaining balanced on a fixed support base, this is called static balance (Gong, 2020; Ha et al., 2019; Tanir, 2018). Since most athletic movements include the ankle–foot complex making contact with the ground, proprioception in the ankles may be crucial for balance control. Athletes achieve complex motor tasks by adjusting their ankle and upper body movements (Han et al., 2015).

Important information regarding the body's position and relationship to its environment is communicated to the brain by the vestibular, visual, and proprioceptive systems. The brain integrates sensory information from various systems

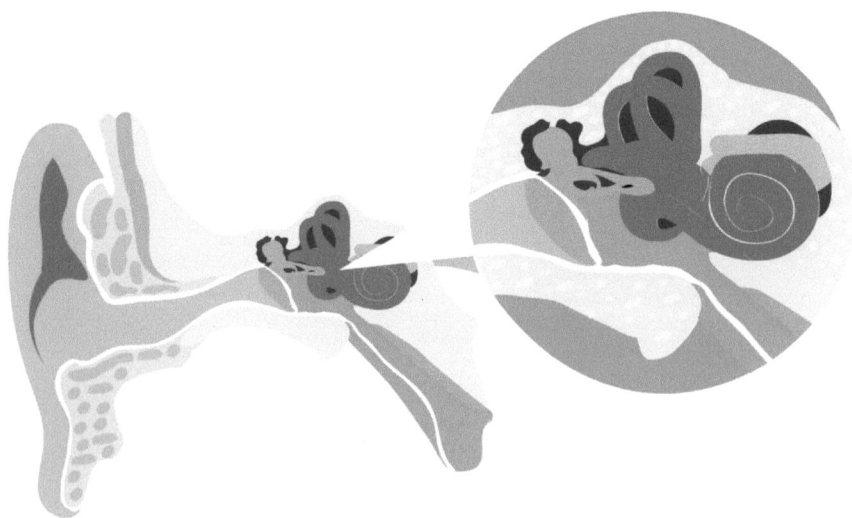

FIGURE 11.2   The vestibular system

to help balance self-awareness, awareness of movement, and perception of space (Khan & Chang, 2013).

Whenever the head moves or changes position, the vestibular system in the inner ear will pick up on it, and help keep balance when doing activities like walking, running, or jumping. Otoliths are tiny crystals that move in reaction to head motions and are contained in the fluid within three semicircular canals that make up the system. The otoliths change position as the head moves, communicating with the brain about its location and motion.

Another essential function of the vestibular system is detecting linear momentum, force, gravity, and leaning motions while the body is in motion. It aids the brain in coordinating movement and maintaining balance by utilizing data from the inner ear and other sensory systems like vision and proprioception. When moving, the vestibular system detects the body's orientation and position based on the direction and speed of movement.

Additionally, it helps keep the head in a neutral position and the body upright so it does not fall. Maintaining equilibrium and coordinating movements would be extremely challenging, if not impossible, without the vestibular system.

In addition, the visual system is responsible for perceiving the surrounding space and the environment's structure.

The visual system's job is to take in data sent by the eyes and make sense of it to depict the world around them. As a result, we can correctly gauge distances

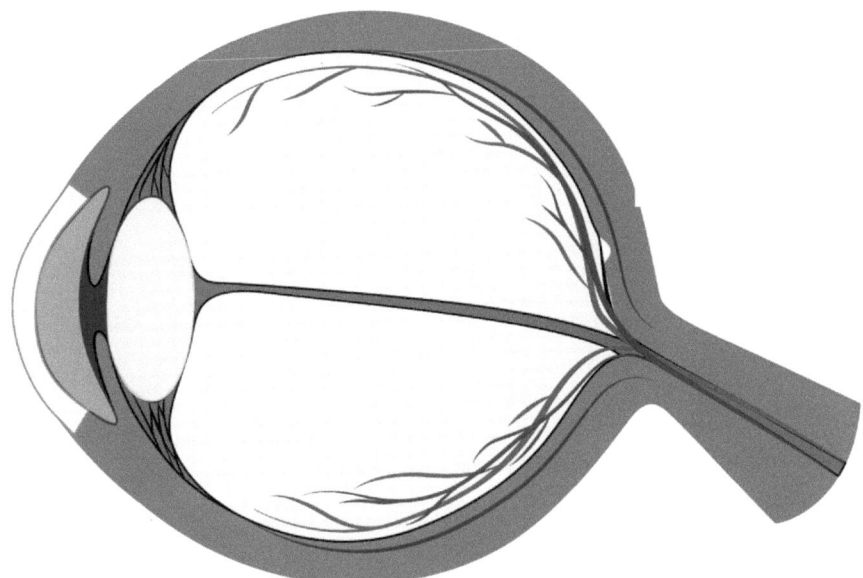

FIGURE 11.3   The visual system

and directions and understand the spatial relationships between various objects. The visual system allows us to recognize familiar places and navigate complicated landscapes. Balance and postural control are also significantly impacted by it, especially in young adults (Gaerlan et al., 2012). The visual system helps the brain keep its balance and prevent falls by providing information about the body's position concerning the environment. Many physically demanding activities, like sports and dancing, rely heavily on the visual system because of the coordination required.

The proprioceptive system also detects the gravitational pull, the weight of an object, and other forces that exert themselves on the musculoskeletal system.

The proprioceptive system detects where various body parts are to one another and how they are moving. This component detects the rate and repetition of the muscle's contract-and-release mechanism and consists of fibers equipped with proprioceptive receptors, including muscle spindles and Golgi tendon organs. When tightening or relaxing the muscles, the Golgi tendon organ detects the tension, whereas the muscle spindle detects the stretch rate. Important for regulating balance and coordination while moving, these proprioceptors pick up on changes in the body's orientation, as well as forces, gravity, and the weight of objects. In weightlifting, for instance, the proprioceptive system detects the barbell's weight, the amount of force needed to lift it, and the body's position, enabling the lifter to make necessary adjustments to their movement and posture to stay balanced and prevent injuries.

A person's visual, vestibular, and proprioceptive systems all collaborate to tell the brain where they are, how they are moving, and how they are oriented in

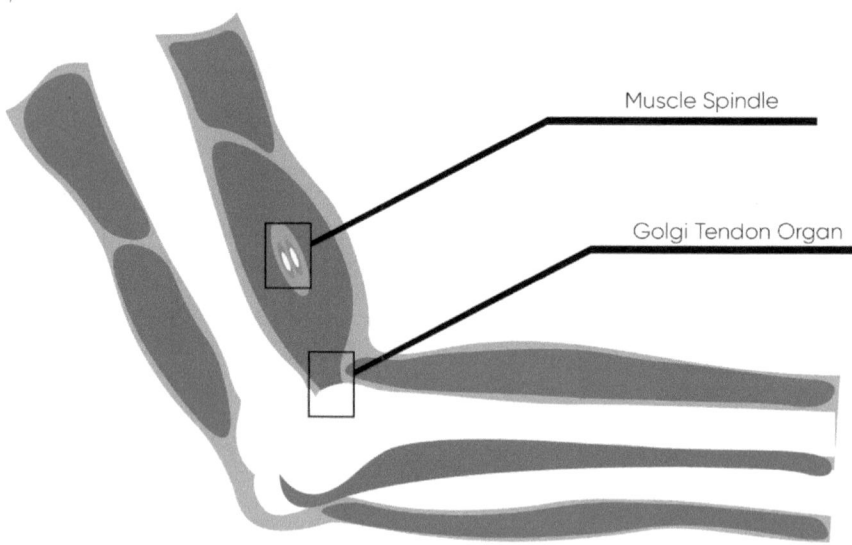

FIGURE 11.4　The proprioceptive system

space. The brain's motor system, which governs and controls the body's movements, reactions, and functions, integrates and processes these sensory inputs. An individual's vestibular system picks up on leaning motions, their visual system on surface structure and obstructions, and their proprioceptive system on ground forces acting on muscles and joints when they walk on an uneven surface. After processing all of this data, the brain instructs the motor system to make necessary adjustments so the body can stay balanced. Balance is crucial for kinesthetic fitness because the sensory and motor systems work together.

Balance and movement

Keeping balance is an automatic reaction that goes unrecognized when a person goes about their daily routine. Still, it is noticeable when people do things like dancing or artistic gymnastics, walk along a narrow path, or stand on one leg. The nervous system's capacity to maintain body position in response to environmental objects and forces is known as balance. This includes locomotor balance, which allows the body to move around, and manipulative balance, which allows the use of implements. Other aspects of fitness, like the ability to control speed, agility, and reaction time, are shown by deliberate responses of the nervous system.

Non-locomotor movements and balance

Static balance, also known as non-locomotor balance, requires coordinated activation of the vestibular, visual, and proprioceptive systems to keep the body in proper alignment while in motion.

During non-locomotor movements, the visual system is vital for tracking stationary and moving objects in the environment and determining how far away stationary objects are, impacting the body's stability. The proprioceptive system, in contrast, allows the body to adapt to stay balanced by providing information

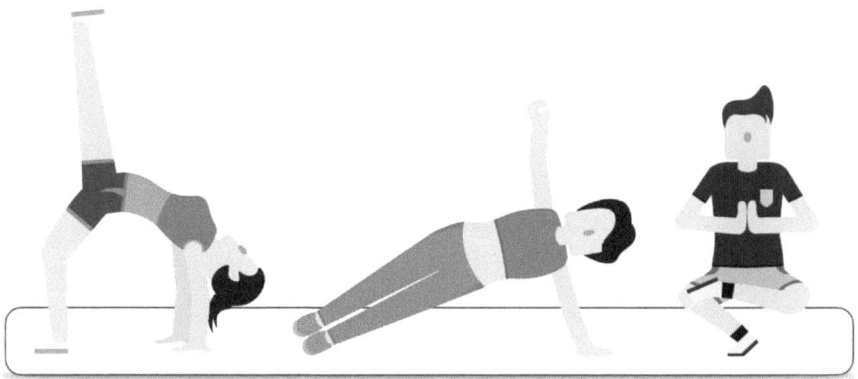

FIGURE 11.5   Balance with non-locomotor movements

about its position, motions, force, gravity, and the weight of things. When we are not moving around, our vestibular system helps us stay upright by sensing forces, gravity, linear momentum, and leaning motions. Maintaining equilibrium while engaging in exercises like yoga requires precisely regulating these systems.

Balance with locomotor movements

Balance with locomotor movements is the ability to stay upright while moving from one location to another in a predetermined area using the limbs. The senses are crucial in helping the body determine the optimal location for the upcoming movements. The visual system determines direction and distance from the body, while the musculoskeletal system perceives the ground's texture. The vestibular sense is responsible for tracking the body's motion when traveling. To keep from falling or hurting oneself, the neurological system modifies motions. Since this kind of balance requires stability even when moving, we call it dynamic balance.

The vault event in artistic gymnastics is an excellent illustration of dynamic balance. The gymnast runs, hops onto the springboard, vaults onto the apparatus, twists, turns, and lands cleanly on the landing mat without using any steps or hops.

Balance with manipulative movements

Several aspects of physical fitness work together to provide a person's manipulative balance. For example, deft hand–eye coordination and mental acuity are

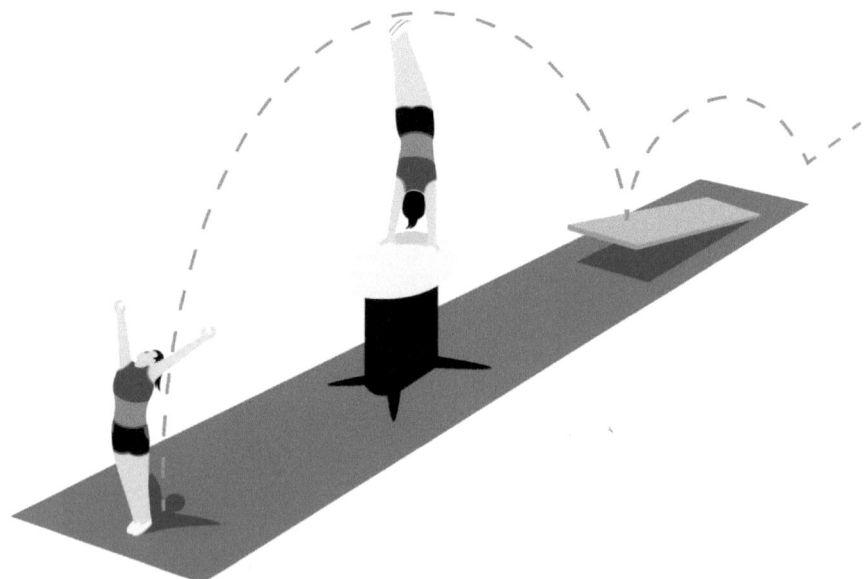

FIGURE 11.6   Balance with locomotor movements

required when juggling balls. While the arms and hands are busy catching and throwing the balls, the eyes keep an eye on their whereabouts. The deft manipulation of the balls also requires precise control over the speed and forces the corresponding muscles to apply in the hands and arms.

To top it all off, the proprioception in the hands and arms tells the brain where the balls are and how they move, aiding balance. In a similar vein, constant readjusting of body position in order to stay balanced while riding a bike or skateboard is required. The lower extremities direct the bike's or skateboard's motion, while the upper body provides stability and balance.

In order to manipulate and control the implementation efficiently while maintaining balance, it is necessary to have high levels of coordination and adjustability across multiple fitness components.

Factors that affect balance

Good balance is essential for most daily tasks, whether sitting, standing, walking, or running. However, the capacity to keep equilibrium can be impacted by many things. Biomechanical concepts like center of gravity and base of support play a role in maintaining equilibrium (Kot & Nawrocka, 2014, 2016).

Where the weight of the body is most uniformly distributed is called its center of gravity (Shoeb et al., 2020). Body instability and the ease of falling occur when the center of gravity is outside the support base. For instance, it becomes challenging to keep balance when the center of gravity moves to support a heavy load on one side of the body.

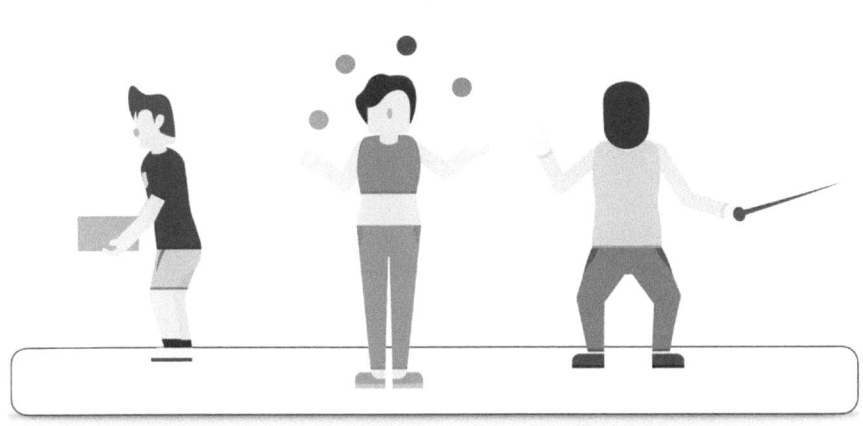

a. Maintaining constant contact with the object

FIGURE 11.7a   Balance with manipulative movements

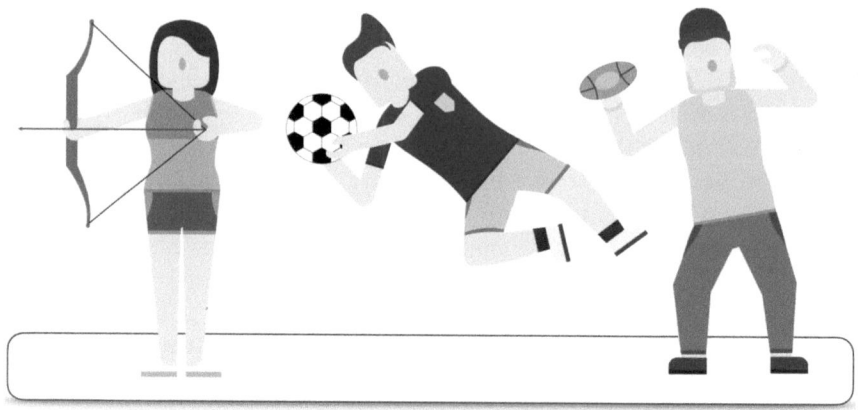

b. Balance while sending or receiving objects

FIGURE 11.7b   Balance with manipulative movements

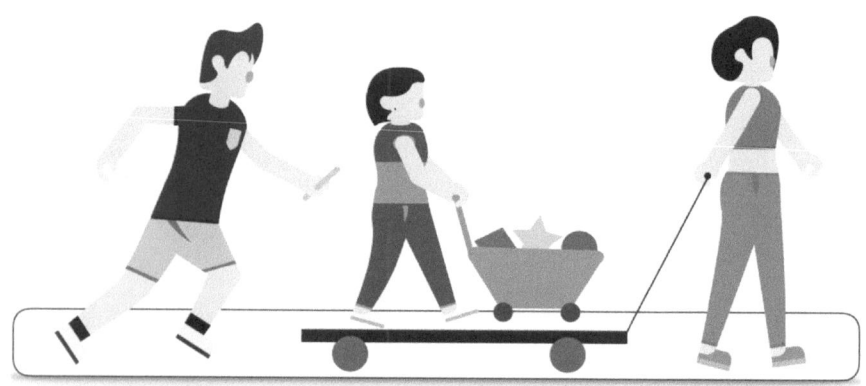

c. Balance while traveling along with the object

FIGURE 11.7c   Balance with manipulative movements

Additionally, when standing, the base of support is the area that includes all the points where the feet contact the supporting surface (Yiou et al., 2017). The ground contact area is the space between the body and the ground, typically the area between the feet (Fernandez & Wada, 2019). Because it controls how stable the body is in the face of outside forces, it plays an essential role in preserving balance. Solid stability and a lower center of gravity result from a broader support base. Standing with feet wide apart instead of close together exemplifies this principle. The former offers a steady foundation, which improves stability and balance.

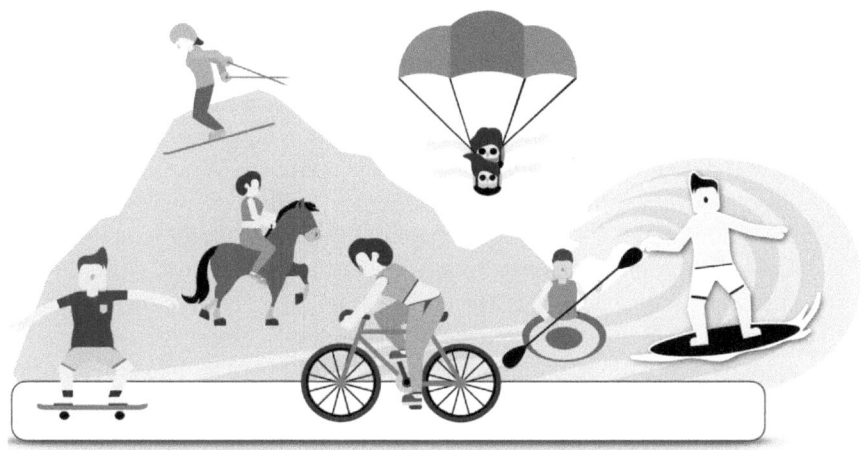

d. Balance while operating or doing tricks with objects capable of transport

FIGURE 11.7d   Balance with manipulative movements

Also, a person's balance can be thrown off if there are issues with the vestibular, visual, or proprioceptive systems (Shirai et al., 2022). For example, problems with the vestibular system in the inner ear, such as ear infections, can affect the ability to maintain balance. Similarly, vertigo, headaches, and trouble keeping balance can be symptoms of a visual impairment. All of the body's sensory organs, including the vestibular system, are affected by aging, which can cause issues with balance.

The neurological system and brain, which act as the body's primary balance regulators, are another vital component. Dizziness and trouble keeping balance can be symptoms of injuries like concussions, brain trauma, and other similar conditions. The vestibular system and other sensory organs that tell the brain where the body is and how it is moving are also vulnerable to damage from these types of injuries (Peterson & Greenwald, 2015; Valovich McLeod & Hale, 2015; Kleffelgaard et al., 2019; Wallace & Lifshitz, 2016).

Finally, musculoskeletal disorders like arthritis and gout can impair balance and mobility by causing pain in the joints, tendons, and muscles of the lower extremities. Medication side effects, low blood pressure, anemia, and the effects of antidepressants, antihistamines, painkillers, and sleeping pills are among medical issues that can impair balance. These drugs have the potential to impair the central nervous system's control of balance, which can cause vertigo and make it hard to stay upright.

Flexibility

Joint flexibility is essential for the health and fitness of adults of all ages (Suga et al., 2021). Increased joint flexibility and reduced injury rates are two potential health benefits of strengthening and stretching exercises (Wiederman, 2018). Assessing muscular strength can help with some health issues, including sarcopenia, functional impairments, frailty, and cardiometabolic risk (Hsu et al., 2021). Conversely, functional impairment and injury to muscles, bones, and joints result from a lack of flexibility (Ibrahim et al., 2018). Osteomuscular and neuromuscular diseases are associated with decreased flexibility and endurance. Muscular power was also formerly considered a component of health-related fitness due to its associations with health (Corbin & Le Masurier, 2014).

The extent to which a joint can move is called its range of motion (ROM). As shown in Figure 11.8, the sample illustration shows that the knee has a potential range of motion from 0 to 141 degrees. With this, the ROM of the knee can fully extend to 0 and flex to 141 degrees.

The knee is just one of many skeletal joint structures that allow the body to move around. Different types of joint structures should broaden the definition of the range of motion (e.g., hinge, pivot, ball-and-socket, ellipsoid, saddle, and

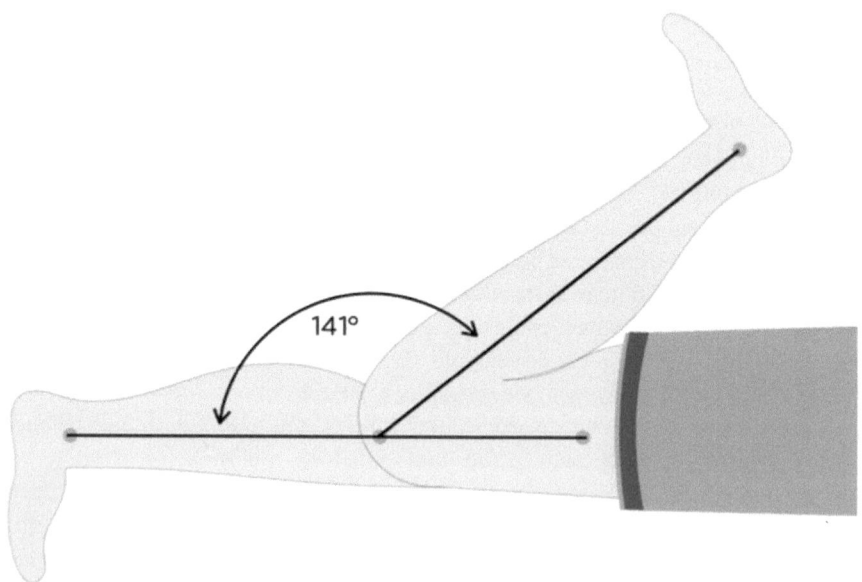

FIGURE 11.8   Range of motion

gliding joints). In this chapter, we will only cover the two main types of joints – the hinge and the ball-and-socket joint – that allow the body to move in its most fundamental ways.

Range of motion in the hinge joints

Joints that allow for flexion and extension, like the knees and elbows, have a limited range of motion. Muscles generate force, which is transmitted to the insertion. A flexed joint is the result of muscle contraction and bone pulling. To create motion, primary muscle tissues pair off in an antagonistic fashion. A contracting muscle tissue, known as the agonist, collaborates with a relaxing and extending muscle tissue, known as the antagonist (Rana et al., 2015).

More than that, the brain controls the relaxation and contraction of flexion and extension muscles, so it is no surprise that the brain is involved in flexibility coordination (Cunningham et al., 2013). Consequently, motor control is thought of as involving flexibility. For hinge joints like the knees and elbows to allow a full range of motion and coordinated motions, the brain ensures the correct muscles work in antagonistic pairs.

Figure 11.9 shows examples of the antagonistic muscle pairs that work to produce flexion-extension movement – the actions that comprise a typical range of motion in the joints.

Range of motion in the ball-and-socket joints

The two most common types of ball-and-socket joints in the human body are the hip and shoulder joints. They allow the limbs to move in a variety of ways, including flexion, extension, abduction, adduction, circumduction, medial rotation, and lateral rotation, as well as bringing the limbs toward and away from the body's midsection (turning away from the midsection of the body) (Yang et al., 2022).

The term *flexibility* describes the extent to which a person's joints can move, from completely extended (as a result of contracting the extensor muscles) to completely flexed (as a result of contracting the flexor muscles) (Hirata et al., 2021). Full abduction, adduction, and circumduction range of motion are all part of a ball-and-socket joint's range of motion regarding flexibility (Moromizato et al., 2016). Flexibility is the ability to increase or decrease the range of motion by adjusting the angle of a joint (Vandervoort & Stathokostas, 2016). On the flip side, not all current flexibility tests capture the entire extended to flexed range of motion (Keogh et al., 2019). As an alternative, they emphasize stretching and reaching to increase the joints' and muscles' suppleness, elasticity, and extensibility (Franchini & Herrera-Valenzuela, 2021).

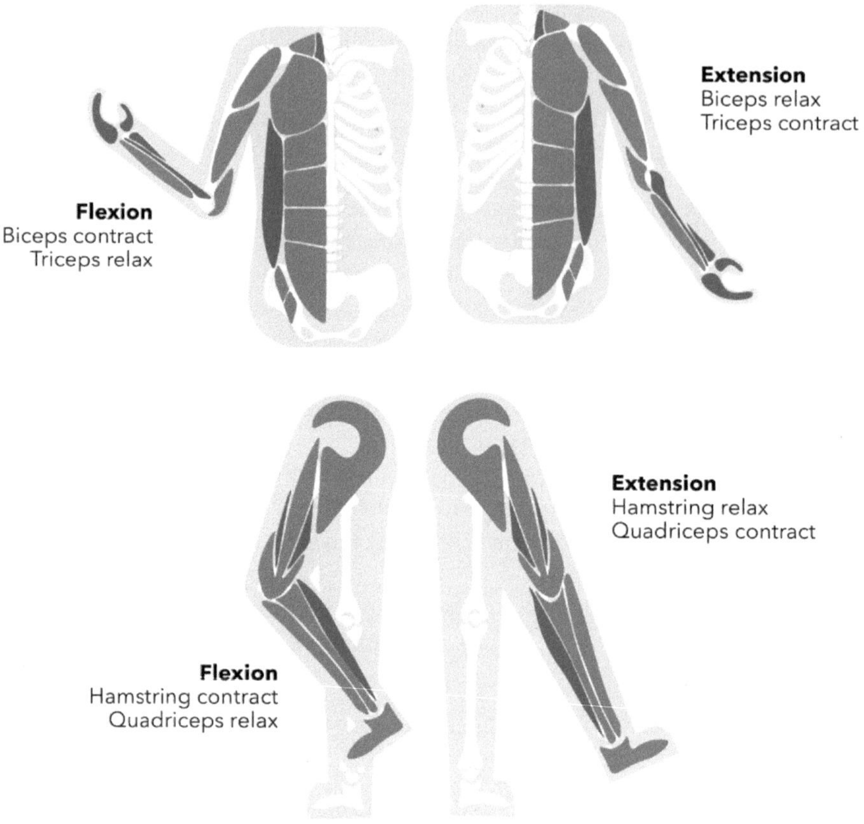

FIGURE 11.9 The antagonistic pairs

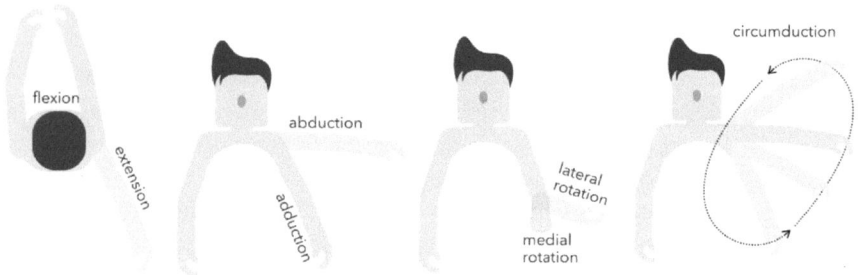

FIGURE 11.10 Movements of the shoulders

What affects flexibility?

The efficiency of movements is affected by the range of motion available in the joint structures. Limitations in flexibility can be caused by the structure of the joints as well as the pliability and malleability of the connective tissues (tendons and ligaments), muscles, and skin surrounding the joints. A thin layer of connective tissues known as fasciae covers and bundles the muscles, nerve fibers, blood vessels, bones, and numerous other organs. Separate from the muscles beneath it, fascia is a clearly defined fibrous covering that encases and connects a bundle of muscles (Fede et al., 2018). Fasciae that are in good health are smooth and affect flexibility. Fasciae can wrinkle and become gluey due to inactivity, exhaustion, or injury, leading to painful and stiff muscles (Knapp, 2016; Wu et al., 2015).

As people age, their body's natural capacity to keep their muscles flexible and mobile declines, because the fibrous tissue that anchors them loosens (Milanović et al., 2013). Furthermore, due to differences in the anatomy of the bones and joints, women generally exhibit greater flexibility and range of motion than men of the same age. Muscle bulge during contraction may limit full flexion, which could limit the range of motion for men. Even women with a lot of muscle mass might feel limited in their movements.

Motor control functions for energy regulation

According to Sreemathi and Murugavel (2017), there are two types of speed – internal speed, which refers to the rate of nerve impulses (reaction time), and external speed, which refers to the velocity of limb movement. The USFD Framework considers these two parts separate but interrelated functions. Moreover, we added the third type of speed related to the space around the body and the environment – agility control. Hence, in the USFD Framework, motor control functions for energy regulation include reaction time, speed control, and agility control.

Figure 11.11 showcases the types of motor control functions for energy regulation. Reaction time is the type of motor control that occurs in the brain in response to stimuli perceived by the receptors – vision, proprioception, and other senses. Speed control is the motor control that occurs externally and is manifested by the musculoskeletal system. Speed control regulates the quality of movement of the body. Lastly, agility control relates to speed control according to the space around the body and the environment. Agility control has the reaction time and speed control aspects as well.

Reaction time

One way to quantify how quickly an organism reacts to an external stimulus is by looking at its reaction time (RT) (Shan et al., 2022). It is the amount of time that elapses between the onset of a stimulus and the subsequent behavioral response, and it is used to describe the amount of time it takes for a person to finish a physical action (Rakpongsiri, 2018). (Daulatabad et al., 2013).

The emergency reaction time, which measures the time it takes for a driver to respond between a risky situation and an emergency operation, has been the subject of multiple studies that have focused on reaction time while driving (Guo

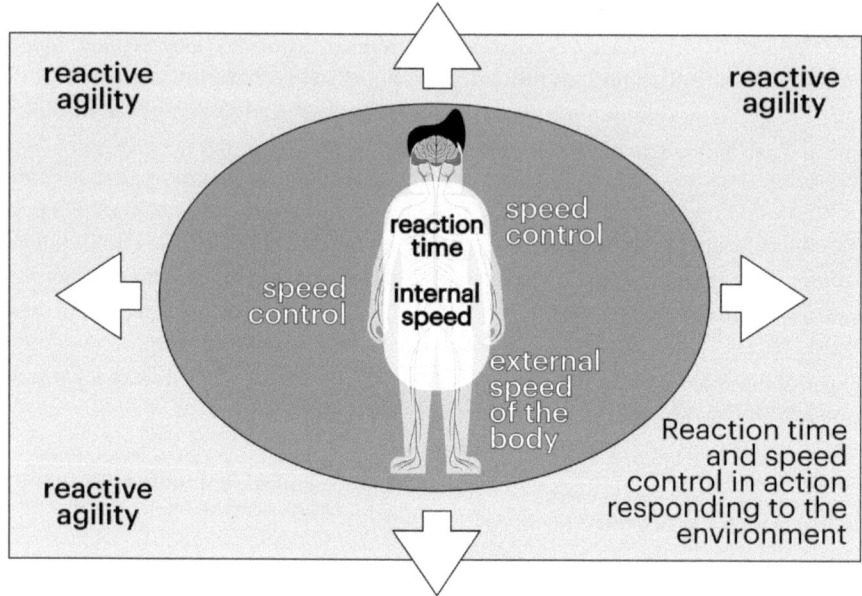

FIGURE 11.11   The motor control functions for energy regulation

et al., 2019; Li et al., 2019; Samani et al., 2022). In order to measure how long it takes for a driver to take over, reaction time is essential. When driving safely, the driver's reaction time (DRT) is paramount (Xing et al., 2015).

Through the use of the senses, the brain responds to its stimuli. The senses of sight, sound, and touch are all considered external stimuli by the brain. The brain can react automatically or voluntarily to data from an outside source. A reflex is an automatic, nonconscious reaction that initiates independently (CK-12 Foundation, 2014). In order to protect the body from potentially dangerous outside stimuli, the brain triggers a series of reflex actions.

Any genuinely voluntary behavior involves some degree of self-awareness, planning, and decision-making. Reaction time is the time it takes for an individual to react voluntarily after being presented with an external stimulus. The time required for a voluntary movement to take place is shown in Figure 11.12.

Types of reaction time

Possible reactions might vary from one to two or more options. Various reaction times are based on the number of available choices and the decisions' accuracy.

1. ***Simple reaction time.*** Simple reaction time occurs when the external stimulus and the situation call for a quick and uncomplicated response (Trueman et al.,

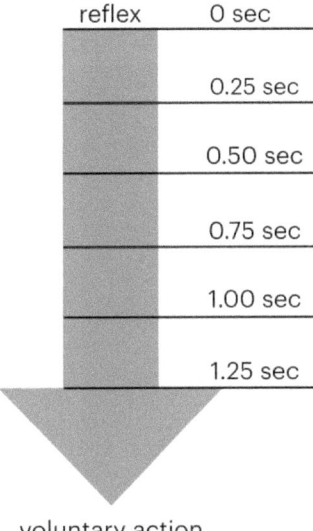

FIGURE 11.12   Reaction time – the time it takes for a voluntary action to occur as a response to an external stimulus

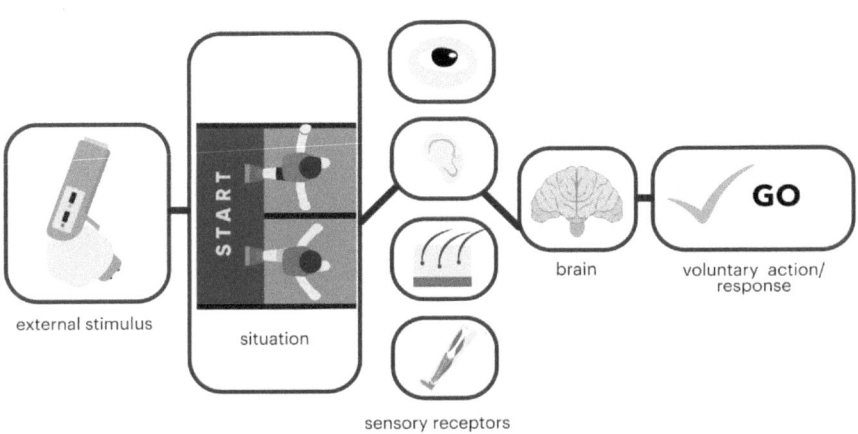

FIGURE 11.13   Simple reaction time model using sprint start as an example

2012; Woods et al., 2015). Shortly after the start gun goes off, an activity (such as swimming or sprinting) occurs in a racing sport. Notice that the only acceptable reaction is to begin swimming, running, or racing. A sprint start is used to illustrate a model for simple reaction time in Figure 11.13.

2. ***Recognition reaction time or go/no-go.*** If the situation and external stimulus call for one correct decision from two response choices, this is called *choice*

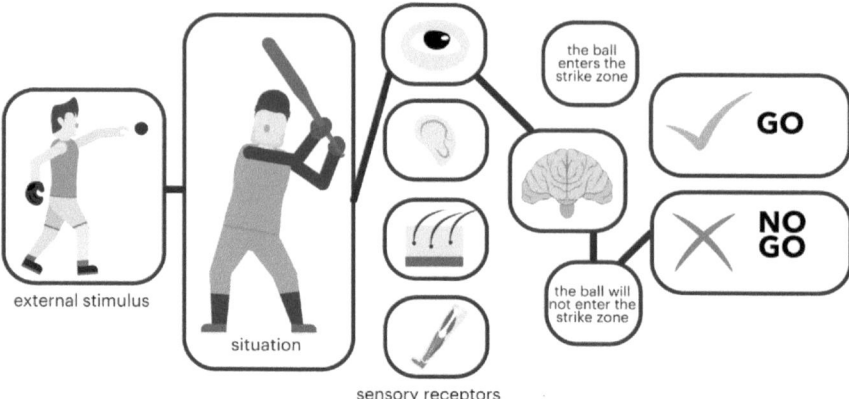

FIGURE 11.14   Go/no-go two-choice reaction time model using baseball batting as an example

reaction time (Trueman et al., 2012; American Psychology Association, 2020). For example, a baseball batter has two response choices to a pitched ball. The batter can either (a) swing the bat after the pitcher releases the ball or (b) hold the position. The correct decision of the batter will depend on the visual cue, i.e., (i) to swing when the ball enters the strike zone or (ii) to hold the position when the ball does otherwise. For this example, the two response choices prompt the batter to go (swing) or not to go (hold). Hence, specialists also call this the *go/no-go* or *recognition reaction time*.

3. ***Choice reaction time.*** Choice reaction time involves decision-making over several external stimuli and corresponding response choices. It is possible to have more than two external stimuli and correct choices associated with them. A classic example is an offensive player who received a basketball during a game. Defensive players are external stimuli aiming to gain possession of the ball and prevent an offensive player from executing a successful shot. The offensive player has several response choices depending on the action of the defensive players: (a) to stay in place and safeguard the ball for a moment, (b) to pass the ball to an open teammate, (c) to take the risk and shoot, (d) to charge against the defending player, or (e) to infiltrate the defense to get under the basket.

Reaction time only works with external stimuli, such as signals or cues the senses perceive. It does not involve internal stimuli, called enteroception, which include hunger, thirst, urge to relieve oneself, awareness of the rate of breathing and heartbeat, feeling the temperature, and internal pain. The brain can recognize enteroceptions that are beneficial for survival. For example, the brain will initiate

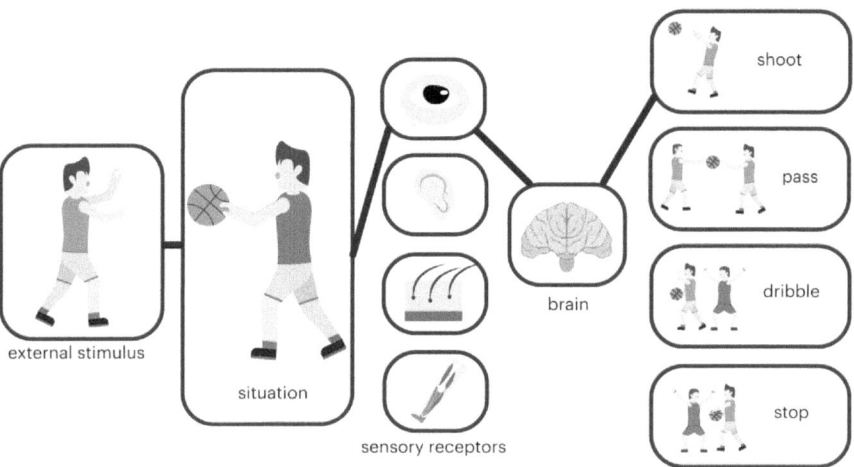

FIGURE 11.15   Multiple choice reaction time model using basketball offense as an
example

thought processes to motivate a person to prepare meals when hungry. Although
in this situation the body has response choices, which include (a) to go hungry or
(b) to grab something to eat, they do not qualify as reaction time.

What affects reaction time?

The amount of time it takes to react to a stimulus is known as reaction time, and
it is a crucial metric in neuroscience and psychology. Multiple factors impact
reaction time. To begin, reaction time can be affected by the stimulus's complexity and the number of response options. A slower reaction time might result from
a few options or complicated stimuli.

Furthermore, as the body gets accustomed to stimuli, processing times for
those stimuli decrease. Also, as people get older, their reaction times become
slower. Males react faster than females, another factor influencing reaction time
(Jain et al., 2015). The stimulus type also influences reaction time; aural stimuli
are processed more quickly than visual ones (Ghuntla et al., 2014).

Additionally, whether a person is right- or left-handed, the dominant hemisphere of the brain is faster at responding than the nondominant hemisphere
(Takeda et al., 2010). Another thing that slows people down is needing more
sleep than usual (Bonnet & Arand, 2003). Finally, a slowed reaction time may
be the outcome of alcohol intoxication, which alters stimulus-response processing. Research studies that evaluate cognitive processes and response times must
comprehend the numerous elements impacting reaction time.

Speed control

A person's *speed* can be defined as their capacity to complete an action within a given time frame. However, let us focus on the definition of fitness that emphasizes optimum speed. For example, according to Mănescu (2017), the essence of athletic speed is the capacity to achieve and sustain a maximal rate of movement while reducing the effects of exhaustion, friction, and air resistance. Elite athletes' maximum peak speed is about 4.5 to 6 seconds (Mohamed & Larion, 2018).

The common understanding of speed in physical fitness is summed up in the adage "the faster, the better," which does not necessarily apply to non-racing sports. In physical fitness, "optimal speed" might mean the fastest possible movements, as if that were the only determinant of performance success. For example, in physical education classes, students take speed tests as part of an extensive fitness evaluation.

In the USFD Framework, the emphasis should instead be on regulating speed. This means that the speed requirement of the task must be the basis of the speed performance – not optimum speed alone. Our perspective is different; we see speed through the motor control for energy regulation lens, emphasizing the control of how fast or slow the movement should go.

Kinesthetic fitness relies heavily on speed control, which stresses the significance of regulating energy expenditure by altering movement speed in response to task demands. While optimum speed is essential for specific sports like sprinting, other sports emphasize maintaining speed and mastering the precision of movement flow. For example, gymnasts rely on control and precision as much as speed to execute their routines properly.

Moreover, in actual life, there is usually no need to rush through tasks. A combination of speed and control is necessary for the efficient and effective completion of many tasks. To avoid making any mistakes, a surgeon doing a delicate operation, for instance, needs complete control and accuracy in their hand and finger movements. In the same way, a chef needs to be precise and controlled when making food so that it stays consistently tasty.

Regulating speed in response to demand is critical to achievement in various contexts, not limited to athletics. Since this aspect of kinesthetic fitness emphasizes control and precision rather than speed, the name "speed control" is appropriate. It also stresses improving the control system's adaptability to meet varying speed demands. In Figure 11.16, the need to regulate speed varies across tasks.

Optimum speed does not apply to all tasks. This is only true when a person wants to cover a certain distance quickly and must use speed and power in a sprint. However, tai chi is best practiced at a slow and controlled pace. Tai chi is a form of martial art that focuses on slow, continuous movements to promote health on all levels (physical, mental, and balance). Smooth and even movement is critical to tai chi, which emphasizes maintaining balance and control.

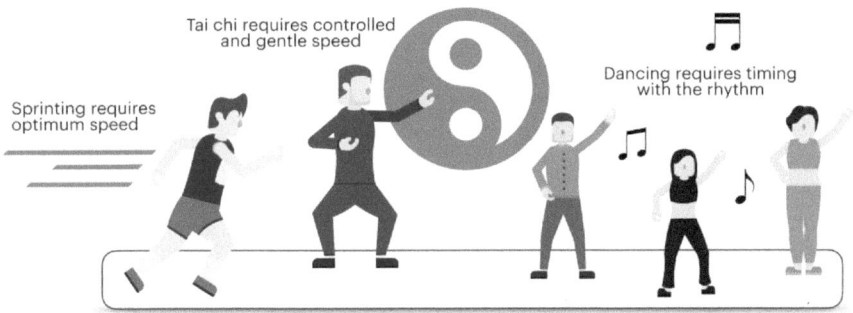

Tai chi requires controlled and gentle speed

Dancing requires timing with the rhythm

Sprinting requires optimum speed

FIGURE 11.16   The speed requirement of the task determines speed control

Meanwhile, dancing calls for precise timing that mirrors the beat and velocity of the music. Depending on the dance style and the individual steps, the tempo of a dance can change. It must be strange to watch tai chi masters execute the martial arts in rapid succession. The same holds for dancers whose timing deviates too much from the beat of the music; it becomes excruciatingly painful to watch.

In each of these activities, speed control is essential for optimal performance. Finding the right balance between speed and control is critical in sprinting to maintain proper form and prevent injuries. For example, tai chi emphasizes the importance of moving slowly and steadily to allow the body to engage in the movements fully and effectively. Meanwhile, speed control is necessary for dancing to execute steps accurately, maintain proper posture and balance, and stay in rhythm with the music.

Based on our observation, we developed a two-dimensional matrix, classifying various activities' speed and control requirements, as shown in Figure 11.17. The vertical axis, which goes from *uncontrolled* to *controlled*, describes how much a person regulates force and energy as they perform their task. Plotting the activity's speed along the horizontal axis from *slow* to *fast* is also meaningful because it shows the pace of the movement.

In Figure 11.17, yoga and tai chi are *slow-controlled speeds* in the top-left quadrant. Football and tennis are dynamic sports that fall under the top-right quadrant and have *fast-controlled speed* because they demand controlled force and rapid motion. Meanwhile, household tasks and gardening are examples of everyday activities that fall into the bottom-left quadrant, *slow-uncontrolled speed*, because they require less control of force and energy and move slower. Activities involving rapid motion and uncontrolled force or energy, such as skydiving and sprinting, fall into the *fast-uncontrolled speed* category in the lower right quadrant. They are fast-uncontrolled in that the speed must be the fastest, as in the running sprints, or it is beyond the performer's control, like roller-coaster rides.

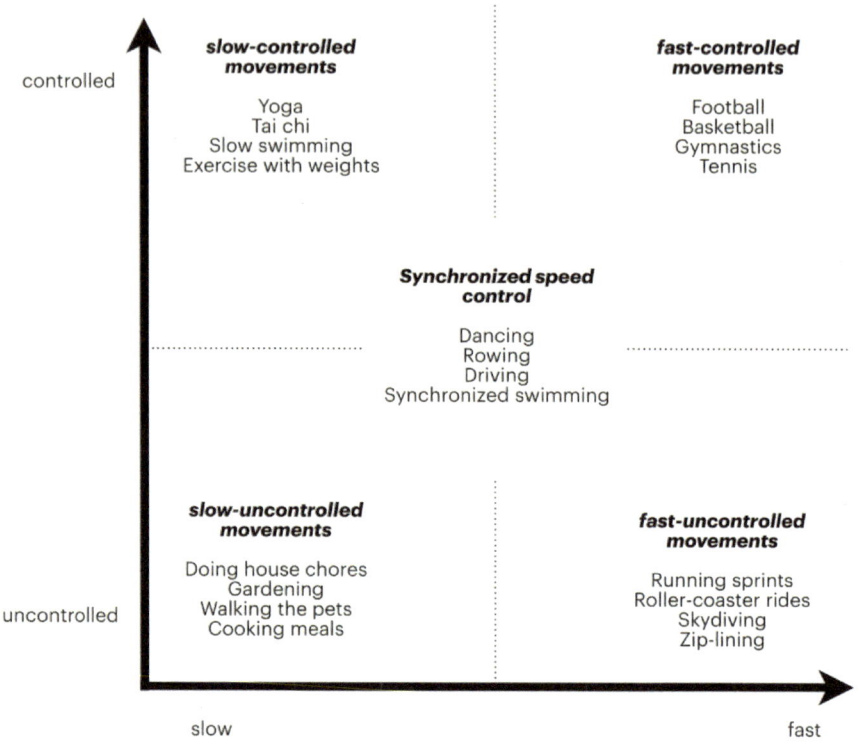

FIGURE 11.17 Two-dimensional matrix categorizing activities based on speed and control level

Synchronized speed control occupies the middle of the matrix. It indicates rhythmic control over speed in activities such as rowing and dancing, which lie on uncontrolled and controlled spectrums. This means that the energy and timing of the movements are synchronized with the timing requirement of the task.

This two-dimensional matrix is helpful for training, rehabilitation, and fitness planning because it helps to understand and categorize activities according to the required control and speed.

Sprinting – speed or power?

The physics definition of speed can be applied to any fast or slow movement and is not necessarily associated with sports or fitness. In contrast, the contemporary fitness definition of speed focuses on the ability of an individual to move as fast as possible, particularly in sports that require sprinting and racing. However, it is essential to note that the ability to move quickly is only sometimes the most critical factor in completing a task or achieving a goal.

Regarding traveling speed, the distance covered and the time taken to cover that distance are essential factors. The formula for speed involves the distance traveled divided by the time taken to travel that distance:

$$speed = \frac{distance}{time}$$

However, this is a different case among humans because the involvement of force generated by muscular contraction and the body's mass also contribute to the rate at which velocity changes. Acceleration, which is the speeding up of an object's velocity, is dependent on the amount of force applied through muscular contraction and the mass of the object:

$$acceleration = \frac{force}{mass}$$

In the fitness context, speed should be emphasized, although optimal speed is only sometimes the most critical factor in completing a task. It is essential to focus on increasing energy output, which can increase power and acceleration, resulting in optimal speed.

Speed control and movements

Establishing a connection between the ability to control speed and physical movements is crucial. Among these motions are locomotor, non-locomotor, and manipulative ones. The capacity to control speed is fundamental for the efficient and effective completion of any given task, regardless of how fast or slow an individual must move.

Non-locomotor movements and speed control

Slow, non-locomotor motions are ideal for yoga and tai chi because of the controlled and sustained nature of the movements. While tai chi's elegant, leisurely motions necessitate balance and coordination, yoga poses are held for lengthy periods and transitioned into the next with slow, deliberate movements. Among the many potential benefits of slow, non-locomotor movements in rehabilitation are improvements in mobility, reduced pain, and enhanced body awareness.

Additionally, dancers frequently use non-locomotor movements to convey their feelings and thoughts. This performance exemplifies the value of control, balance, and rhythm through its painstaking execution. The slow, graceful movements of ballet, for instance, suggest fluidity and elegance; in modern dance, on the other hand, they elicit powerful emotions and create tension.

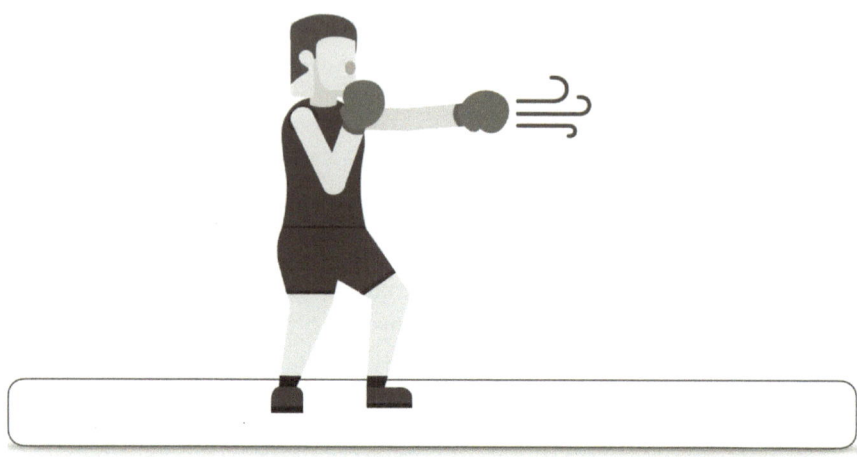

FIGURE 11.18   Quick movement of the arms when punching is essential in boxing

Finally, specific athletic pursuits call for non-locomotor skills. The development of self-awareness, the improvement of balance and coordination, and the expression of emotions through dance all depend on controlled, slow motions. Speed control is fundamental for all movements because the control system adapts the tempo of non-locomotor movements to the task's demands.

Figure 11.18 shows one method of controlling speed in boxing: non-locomotor movements. These are the quick movements of the punching arms. The boxer's arms remain stiff as he delivers a punch. This movement requires kinesthetic fitness, specifically the capacity to control speed precisely. Effective boxing punching requires controlling the speed and trajectory of a blow. Boxing punches and other non-locomotor movements necessitate control of speed.

Locomotor movements and speed control

Locomotor speed is the standard for measuring speed as the body moves from one location to another through locomotor movements. Starting at point A and ending at point B, the test-taker must cover a certain distance. Once the test-taker reaches point B, the time is recorded. Because the task demands maximum speed, test-takers typically sprint. This is seen in sprinting events like the 100-meter, 200-meter, and 400-meter dashes.

Sprinting is not the only locomotor movement that relies on the legs for propulsion. Running, hopping, skipping, leaping, sliding, and galloping are all part of them. The arms can also execute handstand walking, climb ropes or monkey bars, and cartwheel as a means of locomotion. Crawling and climbing on walls or rocks involves using both arms and legs as a locomotor.

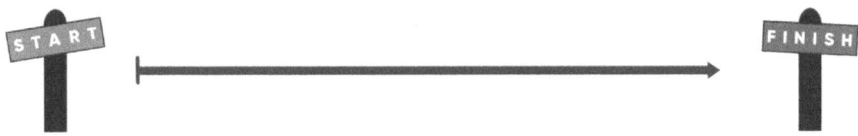

FIGURE 11.19   Speed with locomotor movements

The capacity of the central nervous system to manage the various aspects of coordination necessary to carry out a task involving locomotor speed with efficiency and effectiveness is reflected in locomotor speed control. As previously stated, speed tasks can be rhythmic, optimal, or slow and controlled.

Manipulative movements and speed control

Speed control is integral to kinesthetic fitness when handling objects. Manipulating the object at the required speed is part of the task. In sports like tennis, for instance, a player's serve significantly impacts the final score. Playing it too slowly, the ball might not cross the court; if it is too fast, it could go out of bounds.

The size, shape, and weight of the object being controlled also affect the controllability of speed. These factors affect the object's speed and the force required to move it. Furthermore, speed control can be influenced by the grip and technique employed to manipulate the object. To maintain command of the ball's velocity and course, a baseball pitcher, for instance, must employ the correct grip and throwing technique.

Moving the body in specific ways also impacts the ability to control the speed at which a person manipulates objects. For example, a thrower's body position and movements determine the speed at which the frisbee is released. They can throw the frisbee faster if they wind up and let go the right way. Modifying posture and motions allows for a quicker throw.

The following are instances when the body controls its speed while doing manipulative movements:

Speed control without the object leaving the body. The ability to change the pace of manipulative movement without moving from one location to another is reflected in stationary manipulative speed control (see Figure 11.20). The ability to control speed while stationary and manipulative is essential for basketball players to perform a variety of tricks and maneuvers. Static dribbling drills are joint among basketball players, in which the player remains stationary but changes the ball's speed and direction. The athlete must maintain control of the ball's trajectory and velocity while maintaining a stationary footing.

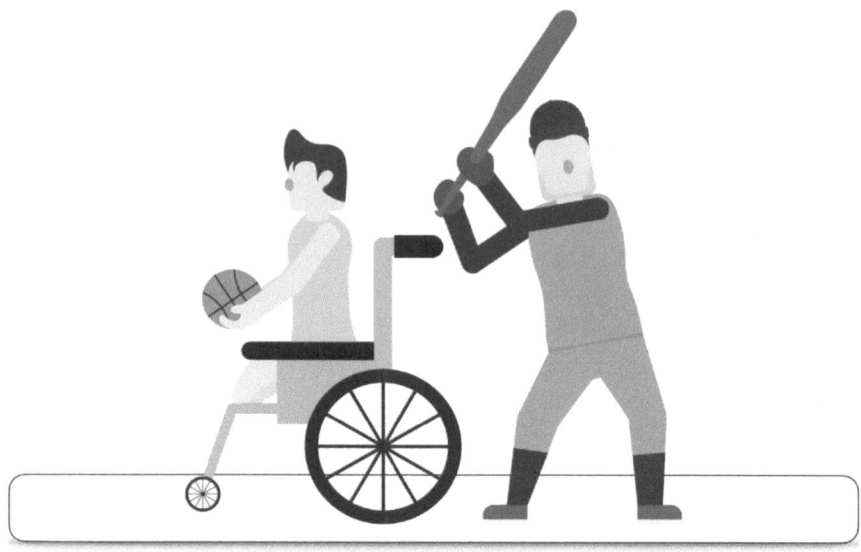

FIGURE 11.20   Speed control without the object leaving the body

Like baseball, manipulating speed at stationary positions is critical for making powerful swings. A batter needs to adjust the speed of their swing to reach the target distance, while a pitcher needs to adjust the force of the pitch to suit their swing. Controlling the speed and timing of the swing while maintaining footing is an absolute must in both sports.

Speed control in propelling objects/implements. In sports involving throwing or propelling an object toward a target, controlling the speed of an object is an essential component (see Figure 11.21). The speed of the implement thrown is defined by the force acting upon it. Hence, one of the most essential skills for these kinds of sports is the ability to regulate the force put on an object.

Take football throw-ins as an example. When a player throws the ball to a teammate, they must regulate the force applied to it. The applied force defines the velocity with which the ball approaches the receiver. Applying excessive force might cause the ball to miss the target or become difficult to catch. Adding extra force might cause the ball to remain inside the goal and be intercepted by the other side.

The same holds in softball and javelin; the speed with which the object approaches the target is determined by the force applied to it. To be precise and accurate in these sports, an individual must control the force used on the object.

Moreover, the object's trajectory toward the target is influenced by some variables, including the force regulation, the release point, the angle of the arm, and the body's position. Athletes can learn to control their force and other performance variables through training and proper technique.

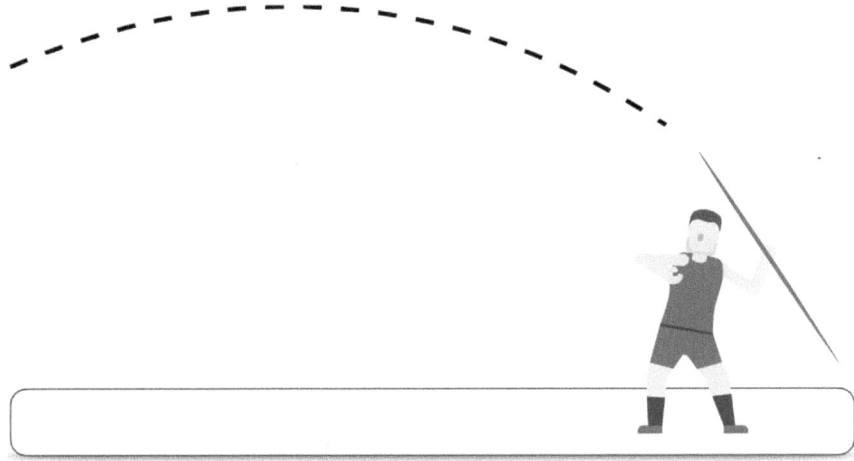

FIGURE 11.21   Speed control in propelling object

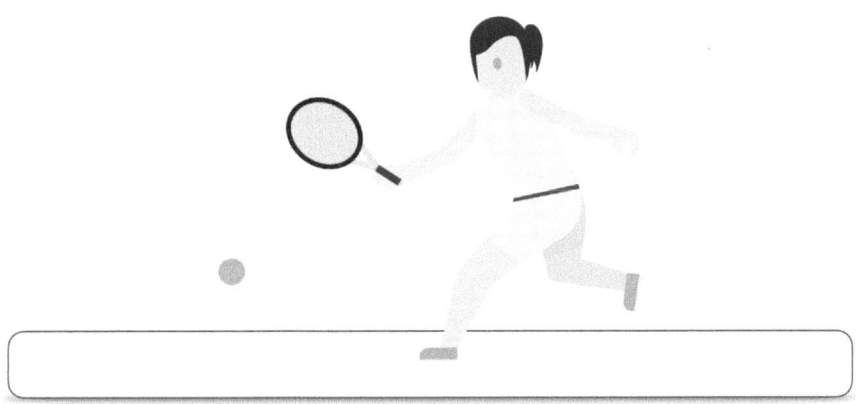

FIGURE 11.22   Speed control in traveling with implements

Speed control in traveling with implements. This is of utmost importance in sports where the implements need management while the player moves. For instance, when playing basketball, players must keep their dribble speed controlled, whether walking or running. They need to exert additional force to maintain the correct height and pace of the ball's bounce as their speed increases. Athletes in tennis face a similar challenge: changing their pace and direction of motion to keep up with the ball and then manipulating its speed and trajectory with the tennis racquet as they smash it back to their opponent.

Controlling locomotion speed with implements is also necessary to, for example, catch and throw baseballs or softballs. If an athlete wants to catch a fly ball, they need to be able to predict its speed and trajectory and adjust their running speed accordingly. The same holds for passing the ball to a teammate; the athlete must precisely control the trajectory and velocity of the throw to ensure it reaches its intended recipient.

The athlete's awareness of their body position and the movement of the implement is crucial for regulating their traveling speed with implements. Maintaining proper posture and control of the implement requires the ability to alter speed and movement. The ability to sense the body's relative position and motion in space, known as proprioception, and integrating visual and motor systems are also required.

Skill and coordination are prerequisites for controlling the speed of travel-along manipulative movements, an essential component of numerous sports. Attaining success in the sport requires fine-tuning the speed and direction of the implement through force adjustment, coordinating the body's movement with the implement, and maintaining proper body position and control.

Speed control in operating a transport implement. It is up to the driver or operator to determine the optimal speed for their transport implement (vehicle) considering the road conditions and other factors when controlling the speed of a mode of transportation. In response to the surface and the resistance, a cyclist, for example, can adjust their pedaling effort to gain speed. Similarly, skateboarders gauge their speed by repeatedly kicking off the floor. By contrast, a skilled kayaker can steer their craft in any direction by balancing and coordinating their strokes with the paddles.

Notably, these situations also call for the driver to have excellent coordination and balance to keep the vehicle under control and avoid obstacles. The ability to set and maintain the vehicle's speed depends on muscular strength, posture, and stamina.

What affects speed control?

Speed control can be affected by multiple factors. The body's mass, extensions, stability, coordination, gravity, and the surface where the movement occurs are all factors in this context.

The body can estimate the force needed to move itself or a limb quickly or put it into action in a specific location or distance. On the other hand, those with stocky frames are more likely to need impressive force development than those with lean frames. All of the body's weight and all of its extensions are affected by this. According to research, male 100km ultramarathoners whose body mass decreased ran faster (Rüst et al., 2012). Based on the results, it seems that a lighter body can move faster with less effort.

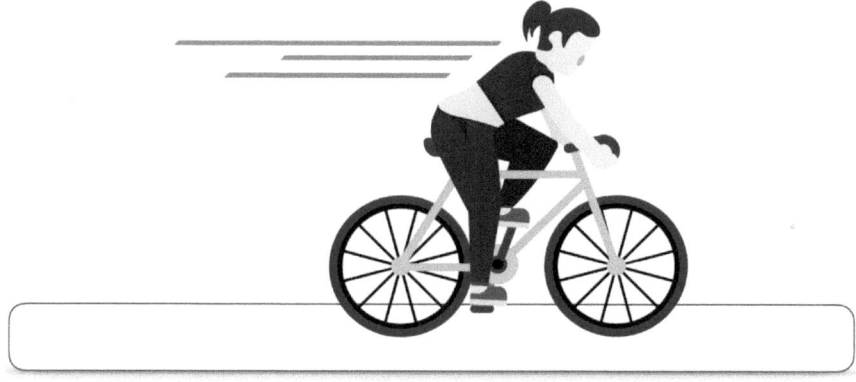

FIGURE 11.23   Speed control in operating a transport implement

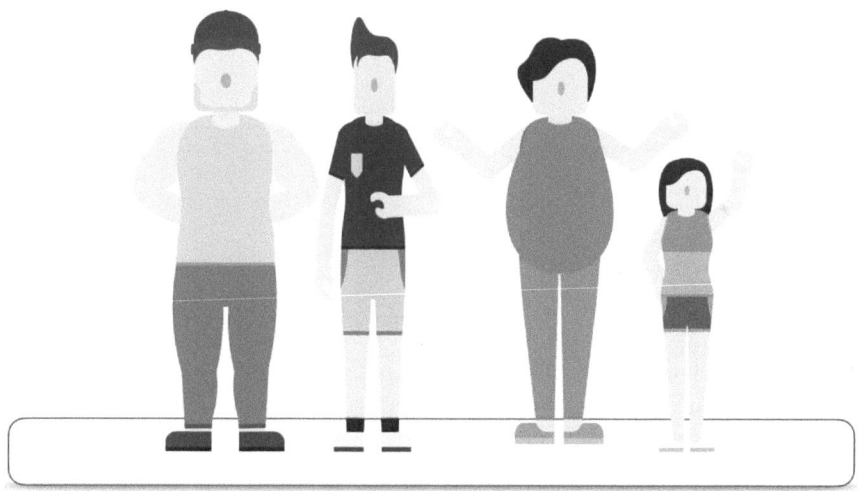

FIGURE 11.24   Body mass, body parts, or extensions affect speed indirectly

Controlling speed relies heavily on balance, a crucial fitness function for health under motor control. However, unsteadiness, drowsiness, and muscle and joint pain can reduce balance. Various factors, such as medical issues, medication, or injury, can impact the systems that interact with the nervous system, leading to this condition. The capacity to control speed is diminished when balance and stability are compromised.

Additionally, speed is linked to coordination, the kinesthetic fitness factor that governs the coordinated sensory and motor activities of various body parts,

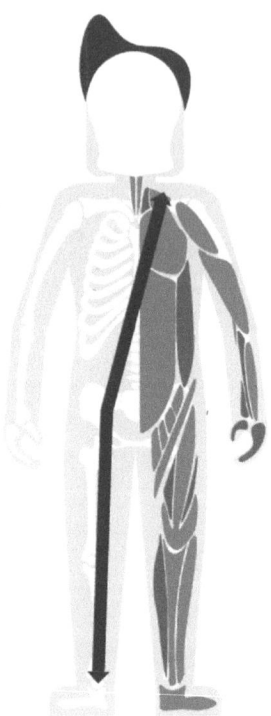

FIGURE 11.25   The kinetic chain

including the limbs, to generate effective motions. In locomotor activities like walking and running, for instance, the legs are supported by the arms swinging. The coordination of the limbs is affected by kinetic chains, which are networks of linked body segments that facilitate mechanical energy transfers between their constituent parts (Latash & Zatsiorsky, 2015). Using kinetic chains influences the pace of walking and running. Because of this, sprinters work on more than just their legs. To maximize their running speed, they also train their core and arms to ensure their legs perfectly coordinate with the rest of the running apparatus.

Moreover, there might be differences in the floor's or ground's slope. Two examples are the steepness of a hill at 30 degrees or the angle of a climbing wall at 90 degrees. As a result of the interaction between gravity and the body's mass, climbing uphill or vertically requires more energy than going downhill, depending on the angle of the activity area. Alterations to the slope also impact gait and balance. Researchers found that the kinetics of the ankle, knee, and hip joints were altered by sloping surfaces (Willwacher et al., 2013).

Finally, the type of floor or activity area affects speed control for safety. Different types of floors can be identified by proprioception (sand, concrete, rubberized floor, slippery floor, etc.). In order to stay safe, the body has to adapt the speed at

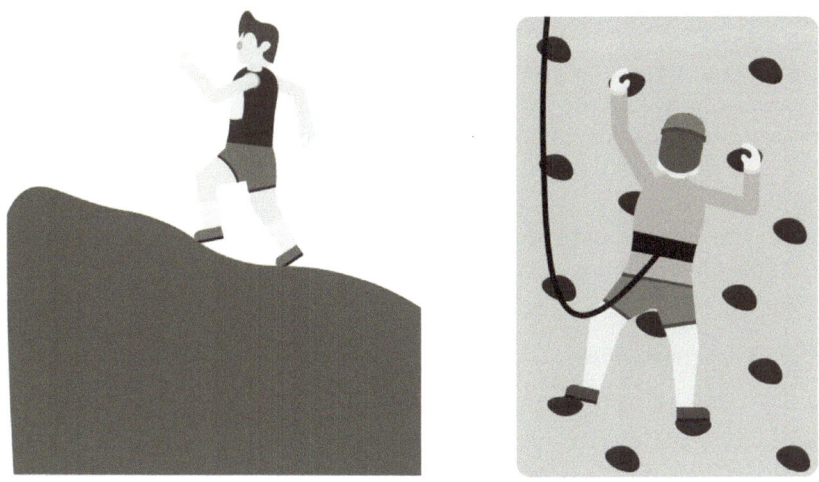

FIGURE 11.26   Uneven, inclined, and upright slopes affect speed

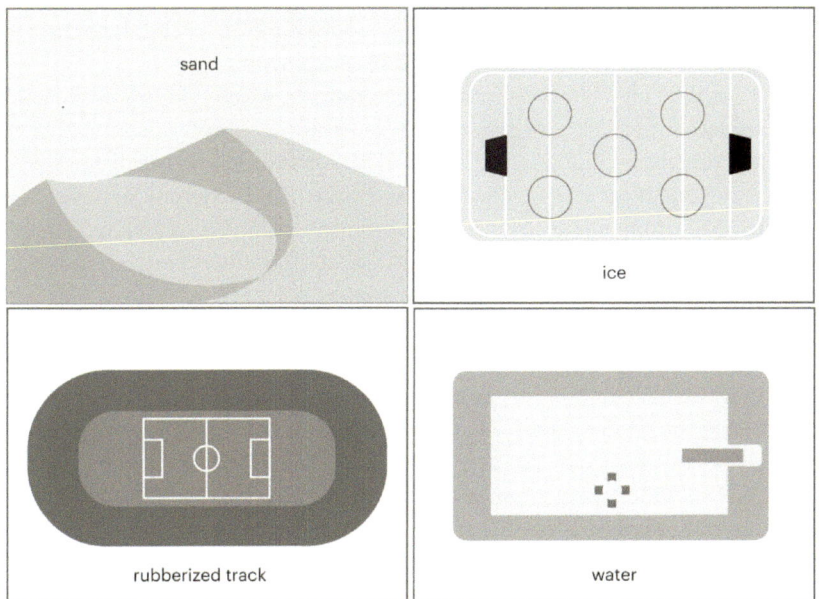

FIGURE 11.27   Different types of surfaces affect the speed of movement

which it moves with the type of surface of the activity area. Moreover, the body can also move around in water. One way to propel through the water is by swimming, a unique form of locomotor movement performed in the water. The speed of a body is affected by hydrodynamics, which is the force acting on it.

Agility

At this point, we will introduce our thoughts on agility, which may differ from the usual definition and how people put it into practice. As a motor control function for energy regulation, agility requires the regulation of force and energy to execute movements. More so, reaction time and speed control are inherent in agility (as illustrated in Figure 11.11). By this, we mean that agility features reactive and speed control aspects. Hence, we are emphasizing reactive agility and agility control in this section.

Active vs reactive agility

Playing a variety of sports like football, basketball, hockey, and swimming requires a certain level of agility, which is defined as the capacity to swiftly change directions while retaining balance and coordination (Saini, 2017; Bloemen et al., 2017; Alia et al., 2019). Agility generally refers to the ability to execute various motor tasks swiftly and precisely in a manner unique to a particular sport (Alia et al., 2019).

The layman's understanding of agility is active agility – the deliberate and conscious execution of change of direction and position movements and does not need stimuli. This is observed in sports training, where players purposefully and deliberately perform drills to improve control in speed, locomotor movements, and direction-changing skills. It is also observed in sports activities where a change of direction is part of the game without an external stimulus – for example, performing a tumble turn in swimming to complete a lap and changing direction in base running in baseball and cricket after a booming bat. Similarly, rhythmic activities like dance performances do not need stimuli to perform a swift change of direction and position as this is planned and deliberate according to the performers' choreography.

From the USFD perspective, agility relates reaction time to the space around the body and the environment. Reactive agility, a critical factor in many sports, especially soccer, has been extensively studied to determine its reliability, validity, and role in athlete performance differentiation. Rebelo (2022) evaluated two reactive agility drills and found the arrow reactive agility test (ARAT) a reliable and valid measure of lower limb reactive agility in elite male volleyball players. Despite their lower reliability, reactive agility tests are more sport specific than nonreactive tests (Tajik et al., 2022).

Moreover, Pojskić and colleagues (2018) validated soccer-specific reactive agility tests, confirming their effectiveness in assessing junior players' performance. Sinkovic and colleagues (2022) created tennis-specific reactive agility tests, proving their reliability and validity in evaluating tennis players. Coh and colleagues (2018) also examined reactive agility skills' independence and stressed the need to assess and train them separately despite shared movement patterns. These studies confirm that reactive agility has been a concept in sports performance for a while now, and there is a need for customized assessments and training to improve athlete performance.

From the studies mentioned previously, the true nature of agility in a sports context is an expanded form of reaction time in that the playing environment has various unpredictable stimuli. For example, in football, stimuli may include the teammates, the ball, the goal, and the opponent's tactics. These stimuli cannot be ignored in the game as they dictate how the football player should move around the playing area, shaping reactive agility. The ability to quickly adapt to changing game situations is crucial, and the eyes, which house 70% of the body's motor function receptors, play a crucial role in this (Hassan et al., 2022).

Agility control

Success in agility may not be defined by "the more agile, the better" – just as it is with speed. Agility is an expanded form of reaction time that requires speed control. A person perceives, reacts, and controls movement to navigate through space. For instance, an office worker knows tables, chairs, and furniture arrangements in an office setting. They are also aware of the walls, doors, and windows. Note that in this context, the stimuli are fixed and stationary. By perceiving the arrangement and design of the office, an office worker can plan and control the movement around the office efficiently. However, if it is the first day of work, the office worker may need some time to get used to the space where they work.

In contrast, the layman's operational definition of agility is optimal agility, meaning that performance success depends on the capacity to shift position and direction swiftly. This is exemplified in the results of agility tests administered in PE classes. To align agility with the fundamental goal of physical fitness, the focus should instead be on agility control.

Agility control is the ability to swiftly and precisely change directions while retaining balance, the expanded version of speed control relating to the environment. Interventions to improve balance can profoundly affect agility, demonstrating the correlation between the two (Dolan, 2013). It is essential for numerous sports and activities dealing with multidirectional movement through space. The vestibular and proprioceptive senses send signals to the brain to regulate the pace of the body's movement relative to the space and multiple directions needed to accomplish the task.

Moreover, being able to control agility helps a person to respond appropriately to various situations in everyday life, which helps avoid injuries. When crossing the street, someone with excellent agility control can swiftly change their gait to sidestep people and other obstacles. In addition, practicing agility control is a way to avoid crashing into other people in a crowded area.

Football and basketball are examples of territory invasion sports requiring players to swiftly change direction and body position to outmaneuver opponents in complex environments. Athletes in these sports can swiftly change directions, make cuts to get an edge, and evade opponents thanks to their agility control. Control over agility is also crucial in gymnastics, dance, and martial arts, among other activities that demand rapid changes of direction and movement. Participating in these pursuits calls for mobility that can adapt to new circumstances or demands.

Movement and agility

Like other fitness aspects, reactive agility and agility control depend on the type of activity and movement. Anyone can hone their abilities to the next level by training their reactive agility and agility control to match particular motions and tasks.

Non-locomotor movements and agility

The capacity to swiftly and efficiently change levels and directions while retaining balance and stability is agility in non-locomotor movements. This skill is crucial for everyday tasks, like picking up an object from the floor, twisting the body to reach an object, and doing household chores.

Good control over non-locomotor movements can prevent injury for older adults, enabling safe and efficient movements while doing daily tasks. One way to lessen the likelihood of injury is for an older person to regulate rapid changes in direction or level.

Furthermore, many athletic and physical pursuits, including gymnastics and dance, require the ability to control agility with non-locomotor movements. Athletes in gymnastics can execute intricate body movements and transitions

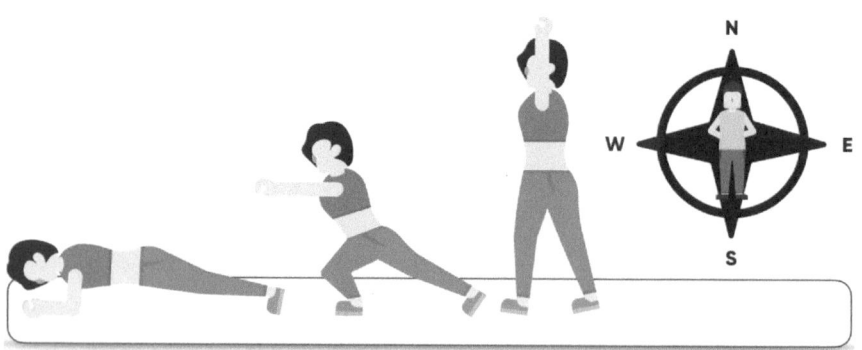

FIGURE 11.28   Change of body position and change of direction

between positions quickly and efficiently because they have agility control with non-locomotor movements. Dancing requires precise and accurate execution of complex footwork and body movements, which requires agility control with non-locomotor movements.

Locomotor movements and agility

Speed in locomotor movements is given by the formula traveling time divided by distance. The arrangement necessitates two locations (A and B) along a horizontal line. The rate of locomotor movement is stated as velocity if the direction is known, such as north. However, agility in locomotor movements is based on multiple directions and pathways; not all are straight lines. Some of these pathways are shown in Figure 11.29.

In addition, linear momentum is the product of a body's mass (kilograms) and speed from A to B. Motion causes a mass to gain momentum (O'Leary, 2011) when moving linearly. A moving body only alters its direction of motion by applying force within a specific time interval to counteract its linear momentum as a reaction to a stimulus (reactive agility). Any force that can induce a change in direction is called an impulse. Hence, being agile means reacting to a stimulus and controlling the impulse during the change of direction of the locomotor momentum, i.e., from point B to point C.

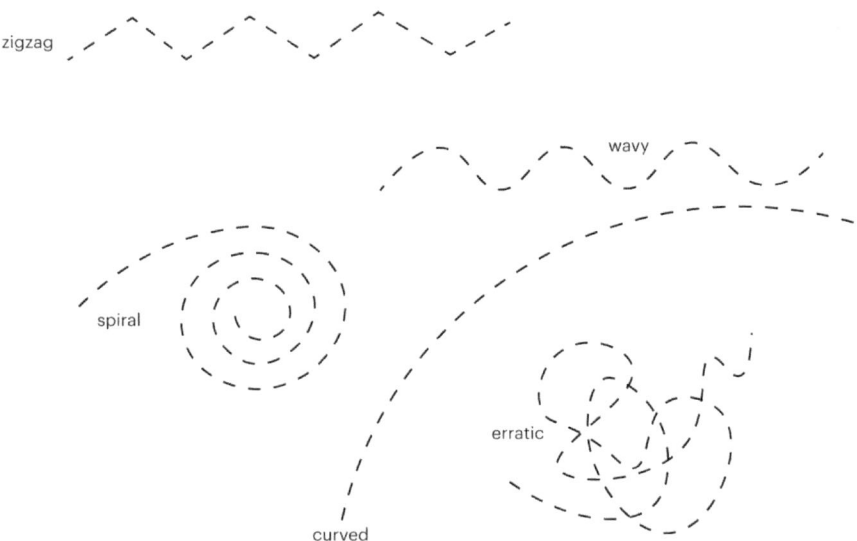

FIGURE 11.29   Pathways for agility control in locomotor movements

Momentum is calculated using the formula:

momentum = velocity × mass

Impulse is calculated using the formula:

impulse = force × time

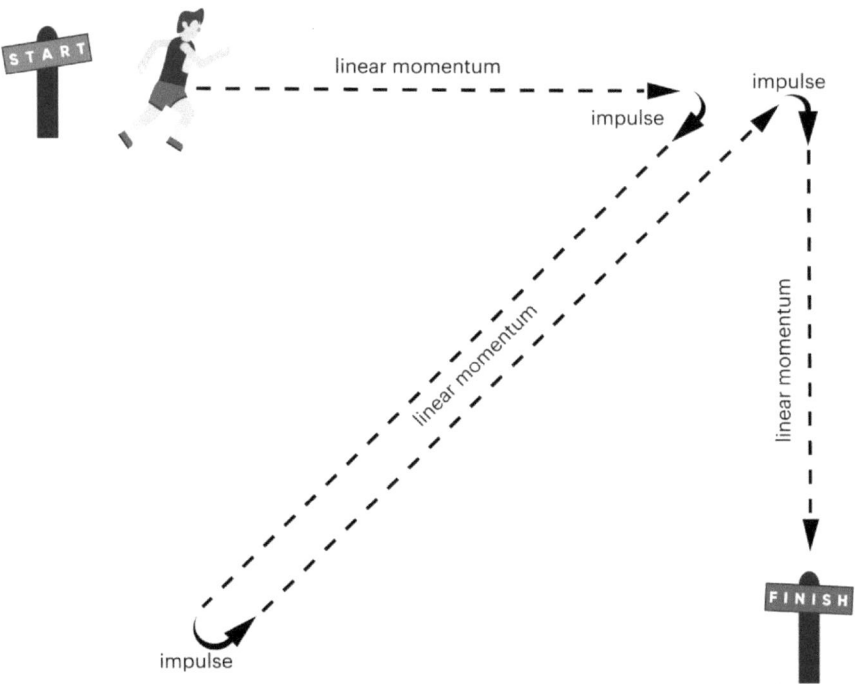

FIGURE 11.30   Linear momentum and impulse in locomotor movements

We still need to learn more about the biomechanical principles that control agility, although it is an essential component of many sports and physical activities. The function of momentum and impulse in determining control of agility is an area that needs further research. Regarding agility control, impulse and momentum affect the pace of changing directions or coming to a complete stop. However, additional studies are required to fully comprehend the function of impulse and momentum in agility control, especially in manipulative and non-locomotor motions.

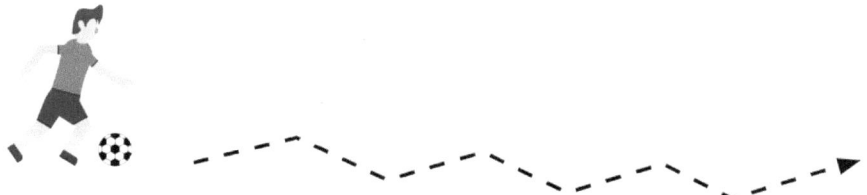

FIGURE 11.31   Traveling along a zigzag pathway

Manipulative movements and agility

Activities involving manipulative agility, like dribbling a football or playing ice hockey, necessitate not only deft control over the object but also the capacity to use reactive agility and agility control while in motion. Furthermore, impulses must be swift and controlled while holding or manipulating an implement. Manipulative movements rely heavily on agility control, necessitating perfect coordination between the manipulator and the object.

Combining locomotor and object control skills is required to travel along a zigzag pathway while using implements. A person must use an implement, like a racket or a bat, to guide an object along a route that twists and turns multiple times. In order to successfully traverse the route, the performer must not only keep the object under control but also react to external stimuli and control their speed and direction. This sounds like complicated coordination work for the brain. Controlling agility in manipulative movements requires various abilities, including spatial awareness, perceptual-motor coordination, and balance. Athletes in sports like cricket, tennis, and baseball frequently use agility control in manipulative movements because of the complexity of the fields they must navigate while holding an implement.

Factors that affect agility

Many factors affect agility, including neuromuscular coordination, mental processes, power and strength of the muscles, body type, shoes, and contact with surfaces. Reactive agility relies heavily on neuromuscular coordination (Zwierko et al., 2022) because it varies with gender and age and can be enhanced by genetics and structured athletic training. Age and gender significantly predict visual-motor performance in reactive agility, emphasizing the beneficial effects of peripheral vision on agility tests (Popowczak et al., 2020).

Moreover, Domenico and colleagues (2022) highlighted the correlation between quick strength and agility and the significance of explosive power. Agility and reactive agility in sports, particularly basketball, can be influenced by anthropometric factors like height, weight, and body fat percentage (Pehar et al., 2018).

Finally, both footwear and playing surfaces influence reactive agility (Latorre et al., 2020). They emphasized the importance of dealing with footwear and playing surfaces for maximizing sports performance outcomes. Taken together, these results highlight the fact that agility is multifaceted and that many factors influence how it manifests and how well it performs in athletic contexts.

Motor control and task performance

Balance is integral to motor control in both stationary and moving situations. The significance of maintaining a steady equilibrium in decreasing the body's resistance to external, internal, and gravitational forces has been emphasized in research (Gong, 2020; Ha et al., 2019; Tanir, 2018). The importance of proprioception and the integration of sensory information for balance maintenance is highlighted by these studies.

Moreover, ankle and upper body movement adjustments are examples of athletes using their proprioceptive sensors to accomplish complex motor tasks (Han et al., 2015). Integrating vestibular, visual, and proprioceptive sensory signals is fundamental for movement control and spatial orientation (Khan & Chang, 2013). Maintaining balance and controlling posture is fundamental to many athletic pursuits, both in and out of the classroom.

Athletes' responsiveness, swiftness, and agility are all parts of kinesthetic fitness, which includes motor control functions for energy regulation. Several functions are crucial to maximizing the amount of energy used during physical activity. Internal speed (reaction time) and external speed (speed of limb movement) are separate forms of speed but have connected roles (Sreemathi & Murugavel, 2017) in the USFD Framework.

Additionally, in many situations, like driving, the ability to respond quickly to stimuli – a form of motor control – is essential for the driver's safety (Guo et al., 2019; Li et al., 2019; Samani et al., 2022). In contrast, speed control is all about controlling speed to the demands of a task. This emphasizes the need to manage energy expenditure. Optimal speed is not the only factor in determining performance success in sports, making this concept particularly significant in specific contexts. For example, accuracy and control are as important as speed for gymnasts to perform their routines correctly.

In conclusion, motor control is an intricate concept critical for task performance in many fields. The integration and efficient functioning of the brain, muscular, and sensory systems are crucial for improving physical activities and general physiological health. This is true regardless of whether a person is trying to maintain balance, optimize reaction time, or control speed. All these facets of motor control affect everyday living and athletic performance, highlighting how vital motor control is for staying active and healthy.

Summary

This chapter explores how kinesthetic fitness can improve physiological health and energy regulation by facilitating efficient motor control. It shows how important it is for the neurological and musculoskeletal systems to work together, such as proprioception and synchronizing visual and vestibular signals, for efficient and effective movement. Maintaining balance in static and dynamic situations is crucial for avoiding injuries and moving around efficiently. The importance of flexibility and a full range of motion in maintaining musculo-skeletal health is emphasized throughout the text, which also delves into how regular physical activity, a balanced diet, and an exercise routine contribute to overall well-being.

Motor control functions – including reaction time, speed control, and agility control – are essential for energy regulation, and this chapter outlines them along with physiological health. In this article, we will examine reaction time and its many facets in light of the importance of responding rapidly and precisely to outside stimuli in contexts such as sports and driving. The focus moves to speed control, arguing that adjusting movement speed based on what is needed for the task is better than going for maximum speed. In sports and daily life, the ability to quickly change directions while keeping balance and coordination is crucial, making agility control a must-have skill.

Many factors affect kinesthetic functions, such as proprioception accuracy, sensory data integration, and individual body mass and extensions. In order to improve physiological health and guarantee efficient energy regulation, this all-inclusive chapter summarizes the core components of kinesthetic fitness, which include motor control, balance, flexibility, reaction time, speed, and agility control.

Review questions

1. What are the motor control elements, and how do they interact to regulate movement?
2. Explain how proprioception affects motor control.
3. What is the significance of the kinetic chain in motor control?
4. Describe the feedback systems involved in motor control and give examples of their use.
5. Discuss the importance of balance in preserving physiological health. How might balance training help with injury prevention?
6. Investigate the significance of flexibility in motor control. What effect does flexibility have on posture and overall well-being?
7. In the context of motor control, define speed control. What is the significance of precision, timing, and adaptability in speed control?

8. Explain the concepts of reactive agility and agility control and give instances of sports or activities in which they are crucial.
9. What function do sensory-motor receptors play in promoting reactive agility? How do they help with quick reactions in shifting game situations?
10. How does response time affect activities such as driving and athletic performance? What are the things that can influence a person's reaction time?

Discussion questions

1. How might learning motor control concepts like balance and flexibility help people's daily lives, especially as they age? What practical solutions are there for maintaining or improving balance and flexibility?
2. Discuss practical training approaches for improving speed control and agility in the context of sports and athletic performance. How can athletes incorporate these approaches into their training regimens to boost their performance in sports?
3. Consider the importance of motor control, particularly reaction time, in professions like medicine (e.g., surgery) and emergency response (e.g., firefighting). How might people in these industries benefit from training that improves their motor control abilities?
4. Investigate the connection between motor control and injury prevention. What practical steps can coaches, physical therapists, and fitness instructors take to lessen the risk of injuries in athletes and clients due to poor motor control?
5. Consider how motor control research can be used to produce assistive technology and equipment for people with physical disability. How might advances in motor control research help improve the quality of life for those with mobility issues?

References

Alia, S. K. S., Fadhilb, M. A. K., & Zulnaidic, H. (2019). Effectiveness of coordination and agility exercises on the performance of basic fencing skills amongst University of Baghdad students. *International Journal of Innovation, Creativity and Change*, 7(3), 117–128. https://ijicc.net/images/vol7iss3/7308_Ali_2019_E_R.pdf

American Psychology Association. (2020). *APA dictionary of psychology*. https://dictionary.apa.org/choice-reaction-time

Bloemen, M. A., Takken, T., Backx, F. J., Vos, M., Kruitwagen, C. L., & de Groot, J. F. (2017). Validity and reliability of skill-related fitness tests for wheelchair-using youth with spina bifida. *Archives of Physical Medicine and Rehabilitation*, 98(6), 1097–1103. https://doi.org/10.1016/j.apmr.2016.08.469

Bonnet, M. H., & Arand, D. L. (2003). Clinical effects of sleep fragmentation versus sleep deprivation. *Sleep Medicine Reviews*, 7(4), 297–310. https://doi.org/10.1053/smrv.2001.0245

CK-12 Foundation. (2014, November 13). *5.1 reflexes: Neurons in action*. https://www.ck12.org/book/human-biology-nervous-system/section/5.1/

Coh, M., Vodičar, J., Žvan, M., Šimenko, J., Stodółka, J., Rauter, S., & Maćkała, K. (2018). Are Change-Of-Direction Speed And Reactive Agility Independent Skills Even When Using The Same Movement Pattern? *Journal of Strength and Conditioning Research, 32*, 1929–1936. https://doi.org/10.1519/JSC.0000000000002553

Corbin, C. B., & Le Masurier, G. C. (2014). *Fitness for life* (6th ed.). Human Kinetics.

Cunningham, D., Machado, A., Yue, G., Carey, J., & Plow, E. (2013). Functional somatotopy revealed across multiple cortical regions using a model of complex motor task. *Brain Research, 1531*, 25–36. https://doi.org/10.1016/j.brainres.2013.07.050

Daulatabad, V. S., Kamble, P. A., & Ps, B. (2013). An appraisal of reaction time in elite sprinters and Its comparison with age-matched controls. *International Journal of Medical Research & Health Sciences, 2*(3), 523–526. http://dx.doi.org/10.5958/j.2319-5886.2.3.092

Dolan, K. (2013). *Reactive agility, core strength, balance, and soccer performance* [Master's Thesis, Ithaca College]. https://core.ac.uk/download/pdf/217288256.pdf

Domenico, F., Altavilla, G., & Raiola, G. (2022). Relationship between rapid strength, reactive and strength and agility in university sports students. *International Journal of Human Movement and Sports Sciences, 10*(1), 98–103. https://doi.org/10.13189/saj.2022.100114

Fede, C., Gaudreault, N., Fan, C., Macchi, V., De Caro, R., & Stecco, C. (2018). Morphometric and dynamic measurements of muscular fascia in healthy individuals using ultrasound imaging: A summary of the discrepancies and gaps in the current literature. *Surgical and Radiologic Anatomy, 40*, 1329–1341. https://doi.org/10.1007/s00276-018-2086-1

Fernandez, I. G., & Wada, C. (2019, March). Cane with millimeter wave radar for base of support measurement. In *2019 IEEE 1st global conference on life sciences and technologies (LifeTech)* (pp. 133–136). IEEE. https://doi.org/10.1109/LifeTech.2019.8884010

Franchini, E., & Herrera-Valenzuela, T. (2021). Developing flexibility for combat sports athletes. *Revista de Artes Marciales Asiáticas, 16*. https://doi.org/10.18002/RAMA.V16I1S.7005

Gaerlan, M. G., Alpert, P. T., Cross, C., Louis, M., & Kowalski, S. (2012). Postural balance in young adults: The role of visual, vestibular and somatosensory systems. *Journal of the American Academy of Nurse Practitioners, 24*(6), 375–381. https://doi.org/10.1111/j.1745-7599.2012.00699.x

Ghuntla, T. P., Mehta, H. B., Gokhale, P. A., & Shah, C. J. (2014). A comparison and importance of auditory and visual reaction time in basketball players. *Saudi Journal of Sports Medicine, 14*(1), 35. https://doi.org/10.4103/1319-6308.131616

Gong, W. (2020). Effects of dynamic exercise utilizing PNF patterns on the balance of healthy adults. *Journal of Physical Therapy Science, 32*(4), 260–264. https://doi.org/10.1589/jpts.32.260

Guo, F., Li, M., Chen, Y., Xiong, J., & Lee, J. (2019). Effects of highway landscapes on drivers' eye movement behavior and emergency reaction time: A driving simulator study. *Journal of Advanced Transportation, 2019*. https://doi.org/10.1155/2019/9897831

Ha, S. Y., Kim, S. Y., & Sung, Y. H. (2019). Effects of visual feedback training using transient Fresnel prism glasses on balance ability in stroke patients without hemispatial neglect. *Journal of Exercise Rehabilitation, 15*(5), 683. https://doi.org/10.12965%2Fjer.1938498.249

Han, J., Anson, J., Waddington, G., Adams, R., & Liu, Y. (2015). The role of ankle proprioception for balance control in relation to sports performance and injury. *BioMed Research International, 2015*. https://doi.org/10.1155/2015/842804

Hassan, A. K., Alhumaid, M. M., & Hamad, B. E. (2022). The effect of using reactive agility exercises with the fitlight training system on the speed of visual reaction time and dribbling skill of basketball players. *Sports, 10*(11), 176. https://doi.org/10.3390/sports10110176

Hirata, K., Kanehisa, H., & Miyamoto, N. (2021). Association between medial gastrocnemius muscle-tendon unit architecture and ankle dorsiflexion range of motion with and without consideration of slack angle. *PLoS One, 16*. https://doi.org/10.1371/journal.pone.0248125

Hsu, C. Y., Chen, L. S., Chang, I. J., Fang, W. C., Huang, S. W., Lin, R. H., Ueng, S. W. N., & Chuang, H. H. (2021). Can anthropometry and body composition explain physical fitness levels in school-aged children? *Children, 8*(6), 460. https://doi.org/10.3390/children8060460

Ibrahim, S., Azhar, A. S., Ather, A. S., & Ahsan, A. S. (2018). Weight training protocol: Impact of diverse and organized exercise on certain components of motor fitness and functional variables amongst males. *International Journal of Pharmaceutical Research & Allied Sciences, 7*(2). https://bit.ly/48jr6K0

Jain, A., Bansal, R., Kumar, A., & Singh, K. D. (2015). A comparative study of visual and auditory reaction times on the basis of gender and physical activity levels of medical first year students. *International Journal of Applied & Basic Medical Research, 5*(2), 124–127. https://doi.org/10.4103/2229-516X.157168

Keogh, J., Cox, A., Anderson, S., Liew, B., Olsen, A., Schram, B., & Furness, J. (2019). Reliability and validity of clinically accessible smartphone applications to measure joint range of motion: A systematic review. *PLoS One, 14*. https://doi.org/10.1371/journal.pone.0215806

Khan, S., & Chang, R. (2013). Anatomy of the vestibular system: A review. *NeuroRehabilitation, 32*(3), 437–443. https://doi.org/10.3233/NRE-130866

Kleffelgaard, I., Soberg, H. L., Tamber, A. L., Bruusgaard, K. A., Pripp, A. H., Sandhaug, M., & Langhammer, B. (2019). The effects of vestibular rehabilitation on dizziness and balance problems in patients after traumatic brain injury: A randomized controlled trial. *Clinical Rehabilitation, 33*(1), 74–84. https://doi.org/10.1177/0269215518791274

Knapp, K. A. (2016). Self-care modalities: Improved performance and decreased injury for female athletes. *Strength & Conditioning Journal, 38*(2), 70–78. https://doi.org/10.1519/SSC.0000000000000205

Kot, A., & Nawrocka, A. (2014, May). Modeling of human balance as an inverted pendulum. In *Proceedings of the 2014 15th international carpathian control conference (ICCC)* (pp. 254–257). IEEE. https://doi.org/10.1109/CarpathianCC.2014.6843607

Kot, A., & Nawrocka, A. (2016). Balance maintaining by human. In *Solid state phenomena* (Vol. 248, pp. 155–160). Trans Tech Publications Ltd. https://doi.org/10.4028/www.scientific.net/SSP.248.155

Latash, M. L., & Zatsiorsky, V. (2015). *Biomechanics and motor control: Defining central concepts*. Academic Press.

Latorre, E., Zúñiga, M., Arriaza, E., Moya, F., & Nikulin, C. (2020). Automatic registration of footsteps in contact regions for reactive agility training in sports. *Sensors (Basel, Switzerland), 20*. https://doi.org/10.3390/s20061709

Li, X., Rakotonirainy, A., & Yan, X. (2019). How do drivers avoid collisions? A driving simulator-based study. *Journal of Safety Research, 70*, 89–96. https://doi.org/10.1016/j.jsr.2019.05.002

Mănescu, C. O. (2017). Aspects regarding speed and acceleration training in football. *Marathon, 9*(1), 37–42. https://marathon.ase.ro/pdf/vol9/6-Catalin.pdf

Milanović, Z., Pantelić, S., Trajković, N., Sporiš, G., Kostić, R., & James, N. (2013). Age-related decrease in physical activity and functional fitness among elderly men and women. *Clinical Interventions in Aging, 8*, 549–556. https://doi.org/10.2147/CIA.S44112

Mohamed, S. A., & Larion, A. (2018). Effect of SAQ training on certain physical variables and performance level for Sabre fencers. *Ovidius University Annals, Series*

Physical Education & Sport/Science, Movement & Health, *18*(1). https://www.anale
fefs.ro/anale-fefs/2018/i1/pe-autori/MOHAMED%20Safwt%20Abbas.pdf

Moromizato, K., Kimura, R., Fukase, H., Yamaguchi, K., & Ishida, H. (2016). Whole-body patterns of the range of joint motion in young adults: Masculine type and feminine type. *Journal of Physiological Anthropology*, *35*. https://doi.org/10.1186/s40101-016-0112-8

O'Leary, D. (2011). *What are Newton's laws of motion?* Crabtree Pub.

Pehar, M., Šišić, N., Sekulić, D., Coh, M., Uljević, O., Spasić, M., Krolo, A., & Idrizovic, K. (2018). Analyzing the relationship between anthropometric and motor indices with basketball specific pre-planned and non-planned agility performances. *The Journal of Sports Medicine and Physical Fitness*, *58*(7–8), 1037–1044. https://doi.org/10.23736/S0022-4707.17.07346-7

Peterson, M., & Greenwald, B. D. (2015). Balance problems after traumatic brain injury. *Archives of Physical Medicine and Rehabilitation*, *96*(2), 379–380. https://www.brain line.org/article/balance-problems-after-traumatic-brain-injury

Pojskić, H., Åslin, E., Krolo, A., Jukic, I., Uljević, O., Spasić, M., & Sekulić, D. (2018). Importance of reactive agility and change of direction speed in differentiating performance levels in junior soccer players: Reliability and validity of newly developed soccer-specific tests. *Frontiers in Physiology*, *9*. https://doi.org/10.3389/fphys.2018.00506

Popowczak, M., Domaradzki, J., Rokita, A., Zwierko, M., & Zwierko, T. (2020). Predicting visual-motor performance in a reactive agility task from selected demographic, training, anthropometric, and functional variables in adolescents. *International Journal of Environmental Research and Public Health*, *17*. https://doi.org/10.3390/ijerph17155322

Rakpongsiri, K. (2018). iRIS-RT: Eye fatigue and reaction time detector. *ECTI Transactions on Computer and Information Technology (ECTI-CIT)*, *12*(1), 42–51. https://doi.org/10.37936/ecti-cit.2018121.95077

Rana, M., Yani, M., Asavasopon, S., Fisher, B., & Kutch, J. (2015). Brain connectivity associated with muscle synergies in humans. *The Journal of Neuroscience*, *35*, 14708–14716. https://doi.org/10.1523/JNEUROSCI.1971-15.2015

Rebelo, A. (2022). Absolute reliability, relative reliability, and criterion-related validity of two reactive agility tests using two types of stimuli in elite male volleyball players. *Polish Journal of Sport and Tourism*, *29*, 24–29. https://doi.org/10.2478/pjst-2022-0011

Rüst, C. A., Knechtle, B., Knechtle, P., Wirth, A., & Rosemann, T. (2012). Body mass change and ultraendurance performance: A decrease in body mass is associated with an increased running speed in male 100-km ultramarathoners. *The Journal of Strength & Conditioning Research*, *26*(6), 1505–1516. https://doi.org/10.5812%2Fasjsm.34547

Saini, H. K. (2017). Effect of plyometric and circuit training programme on agility of male basketball players of Punjab. *Hill Quest*, *4*(1), 101–109. https://bit.ly/3SpTxOR

Samani, A. R., Mishra, S., & Dey, K. (2022). Assessing the effect of long-automated driving operation, repeated take-over requests, and driver's characteristics on commercial motor vehicle drivers' driving behavior and reaction time in highly automated vehicles. *Transportation Research Part F: Traffic Psychology and Behaviour*, *84*, 239–261. https://doi.org/10.1016/j.trf.2021.10.015

Shan, R., Nazir, A., Bhat, J. H., Sharma, V., Gupta, M., & Raj, D. (2022). Is there a difference in auditory reaction time between men and women? *Journal of Cardiovascular Disease Research*, *13*(4), 1113–1119. https://www.jcdronline.org/admin/Uploads/Files/62f7cd45c6d6b9.59096146.pdf

Shirai, N., Yamamoto, S., Osawa, Y., Tsubaki, A., Morishita, S., & Narita, I. (2022). Dysfunction in dynamic, but not static balance is associated with risk of accidental falls in hemodialysis patients: A prospective cohort study. *BMC Nephrology*, *23*(1), 1–7. https://doi.org/10.1186/s12882-022-02877-6

Shoeb, M., Mishra, A., Yadav, K. K., Kumar, S., & Yadav, S. (2020). Effect of BAPS board versus Frenkel exercise on balance in stroke patient's – a pilot study. *International Journal for Research in Applied Science & Engineering Technology*, 8(11). http://doi.org/10.22214/ijraset.2020.6397

Sinkovic, F., Foretić, N., & Novak, D. (2022). Reliability, validity and sensitivity of newly developed tennis-specific reactive agility tests. *Sustainability*, *14*(20). https://doi.org/10.3390/su142013321

Sreemathi, A., & Murugavel, K. (2017). Comparative effect of two different frequency of plyometric training on explosive power parameters of college women players. *International Journal of Physiology, Nutrition and Physical Education*, 2(2), 72–76. https://www.journalofsports.com/pdf/2017/vol2issue2/PartB/2-2-14-125.pdf

Suga, T., Terada, M., Tomoo, K., Miyake, Y., Tanaka, T., Ueno, H., Nagano, A., & Isaka, T. (2021). Association between plantar flexor muscle volume and dorsiflexion flexibility in healthy young males: Ultrasonography and magnetic resonance imaging studies. *BMC Sports Science, Medicine and Rehabilitation*, *13*(1), 1–8. https://doi.org/10.1186/s13102-021-00233-z

Tajik, M., Azarbayjani, M., & Peeri, M. (2022). A review of reactive and non-reactive agility tests concerning neurologic aspects. *Thrita*, *11*(1). https://doi.org/10.5812/thrita-129744

Takeda, K., Shimoda, N., Sato, Y., Ogano, M., & Kato, H. (2010). Reaction time differences between left- and right-handers during mental rotation of hand pictures. *Laterality*, *15*(4), 415–445. https://doi.org/10.1080/13576500902938105

Tanir, H. (2018). The effect of balance and stability workouts on the development of static and dynamic balance in 10–12-year-old soccer players. *Journal of Education and Training Studies*, 6(9), 132–135. https://doi.org/10.11114/jets.v6i9.3499

Trueman, R. C., Brooks, S. P., & Dunnett, S. B. (2012). Choice reaction time and learning. In N. M. Seel (Ed.), *Encyclopedia of the sciences of learning*. Springer. https://doi.org/10.1007/978-1-4419-1428-6_594

Valovich McLeod, T. C., & Hale, T. D. (2015). Vestibular and balance issues following sport-related concussion. *Brain Injury*, *29*(2), 175–184. https://doi.org/10.3109/02699052.2014.965206

Vandervoort, A., & Stathokostas, L. (2016). The flexibility debate: Implications for health and function as we age. *Annual Review of Gerontology and Geriatrics*, *36*, 169–192. https://doi.org/10.1891/0198-8794.36.169

Wallace, B., & Lifshitz, J. (2016). Traumatic brain injury and vestibulo-ocular function: Current challenges and future prospects. *Eye and Brain*, 153–164. https://doi.org/10.2147/EB.S82670

Wiederman, B. (2018). Don't buy this article on preventing elbow injuries in youth baseball players. *AAP Journal Blogs*. https://aap2.silverchair-cdn.com/aap2/content_public/autogen-pdf/cms/2757/2757.pdf

Willwacher, S., Fischer, K. M., Benker, R., Dill, S., & Brüggemann, G. P. (2013). Kinetics of cross-slope running. *Journal of Biomechanics*, *46*(16), 2769–2777. https://doi.org/10.1016/j.jbiomech.2013.09.006

Woods, D. L., Wyma, J. M., Yund, E. W., Herron, T. J., & Reed, B. (2015). Factors influencing the latency of simple reaction time. *Frontiers in Human Neuroscience*, *9*, 131. https://doi.org/10.3389/fnhum.2015.00131

Wu, W. T., Hong, C. Z., & Chou, L. W. (2015). The Kinesio taping method for myofascial pain control. *Evidence-Based Complementary and Alternative Medicine*, *2015*. https://doi.org/10.1155/2015/950519

Xing, C. F., Yang, L., & Zhang, Y. H. (2015). Study of driver's reaction time (DRT) during car following. In *Applied mechanics and materials* (Vol. 713, pp. 2089–2092). Trans Tech Publications Ltd.

Yang, Y., Zou, L., & Li, Z. (2022). A meta-analysis of CT as a tool for diagnosing and treating shoulder joint Bankart injuries. *Computational and Mathematical Methods in Medicine, 2022.* https://doi.org/10.1155/2022/9137706

Yiou, E., Caderby, T., Delafontaine, A., Fourcade, P., & Honeine, J. L. (2017). Balance control during gait initiation: State-of-the-art and research perspectives. *World Journal of Orthopedics, 8*(11), 815. https://doi.org/10.5312%2Fwjo.v8.i11.815

Zwierko, T., Nowakowska, A., Jedziniak, W., Popowczak, M., Domaradzki, J., Kubaszewska, J., Kaczmarczyk, M., & Ciechanowicz, A. (2022). Contributing factors to sensorimotor adaptability in reactive agility performance in youth athletes. *Journal of Human Kinetics, 83,* 39–48. https://doi.org/10.2478/hukin-2022-0067

12

BODY COMPOSITION

Oliver Napila Gomez and Nguyen Tra Giang

This chapter goes into the numerous implications of body composition in human physiology. Body composition, from atomic to whole-body levels, gives critical insights into nutritional status, energy regulation, and health prediction, outperforming standard metrics such as body mass index (BMI). It is essential for sustaining homeostasis, with minerals, bone mass, water content, and essential lipids contributing to internal equilibrium. Mineral balance, water homeostasis, and bone health are critical physiological processes these elements regulate. Furthermore, body composition influences metabolic rate, energy storage, and overall health by utilizing glycogen, nonessential lipids, and protein. Understanding and managing body composition is critical for encouraging wellness, preventing metabolic diseases, and obtaining optimal health outcomes.

Outcomes

By the end of this chapter, you will be able to

- explore body composition, from atomic to whole-body levels, as well as its significance as a critical driver of nutritional status, health, and energy regulation
- explain homeostasis and its relationship to body composition, examining the crucial functions that soft mineral tissues, bone mass, water content, and essential lipids play in maintaining internal equilibrium
- recognize the impact of body composition on energy regulation, with a focus on glycogen, nonessential lipids, and protein

DOI: 10.4324/9781003502937-14

- investigate the health implications of body composition changes, such as the hazards of obesity, malnutrition, and metabolic illnesses
- apply knowledge of body composition in real-world circumstances, making educated decisions about diet, health, and fitness

What is body composition?

Body composition is used by nutritionists to measure nutritional status and to track dietary therapy. Nutrient imbalances can drastically affect body composition, leading to malnutrition or obesity (Kuriyan, 2018). Furthermore, newborn body composition is an essential predictor of fetal adaptation and illness programming, stressing the importance of early-life body composition in long-term health consequences (Demerath & Fields, 2014). Researchers have discovered that body composition is a reliable predictor of various health disorders, including cardiovascular disease, diabetes, cancer, osteoporosis, and osteoarthritis (Turk et al., 2018; Kuriyan, 2018). Unlike the traditional reliance on body mass index (BMI), research suggests that body composition, which considers factors such as excess fat and low lean body mass, provides precise insights into mortality risk (Lee et al., 2018).

Nutritionists examine body composition to determine nutritional status and track improvement during dietary treatments (Holmes & Racette, 2021; Kuriyan, 2018; Prado et al., 2013). Nutrient imbalances change body composition. For example, muscle wasting and stunting cause a malnourished body composition, while overnutrition causes obesity (Kuriyan, 2018). With this, the body mass index (BMI) is more of a nutritional status indicator rather than body composition (Prado et al., 2013).

Moreover, infant body composition is crucial to fetal adaptability and illness programming (Demerath & Fields, 2014). Body composition predicts cardiorespiratory diseases better than BMI, as cardiorespiratory comorbidity and shorter lifespans are linked to poor body composition (Turk et al., 2018). Aside from cardiovascular disease, diabetes, malignancies, osteoporosis, and osteoarthritis are related to body composition (Kuriyan, 2018). Body composition is the main component differentiating type 2 diabetes pathophysiology between Japanese and Caucasians in a study (Møller et al., 2014), while inflammatory arthritis begins with poor body composition (Turk et al., 2018). It is linked with low back, knee, and foot problems in obesity–musculoskeletal disease research (Brady et al., 2015).

Body composition is also a relevant indicator of health. Lee and colleagues (2018) suggested that excess fat mass increases the risk of mortality. Additionally, low lean body mass, rather than low fat mass, may be responsible for the increased mortality risk in individuals with lower body mass index (BMI). Body composition refers to the components of a person's body form and structure.

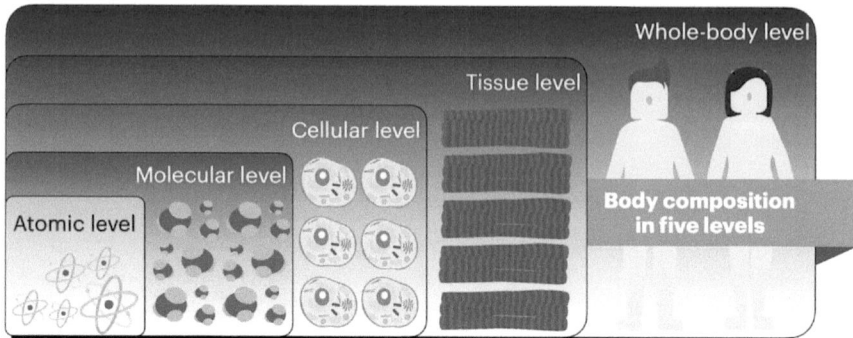

FIGURE 12.1   Body composition in five levels

Researchers (Wang et al., 1992; Zemel & Barden, 2004; Weber et al., 2012) offer a model framework to help understand what constitutes body composition in five levels (see Figure 12.1). This model framework perceives body composition at atomic, molecular, cellular, tissue, and whole-body levels.

The body mass

From the model (Figure 12.1), we will pay attention to the whole-body level, of which the most common indicator that people know is body mass, which may also refer to a person's body size or weight (Yilmaz, 2013). Weight is a convenient indicator of body composition since it is straightforward to measure and generally available. It gives a basic and quick evaluation of an individual's body mass.

While body weight alone does not give precise information regarding fat and lean mass distribution, it is a helpful initial screening tool. It is often employed in population-level research and clinical settings owing to its simplicity and practicability. Nevertheless, body weight is somewhat imprecise because some compartments of the total body composition, including the relative proportion of fat and fat-free mass, still need to be discovered.

The 2C model

Body fat refers to the subcutaneous and visceral fat stored under the skin (Balasunder, 2014) and around/inside the belly (including intestines, liver, kidneys, pancreas, and heart). Fat-free or lean mass refers to the total body weight minus bone and fat, thus representing the skeletal muscle mass (Kiss et al., 2016; Sandberg et al., 2021). Lean mass includes muscles, vital organs, the mineral content of soft tissues, and the body's water content. Hence, a model of body composition

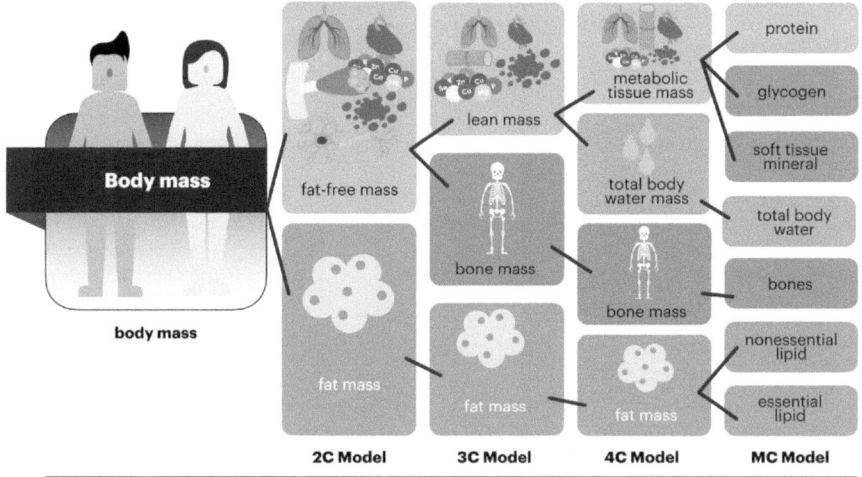

FIGURE 12.2   Simplified presentation of the models of body composition

called the two-compartment (2C) model is expressed as a mathematical formula that divides the amount of fat against the amount of fat-free mass of the body (Zemel & Barden, 2004; Weber et al., 2012; Kuriyan, 2018).

The 3C model

The 2C model is still vague when defining what constitutes the fat and fat-free mass of the body. For instance, bones are part of the fat-free mass. However, the composition of the skeleton is different from the soft lean mass.

As a resolution, the three-compartment (3C) model further splits up the fat-free mass into two compartments – the lean body mass (soft tissues and vital organs) and the hard compartment (bones and teeth).

The 4C model

The average total water content of the body is 60% relative to a person's body mass. The total water content is another separate compartment in the existing compositions of the body. The four-compartment (4C) model divides body composition into fat mass, bone mass, total water content, and desiccated metabolic tissues.

The MC model

The dried-out metabolic tissues consist of protein, glycogen, and soft tissue minerals (electrolytes such as sodium, potassium, calcium, bicarbonate, magnesium, chloride, and phosphate). Moreover, the fat mass includes nonessential lipids obtained from food that the body can manufacture from food, and essential lipids obtained from food that the body cannot manufacture. The multi-compartment (MC) model rationalizes that the body comprises protein, glycogen, soft tissue minerals, bone mass, total water content, nonessential lipids, and essential lipids.

Body composition for homeostasis and energy regulation

In our framework, body composition is shared by two components – homeostasis and energy regulation. As previously mentioned, this function consists of the musculoskeletal and endocrine systems regulating the proportions of fat, muscle, and other body components.

Based on the MC, we reckoned that the body composition for homeostasis includes soft tissue minerals, bone mass, total body water, and essential lipids. In contrast, the body composition for energy regulation includes protein, glycogen, and nonessential lipids.

Body composition for homeostasis

Homeostasis, a dynamic self-regulating process that allows organisms to maintain internal stability while adjusting to external changes, emphasizes a key concept in physiology that emphasizes flexibility over stagnation. It is caused by the intricate interaction of many feedback systems and disruptions to this delicate balance result in disease. At the same time, therapy attempts to restore these crucial conditions by nature's laws (Billman, 2020).

Through a complicated and painstakingly regulated process, the body maintains the internal conditions required for health. This delicate balance of many

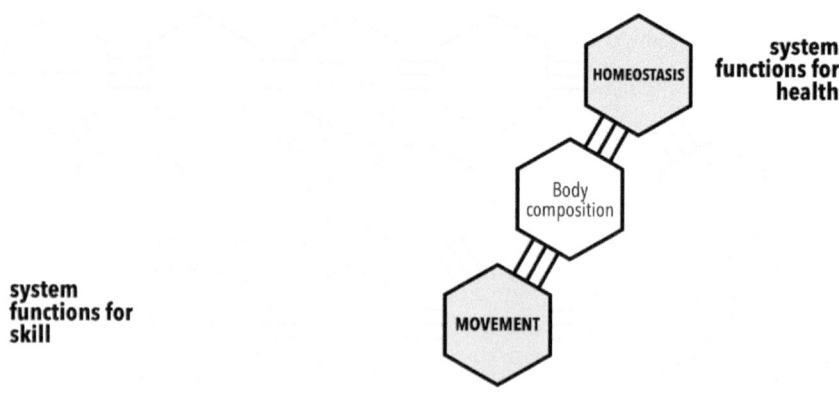

FIGURE 12.3   Body composition – shared by homeostasis and energy regulation

physiological factors is critical for maintaining homeostasis, with body composition playing a critical role in achieving this balance. The USFD defines critical body composition components for homeostasis as soft tissue minerals, bone mass, total body water, and essential lipids. Let us go into detail in this investigation of these elements.

Soft mineral tissues

Mineral homeostasis is preserving normal circulation levels of calcium and phosphate ions, which are necessary for various physiological processes (Shore et al., 2013). Mineral homeostasis strictly preserves a specific element's internal equilibrium in tissues (Hermans et al., 2013). Mineral homeostasis refers to the phosphate and calcium ions in extracellular fluid required for normal physiological function (Öhrnell Malekzadeh, 2017).

Calcium, magnesium, potassium, sodium, and phosphorus are critical minerals that help the body maintain homeostasis. Calcium is vital in neuromuscular conduction, bone mineralization, and enzyme secretion (Bharill & Wu, 2023). It is a crucial mineral for general health, promoting various physiological activities.

Magnesium's importance stems from its function in manufacturing vitamin D, which is required for its activation (Gong et al., 2022). This emphasizes its role in bone health and calcium absorption control.

Moreover, by counteracting the effects of calcium ions, potassium is necessary for enhancing cell membrane permeability (Szczuko et al., 2022). It is essential for excitable tissues, including skeletal muscles, cardiac muscles, and neurons, to ensure optimal function (Hoque et al., 2020).

Sodium is essential for managing bodily water content and maintaining fluid balance, particularly in the extracellular fluid (Minegishi et al., 2020; Dharmawan et al., 2023). It is required for proper hydration and electrolyte balance.

Phosphorus, mainly in the form of inorganic orthophosphate, is essential to all life's metabolism (Nicholls et al., 2023). It stores genetic information, constructs cellular membranes, phosphorylates metabolites, and controls enzymes. Phosphorylated nucleotides, such as adenosine triphosphate (ATP), are essential energy carriers that aid in various metabolic activities (Nicholls et al., 2023).

Water

The efficient dissipation of excess body heat depends mainly on evaporative cooling; hence, maintaining body water homeostasis is critical for preventing hyperthermia (Sladek & Johnson, 2013). This delicate water homeostasis depends on managing water intake and renal water loss (Sladek & Johnson, 2013). Furthermore, abnormalities in the genes responsible for brain ion and water homeostasis underpin various human disorders, with many of these genes primarily expressed in glial cells, emphasizing the critical function of glia in maintaining ion and water equilibrium in the brain (Min & van der Knaap, 2018).

The hypothalamic osmostat orchestrates the sense of thirst and the production of vasopressin to limit water loss in humans. Although thirst and water retention are physically connected, their regulation happens independently (Gáliková et al., 2018). The exact management of water homeostasis is required to maintain proper central nervous system (CNS) function (Salman et al., 2022). Any disruption in this process can result in sudden and potentially fatal increases in intracranial or intraspinal pressure and the accumulation of toxic waste products (Salman et al., 2022). This complicated network of water balance and its repercussions highlight the fundamental need for maintaining water homeostasis for general health and the appropriate functioning of vital body systems.

Water is essential for the regulation of physiological processes and the maintenance of homeostasis inside the human body. It is required for many processes, including metabolic reactions, nutrition and waste movement, temperature regulation, cell structure, osmotic equilibrium, and cellular hydration (Lorenzo et al., 2019). Water's involvement in thirst perception, a critical regulatory mechanism for maintaining body fluid balance, is vital to its contribution to homeostasis. This hunger sense might arise in two ways: as a reactive response to present shortfalls or an anticipatory response to prevent future imbalances. These processes are controlled by complex brain mechanisms (Gizowski & Bourque, 2018).

One serious consequence of insufficient water consumption and resulting dehydration is the possibility of prerenal damage, which might progress to intrinsic renal failure, complicating patient care (Mahesh et al., 2018). Chronic dehydration has serious dangers, such as increased susceptibility to kidney stones, urinary tract infections, hypertension, and, in extreme situations, the risk of having a stroke (Blancaflor et al., 2022).

The interaction of water and homeostasis is dynamic, highlighting the body's incredible ability to manage its internal environment. Water's contribution to fluid balance via thirst perception is critical in preventing departures from the body's ideal set points. This regulatory function assists the body in adapting to changing situations such as temperature changes, physical exercise, and nutritional intake. Furthermore, chronic dehydration's catastrophic implications highlight the need for water to avoid life-threatening illnesses and emphasize the importance of hydration.

Water's significance in homeostasis goes beyond its status as an essential beverage; it is a crucial component of the intricate machinery that guarantees the body's internal milieu remains stable and favorable to good physiological performance. Recognizing water's vital function in sustaining homeostasis emphasizes the significance of appropriate hydration in maintaining general health and well-being.

Bone mass

Bone homeostasis is a dynamic process involving a delicate balance of osteoblasts responsible for bone creation and osteoclasts responsible for bone destruction (Lin et al., 2023; Enoki et al., 2017). This balance between bone production and resorption is critical for these cells' appropriate functional functioning (Feng et al., 2022). Disruptions in this balance frequently result in debilitating bone illnesses such as osteoporosis, osteoarthritis, and osteosclerosis (Feng et al., 2022). Furthermore, vitamin D has emerged as an essential regulator of calcium delivery to the skeletal system, emphasizing its significance in maintaining bone and calcium homeostasis (Bouillon & Suda, 2014).

Furthermore, bones play a diverse role in the body, giving structural support, protecting internal organs, facilitating movement, storing vital minerals such as calcium and phosphorus, and acting as a location for hematopoiesis (Balogh et al., 2018). The process of bone remodeling, which is managed by interactions between osteoclasts and osteoblasts and regulated by proteins such as RUNX2[1] and TGF-β1,[2] is critical for skeletal integrity and metabolic equilibrium (Balogh et al., 2018; Tang & Alliston, 2013). TGF-β emerges as a prominent figure in this delicate dance of bone homeostasis, monitoring the bone matrix's recruitment, differentiation, function, and quality throughout the remodeling phases (Tang & Alliston, 2013). Understanding and maintaining this equilibrium is critical not only for bone health but also for overall well-being.

Essential fats

Lipid homeostasis is the preservation of a steady lipid content and metabolic activity in the blood and tissues, which is required for appropriate physiological functioning, and it is regulated by factors such as dietary fat, organ function, and organ control (Li et al., 2023). This control is accomplished through a well-balanced process that includes intestinal absorption, endogenous production, metabolism, and lipoprotein transport (Zhang et al., 2023). Lipoprotein lipase is essential for releasing fatty acids from circulating triacylglycerol, which helps maintain lipid homeostasis (Riaz, 2014). The liver, pancreas, and adipose tissues work together to maintain lipid homeostasis, and the metabolic functions of adipose tissues have received increased attention due to hormone discoveries such as leptin and adiponectin (Al-Mrabeh, 2021).

Essential fats, an important component of the human diet, play an important role in general health and are required for appropriate physiological and biological activities (Kamaludin et al., 2021). Because the human body cannot generate these fats from other fats, they must be included in our diet to promote optimal health (Robinson, 2021).

These necessary fats are divided into omega-3 and omega-6 fatty acids (Strzelczyk et al., 2023). They are necessary since they cannot be manufactured internally and must be obtained through diet.

Essential fats are carefully stored throughout the body in numerous tissues and organs, in addition to their dietary relevance. The storage locations include the bone marrow, heart, lungs, liver, spleen, kidneys, intestines, muscles, and lipid-rich tissues (Andrei & Andrei, 2018). Notably, essential fats are absorbed into vital tissues and organs such as the brain, kidney, heart, lungs, liver, and mammary glands rather than stored in storage form (Bakinde, 2021).

Furthermore, the distribution of essential fats might differ by gender, with women often having somewhat bigger stores due to hormonal dynamics and the demands of pregnancy (Kumala et al., 2022). Essential fats are necessary dietary components that support a wide range of physiological processes, and their strategic storage throughout the body emphasizes their critical role in homeostasis and general health. Understanding the significance of these fats and incorporating them into our diet is critical for overall health.

Other ways body composition supports homeostasis

Body composition, influenced by genetics, environment, and lifestyle, is crucial to maintaining homeostasis. This balance is essential for several reasons, including its effect on metabolic homeostasis, redox balance, and other physiological processes (Holmes & Racette, 2021).

On the one hand, appropriate body composition promotes improved redox (oxidative stress) homeostasis. Nevertheless, differences in body composition, such as being underweight or overweight, can impair redox balance at rest and during exercise (Margaritelis et al., 2019). This underlines the significance of body composition for overall physiological stability.

Obesity, on the other hand, disrupts metabolic homeostasis by lowering insulin sensitivity, changing lipid metabolism, and raising inflammation (Tee et al., 2023). However, changes in body composition, particularly an increase in fat content, help to maintain homeostasis by improving energy storage efficiency even during pregnancy (Abeysekera et al., 2016). This adaptation maintains a consistent environment for the developing fetus and mother.

Furthermore, body composition is vital in promoting homeostasis through regulating weight and balancing energy expenditure. Notably, changes in body composition, such as a decrease in fat mass, trigger adaptive thermogenesis, which influences energy expenditure during weight loss and maintenance (Rosenbaum & Leibel, 2016). This process, which adjusts energy expenditure in response to changes in body composition and weight, is part of the body's efforts to maintain energy homeostasis.

Regarding food metabolism, body composition can influence the fermentation of nondigestible carbohydrates in the colon, forming short-chain fatty acids

(SCFAs). These SCFAs influence energy balance and metabolic activity by regulating appetite and energy intake homeostasis (Byrne et al., 2015).

Furthermore, myostatin, a component in muscle growth and metabolism, regulates body composition (Mosler et al., 2014). Inhibiting myostatin with exercise training results in considerable changes in body composition, boosting muscle growth, lowering fat, and enhancing metabolism – all of which contribute considerably to muscle homeostasis.

Similarly, syndecan-1 (SDC1) impairment has far-reaching implications on several areas of body composition and metabolic function (Jaiswal et al., 2020). Syndecan-1 is a heparan sulfate proteoglycan (HSPG) present on cell surfaces, primarily epithelial and plasma cells, and plays an essential role in cell adhesion, signaling, and overall cellular activity. Its absence affects body fat, lean mass, feeding behavior, energy expenditure, glucose tolerance, and insulin resistance, among other things.

Also, in collaboration with the Bmal1 gene, skeletal muscle is essential in regulating glucose metabolism, substrate use, and overall metabolic health (Harfmann et al., 2016). The Bmal1 gene regulates circadian rhythms and physiological processes, emphasizing the importance of time in homeostasis maintenance.

These complex processes make body composition crucial to the intricate web of factors contributing to homeostasis. Its impact on metabolic processes, redox balance, and various physiological activities emphasizes its importance in maintaining stable internal conditions necessary for health. As scientists continue to unravel the complexities of body composition, we gain important insights into how it contributes to the delicate balance of homeostasis – a never-ending quest for overall well-being.

Body composition for energy regulation

The body composition for energy regulation includes glycogen, nonessential lipids, and protein.

Glycogen

Glycogen is a vital glucose storage molecule found in many mammalian organs, including the liver and the brain, where it plays essential roles in energy control and metabolic activities. Glycogen is vital in the liver for maintaining blood glucose levels. During glucose deficiency, such as fasting or high energy needs, the liver can convert glycogen into glucose molecules via a series of enzyme processes. This glucose release into the bloodstream aids in blood glucose regulation, delivering a consistent energy supply to the body (Waitt et al., 2017).

Glycogen is a rapidly available energy substrate in skeletal muscles, especially during high-intensity exercise. Muscle contraction demands significant energy during activities such as exercise, and muscle glycogen reserves provide an immediate source of glucose for ATP generation. This is necessary to maintain muscular function and performance during severe physical activities (Adeva-Andany et al., 2016).

Glycogen plays a unique role in the brain as an emergency energy source for neurons, especially when glucose availability is low. While glucose is the brain's principal energy source under normal conditions, glycogen in the brain can be broken down into glucose molecules to support neuronal function when blood glucose levels decrease or energy needs increase. This system aids in maintaining brain function and ensures neurons have access to energy even under challenging circumstances (Waitt et al., 2017).

Furthermore, glycogen in the brain has been linked to sustaining learning and memory processes, implying a role in cognitive tasks other than energy provision (Waitt et al., 2017). Glycogen metabolism defects, common in glycogen storage disorders, can have a variety of metabolic and clinical repercussions. These illnesses can interfere with adequately regulating blood glucose levels in the liver, decrease muscle function during physical activity, and impact brain function, emphasizing the importance of glycogen in total energy balance and metabolic homeostasis (Kanungo et al., 2018).

The distribution of glycogen in distinct cellular pools in skeletal muscles, particularly intramyofibrillar glycogen, can alter muscular performance and fatigue. Muscular glycogen is the principal energy source during high-intensity exercise and is essential for muscle contraction maintenance. The rate of glycogen use and availability during physical activities can alter muscular function and endurance (Ørtenblad et al., 2013).

Furthermore, glycogen's involvement in muscle goes beyond just providing energy. It can also affect muscular excitability and calcium kinetics during muscle contractions, which affect muscle function and fatigue development. As a result, glycogen concentration and distribution within muscle fibers are essential factors in defining an individual's physical capabilities and endurance (Vigh-Larsen et al., 2021).

Nonessential lipids

Nonessential fats' role in energy regulation is a complicated and intricate component of human physiology. Nonessential lipids, especially triacylglycerols, are essential energy storage within the body. These lipids comprise a considerable amount of an individual's overall body composition, ranging from 10% to 25% in males and 15% to 35% in females (Almasoudi, 2022). These energy storage molecules, sometimes known as fat mass, are essential in maintaining energy balance and metabolic homeostasis (MacDonald, 2015).

Nonessential fats are distinct in that the body generates them and they are not considered necessary dietary components; thus, they are called *nonessential fats*.

The body can produce these lipids, most notably through de novo lipogenesis, which transforms extra carbs and proteins into triacylglycerols for storage. The fact that nonessential lipids are produced endogenously emphasizes their role in energy control and metabolic function.

However, the consequences of excessive nonessential fat storage within the body must be considered. Nonessential fat consumption has increased significantly in modern culture, partly due to changes in animal husbandry practices, such as chicken meat production (Alders, 2017). Concerns about the influence of this increase in nonessential fat consumption on general health and well-being have been expressed.

Adiposity increases significantly as nonessential fats accumulate when calorie intake continuously exceeds energy expenditure (Hussain, 2016). Adiposity is the excessive body storage of energy as fat, primarily in adipose tissue. Overweight and obesity result from this long-term calorie surplus (Hussain, 2016). Obesity and overweight are linked to a variety of health problems, including cardiovascular disease, diabetes, and metabolic syndrome, underscoring the vital function of nonessential lipids in energy regulation and its consequences for health.

Protein

Protein has many functions in human biology, including energy control, growth, and the appropriate operation of many biological systems. Recognizing its relevance in overall health highlights the importance of getting appropriate protein into a diet to support a well-balanced and healthy life.

To begin, protein refers to a wide variety of proteins found in serum, and its quantification is critical for understanding human physiology (Zhang et al., 2023). Aside from its role as a complete protein, it can be divided into muscle and non-muscle proteins (MacDonald, 2015). These proteins are not only structural parts of tissues in animals, such as muscles, nails, hair, and skin (Mehmood, 2017), but they also serve as the foundation for many cellular components (Service, 2015). Proteins, for example, make up cell receptors essential for signal transduction (Jarouliya & Keservani, 2019).

Furthermore, protein is a vital element in human growth and development. It promotes strength and overall health by interacting with other vital nutrients such as carbs and lipids. The type and amount of protein consumed substantially impact health, emphasizing the necessity of adopting informed dietary decisions (Hodgson, 2016). It is vital in many biological processes, including transcription, cell differentiation, cell growth, storage, cell division, and cell signaling (Singh, 2016). The importance of it in human nutrition cannot be emphasized (Thanigaivel et al., 2016).

It is necessary to sustain a healthy human body with protein, contributing to its composition and function throughout life. A well-balanced diet that promotes the development and maintenance of thousands of encoded proteins and nitrogenous substances is critical for general health. The protein demand is defined by the body's need to achieve the necessary structure and function (Barik, 2016).

Other ways body composition supports energy regulation

Body composition is essential in energy regulation because it influences numerous aspects of metabolism and the body's ability to maintain a balanced energy state. Let us explore the complex relationship between body composition and energy control using information from diverse scientific investigations.

The hormone irisin, released by muscle tissue during exercise, is a significant factor in the relationship between body composition and energy control. Irisin has been proven to contribute significantly to energy regulation, but its interaction with body composition is complicated. The existence of fat mass can alter the relationship between irisin and resting energy expenditure, demonstrating the subtle linkages between body composition and energy regulation (Pardo et al., 2014). This interaction demonstrates how different bodily components might influence energy consumption.

Body composition, which includes fat and lean mass (water, bone, organs, and mostly muscle), is significantly linked to cardiorespiratory fitness (Nogueira et al., 2016). This organization highlights the importance of body composition in energy regulation, as cardiorespiratory fitness is essential in determining the body's ability to use energy resources efficiently.

Skeletal muscle mass is a vital body composition component influencing metabolic rate. Cameron and colleagues (2016) state that lean muscular tissue has a greater metabolic rate than fat tissue. This research emphasizes the importance of maintaining lean muscle mass in energy control.

Furthermore, losing lean muscle mass during weight loss might result in metabolic adaptation, in which the body's metabolism slows down dramatically in people who lose a large quantity of lean muscle mass (Fothergill et al., 2016). This occurrence emphasizes the importance of maintaining lean muscle mass to maintain a good metabolic rate and energy balance when losing weight.

In another context, estrogen shortage, which is common in postmenopausal women and men, can result in metabolic dysfunction, such as obesity and type 2 diabetes (Mauvais-Jarvis et al., 2013). Estrogen, primarily through receptors such as ERα or estrogen receptor alpha, regulates food intake and energy expenditure in several brain regions. This emphasizes the importance of estrogen in regulating energy balance and glucose homeostasis.

Moreover, the peptide neurotransmitter neuropeptide Y (NPY) regulates appetite, food intake, and energy balance. Insulin signaling in NPY-expressing neurons is required for appetite and energy expenditure regulation. Impaired signaling in this route can result in insulin resistance, decreasing glucose absorption in skeletal muscle (Loh et al., 2017). This change in glucose regulation reveals how insulin–NPY signaling affects overall energy balance and contributes to metabolic illness development.

Aging and sarcopenia, defined by muscle loss and dysfunction caused by aging and chronic diseases, considerably impact energy control (Biolo et al., 2014). Sarcopenia, or the progressive loss of muscle mass and function, is expected among the senior population and people with chronic diseases, and it affects muscle strength and physical performance, leading to less physical activity and an increased vulnerability to metabolic imbalances. Insulin resistance, hormonal disturbances, and decreased glucose utilization are all examples of imbalances that alter energy balance and raise the risk of morbidity and mortality (Gungor et al., 2021).

Body composition and task performance

Body composition has a significant impact on dietary status and physical capacity. When the fat-to-muscle mass ratio is optimal, a person is in a better position to function at their physical best. Nutrient imbalances can significantly impact physical capacities and task performance, resulting in starvation or obesity. Conditions like obesity and malnutrition, which alter body composition due to food imbalances, directly impair athletic capacities (Kuriyan, 2018).

Consequently, how quickly the body uses energy and how much it stores is greatly influenced by how it is composed. A higher percentage of muscle mass is associated with a higher metabolic rate, affecting energy levels and endurance when engaging in physical activities (Holmes & Racette, 2021; Prado et al., 2013). The significance of muscle mass in sustaining a high energy level, which is necessary for efficient task performance, is highlighted by this relationship.

Moreover, supporting and carrying out physical activities requires a well-balanced physique with sufficient muscle strength and bone mass. Fractures are likely to occur, and performance on tasks is impaired in those with poor body composition, which includes low bone density and muscular atrophy, which can cause crippling diseases like osteoporosis (Turk et al., 2018; Kuriyan, 2018). As a result, being physically functional depends on having strong bones and muscles.

Similarly, how well the heart and lungs work depends on body composition, especially the fat-to-muscle ratio. Loss of pulmonary function and cardiovascular efficiency due to obesity reduces endurance and the ability to engage in strenuous physical activity for lengthy periods (Turk et al., 2018). The importance of maintaining a balanced body composition for maintaining cardiorespiratory health and athletic endurance is underscored by this relationship.

It is well established that specific body compositions are associated with an increased risk of diseases like diabetes, cardiovascular disease, and some types of cancer (Kuriyan, 2018). The capacity to carry out routine activities effectively may be impaired due to these disorders' effects on mobility and physical function. So, a healthy body composition is crucial to keep sickness at bay and movement intact.

Moreover, body composition can predict mortality risk more accurately than body mass index alone. Factors including poor lean body mass and excess fat mass are linked to an increased risk of mortality (Lee et al., 2018). Maintaining a healthy body composition for overall health and task performance is vital since it is associated with higher functional capability and a lower mortality risk.

Lastly, strength and power-requiring abilities are strongly correlated with muscle mass, an essential component of body composition. The significance of keeping muscles healthy for optimal job performance is highlighted because reduced muscle mass might decrease efficiency.

Summary

Body composition, a fundamental element of human physiology, is critical in determining nutritional status, controlling energy, and predicting health outcomes. It provides a comprehensive view of a person's body structure, from the atomic and molecular to the cellular, tissue, and whole-body levels. Body composition, as opposed to simple metrics like body weight or BMI, which only examine overall mass, provides specific insights into fat distribution and lean muscle mass, providing an accurate assessment of an individual's health.

The significance of body composition in sustaining homeostasis is critical. Minerals, bone mass, water content, and vital lipids contribute to internal stability. Mineral homeostasis, for example, balances calcium and phosphate ions, which are essential for many physiological functions. Water homeostasis regulates temperature and prevents issues like intracranial pressure increases. Bone mass also provides structural support, protects organs, and aids in mineral storage and hematopoiesis. Essential lipids, such as omega-3 and omega-6 fatty acids, help with various biological activities and general health.

Body composition components such as glycogen, nonessential lipids, and protein are essential in energy control. Glycogen acts as a quick supply of glucose during times of high energy demand and aids in the maintenance of blood glucose levels. Nonessential lipids impact adiposity and energy storage and must be balanced to maintain a healthy metabolic state. Protein, which is essential for cellular functioning and growth, has an impact on metabolism, cell signaling, and general health. Skeletal muscle mass, a component of body composition, has a higher metabolic rate than adipose tissue and is essential for maintaining a healthy metabolism. Understanding and regulating body composition is critical for fostering well-being, minimizing health problems, and keeping optimal metabolic balance.

Review questions

1. Why is body composition considered an essential indicator of nutritional status and health?
2. How does body composition differ from body mass index (BMI), and why is it frequently regarded as a more exact health measure?
3. What are the essential components of body composition at the atomic, molecular, cellular, tissue, and whole-body levels?
4. Explain the concept of homeostasis regarding body composition. How do soft mineral tissues, bone mass, water content, and vital lipids contribute to homeostasis?
5. What role do minerals like calcium, magnesium, potassium, sodium, and phosphorus play in mineral homeostasis and overall health?
6. How does the body regulate water homeostasis, and why is it essential for internal stability and good central nervous system function?
7. What role does glycogen play in energy control, and how does it differ across the liver, muscles, and brain?
8. Describe the activities of nonessential lipids in the body and analyze the probable health consequences of excessive fat storage.
9. How can protein help with energy control, growth, and overall health? What are the implications of a low protein intake?
10. Investigate the relationship between body composition and energy balance, considering parameters such as irisin, skeletal muscle mass, hormonal impacts, and aging-related muscle loss (sarcopenia).

Discussions questions

1. How can individuals use their knowledge of their body composition to make informed nutritional and fitness decisions to improve their overall health?
2. How can healthcare practitioners use body composition analysis in a clinical environment to personalize food and exercise advice for patients with specific health objectives or conditions?
3. Discuss the practical consequences of understanding the effects of minerals, such as calcium, magnesium, potassium, sodium, and phosphorus, on health. How can people improve their mineral intake for improved health?
4. Investigate practical ways for achieving water balance and proper hydration in daily life. How can people ensure they are getting enough water into their bodies?
5. Discuss practical dietary recommendations for reaching an optimum protein intake, considering the role of protein in energy regulation and metabolic health. How can people improve their health by incorporating protein-rich foods into everyday diets?

Notes

1 RUNX2, or runt-related transcription factor 2, is a protein that is essential for bone formation and homeostasis. It is a transcription factor that influences gene expression in numerous biological processes. RUNX2 is a master regulator of osteoblast development and function in bone biology.
2 Transforming growth factor-beta 1 (TGF-β1) is a multifunctional cytokine, or signaling protein, that plays a critical role in various biological processes, including cell growth, differentiation, immune response regulation, and tissue development. TGF-β1 is part of a larger family of growth factors known as the transforming growth factor-beta superfamily, which includes different isoforms of TGF-β and other related proteins.

References

Abeysekera, M. V., Morris, J. A., Davis, G. K., & O'Sullivan, A. J. (2016). Alterations in energy homeostasis to favour adipose tissue gain: A longitudinal study in healthy pregnant women. *Australian and New Zealand Journal of Obstetrics and Gynaecology, 56*(1), 42–48. https://doi.org/10.1111/ajo.12398

Adeva-Andany, M. M., González-Lucán, M., Donapetry-García, C., Fernández-Fernández, C., & Ameneiros-Rodríguez, E. (2016). Glycogen metabolism in humans. *BBA Clinical, 5*, 85–100. https://doi.org/10.1016/j.bbacli.2016.02.001

Al-Mrabeh, A. (2021). β-Cell dysfunction, hepatic lipid metabolism, and cardiovascular health in type 2 diabetes: New directions of research and novel therapeutic strategies. *Biomedicines, 9*(2), 226. https://doi.org/10.3390/biomedicines9020226

Alders, R. (2017). Plenary 1: Nutrition, health and the environment: A global perspective. *Journal of Nutrition & Intermediary Metabolism, 8*, 60e121.

Almasoudi, S. (2022). *Salivary α-amylase gene 1 (AMY1) copy number variation and association with inter-individual differences in body composition and response to carbohydrates intake* [Doctoral dissertation, University of Stirling]. http://hdl.handle.net/1893/34548

Andrei, I., & Andrei, E. G. (2018). Adipose tissue. In *International scientific conference "strategies XXI"* (Vol. 1, pp. 19–22). "Carol I" National Defence University. https://www.proquest.com/openview/9c5a8e25e6c7fa82e9aca7b287b58161/1?pq-origsite=gscholar&cbl=2026346

Bakinde, T. S. (2021). Correlates of body composition and motor performance variables of University of Ilorin male handball players. *International Journal of Research in Education, 1*(2), 75–85. https://doi.org/10.26877/ijre.v1i2.8180

Balasunder, J. (2014). *Pharmacotherapeutic analysis of prescribing pattern of drugs in metabolic syndrome* [Doctoral dissertation, Rajiv Gandhi University of Health Sciences]. https://www.proquest.com/openview/9a939baaf0898caad8015e8a162f7baf/1?pq-origsite=gscholar&cbl=2026366&diss=y

Balogh, E., Paragh, G., & Jeney, V. (2018). Influence of iron on bone homeostasis. *Pharmaceuticals, 11*(4), 107. https://doi.org/10.3390/ph11040107

Barik, N. K. (2016). Potential in improving nutritional security through aquaculture development in India: A regional level analysis. *Agricultural Economics Research Review, 29*, 99–109. http://doi.org/10.5958/0974-0279.2016.00037.9

Bharill, S., & Wu, M. (2023). Hypocalcemia and hypercalcemia in children. *Pediatrics in Review, 44*(9), 533–536. https://doi.org/10.1542/pir.2022-005578

Billman, G. E. (2020). Homeostasis: The underappreciated and far too often ignored central organizing principle of physiology. *Frontiers in Physiology, 11*, 200. https://doi.org/10.3389/fphys.2020.00200

Biolo, G., Cederholm, T., & Muscaritoli, M. (2014). Muscle contractile and metabolic dysfunction is a common feature of sarcopenia of aging and chronic diseases: From sarcopenic obesity to cachexia. *Clinical Nutrition*, *33*(5), 737–748. https://doi. org/10.1016/j.clnu.2014.03.007

Blancaflor, E., Cruz, M. R. A. D., Dionisio, N. M. E., Española, J. M. V., Maranan, J. W. J., & Miraflores, J. M. (2022, December). An IoT design of a dehydration indicator system based on urine color. In *2022 5th international conference on computing and big data (ICCBD)* (pp. 118–122). IEEE. https://doi.org/10.1109/ICCBD56965.2022. 10080279

Bouillon, R., & Suda, T. (2014). Vitamin D: Calcium and bone homeostasis during evolution. *BoneKEy Reports*, *3*. https://doi.org/10.1038%2Fbonekey.2013.214

Brady, S. R., Mamuaya, B. B., Cicuttini, F., Wluka, A. E., Wang, Y., Hussain, S. M., & Urquhart, D. M. (2015). Body composition is associated with multisite lower body musculoskeletal pain in a community-based study. *The Journal of Pain*, *16*(8), 700–706. https://doi.org/10.1016/j.jpain.2015.04.006

Byrne, C. S., Chambers, E. S., Morrison, D. J., & Frost, G. (2015). The role of short chain fatty acids in appetite regulation and energy homeostasis. *International Journal of Obesity*, *39*(9), 1331–1338. https://doi.org/10.1038/ijo.2015.84

Cameron, J. D., Sigal, R. J., Kenny, G. P., Alberga, A. S., Prud'homme, D., Phillips, P., Doucette, S., & Goldfield, G. (2016). Body composition and energy intake – skeletal muscle mass is the strongest predictor of food intake in obese adolescents: The HEARTY trial. *Applied Physiology, Nutrition, and Metabolism*, *41*(6), 611–617. https://doi.org/10.1139/apnm-2015-0479

Demerath, E. W., & Fields, D. A. (2014). Body composition assessment in the infant. *American Journal of Human Biology*, *26*(3), 291–304. https://doi.org/10.1002/ ajhb.22500

Dharmawan, A., Dharmawan, A., Setiawati, Y., & Yurista, S. (2023). The relationship between hypertension factors and the severity of hypertension: A literature. *International Journal of Creative Thoughts*, *11*(7), e629–e633.

Enoki, Y., Sato, T., Kokabu, S., Hayashi, N., Iwata, T., Yamato, M., Usui, M., Matsumoto, M., Tomoda, T., Ariyoshi, W., Nishihara, T., & Yoda, T. (2017). Netrin-4 promotes differentiation. *In Vivo*, *31*(5), 793–799. https://iv.iiarjournals.org/content/31/5/793.short

Feng, C., Xu, Z., Tang, X., Cao, H., Zhang, G., & Tan, J. (2022). Estrogen-related receptor α: A significant regulator and promising target in bone homeostasis and bone metastasis. *Molecules*, *27*(13), 3976. https://doi.org/10.3390/molecules27133976

Fothergill, E., Guo, J., Howard, L., Kerns, J. C., Knuth, N. D., Brychta, R., Chen, K. Y., Skarulis, M. C., Walter, M., Walter, P. J., & Hall, K. D. (2016). Persistent metabolic adaptation 6 years after "the biggest loser" competition. *Obesity*, *24*(8), 1612–1619. https://doi.org/10.1002/oby.21538

Gáliková, M., Dircksen, H., & Nässel, D. R. (2018). The thirsty fly: Ion transport peptide (ITP) is a novel endocrine regulator of water homeostasis in Drosophila. *PLoS Genetics*, *14*(8), e1007618.

Gizowski, C., & Bourque, C. W. (2018). The neural basis of homeostatic and anticipatory thirst. *Nature Reviews Nephrology*, *14*(1), 11–25. https://doi.org/10.1038/ nrneph.2017.149

Gong, R., Liu, Y., Luo, G., & Yang, L. (2022). Dietary magnesium intake affects the vitamin D effects on HOMA-β and risk of pancreatic β-cell dysfunction: A cross-sectional study. *Frontiers in Nutrition*, *9*, 849747. https://doi.org/10.3389/fnut.2022.849747

Gungor, O., Ulu, S., Hasbal, N. B., Anker, S. D., & Kalantar-Zadeh, K. (2021). Effects of hormonal changes on sarcopenia in chronic kidney disease: Where are we now and what can we do? *Journal of Cachexia, Sarcopenia and Muscle*, *12*(6), 1380–1392. https://doi.org/10.1002/jcsm.12839

Harfmann, B. D., Schroder, E. A., Kachman, M. T., Hodge, B. A., Zhang, X., & Esser, K. A. (2016). Muscle-specific loss of Bmal1 leads to disrupted tissue glucose metabolism and systemic glucose homeostasis. *Skeletal Muscle*, *6*(1), 1–13.

Hermans, C., Conn, S. J., Chen, J., Xiao, Q., & Verbruggen, N. (2013). An update on magnesium homeostasis mechanisms in plants. *Metallomics*, *5*(9), 1170–1183. https://doi.org/10.1039/c3mt20223b

Hodgson, K. (2016). *Keep you and your family lean with lean protein*. Virginia Tech. https://vtechworks.lib.vt.edu/bitstream/handle/10919/75383/348-672.pdf?sequence=1&isAllowed=y

Holmes, C. J., & Racette, S. B. (2021). The utility of body composition assessment in nutrition and clinical practice: An overview of current methodology. *Nutrients*, *13*(8), 2493. https://doi.org/10.3390/nu13082493225

Hoque, M. A., Alam, H. S. K., Sayeed, M. A., Al Mamun, M. A., & Islam, M. N. (2020). Electrolyte changes in malnourished under-5 children with or without diarrhoea. *Journal of Shaheed Suhrawardy Medical College*, *12*(1), 50–53. http://www.banglajol.info/index.php/JSSMC

Hussain, R. (2016). *Prevalence of overweight and obesity among AA. Himandhoo school of age 6–17 year and their knowledge, attitude and practice towards overweight and obesity* [Thesis, The Maldives National University]. http://saruna.mnu.edu.mv/jspui/bitstream/123456789/1617/1/Ramiz%20Hussain%20May%202016.pdf

Jaiswal, A. K., Sadasivam, M., Aja, S., & Hamad, A. R. A. (2020). Lack of Syndecan-1 produces significant alterations in whole-body composition, metabolism and glucose homeostasis in mice. *World Journal of Diabetes*, *11*(4), 126. https://doi.org/10.4239%2Fwjd.v11.i4.126

Jarouliya, U., & Keservani, R. K. (2019). Protein function as cell surface and nuclear receptor in human diseases. In *Medicinal chemistry with pharmaceutical product development* (pp. 1–32). CRC Press.

Kamaludin, K., Subarjah, H., & Pitriani, P. (2021). The influence of superset training model and circuit training on fat mass changes and muscle mass increase in men. *Competitor*, *13*(3), 362–370. https://dx.doi.org/10.26858/cjpko.v13i3.22807

Kanungo, S., Wells, K., Tribett, T., & El-Gharbawy, A. (2018). Glycogen metabolism and glycogen storage disorders. *Annals of Translational Medicine*, *6*(24). https://doi.org/10.21037%2Fatm.2018.10.59

Kiss, T., Bluth, T., & de Abreu, M. G. (2016). Perioperative complications of obese patients. *Current Opinion in Critical Care*, *22*(4), 401–405. https://doi.org/10.1097/MCC.0000000000000322

Kumala, S. H., Widiretnani, S., & Moelyo, A. G. (2022). The relationship between triceps skinfold thickness and age of menarche adolescent girls in Surakarta city junior high school. *Smart Medical Journal*, *5*(3), 142–147. https://doi.org/10.13057/smj.v5i3.64665

Kuriyan, R. (2018). Body composition techniques. *The Indian Journal of Medical Research*, *148*(5), 648–658. https://doi.org/10.4103/ijmr.IJMR_1777_18

Lee, D. H., Keum, N., Hu, F. B., Orav, E. J., Rimm, E. B., Willett, W. C., & Giovannucci, E. L. (2018). Predicted lean body mass, fat mass, and all cause and cause specific mortality in men: Prospective US cohort study. *BMJ*, *362*. https://doi.org/10.1136/bmj.k2575

Li, X., Qi, B., Zhang, S., & Li, Y. (2023). Foodomics revealed the effects of ultrasonic extraction on the composition and nutrition of cactus fruit (Opuntia ficus-indica) seed oil. *Ultrasonics Sonochemistry*, *97*, 106459. https://doi.org/10.1016/j.ultsonch.2023.106459226

Lin, Y., Wang, Z., Liu, S., Liu, J., Zhang, Z., Ouyang, Y., Su, Z., Chen, D., Guo, L., & Luo, T. (2023). Roles of extracellular vesicles on macrophages in inflammatory bone diseases. *Molecular and Cellular Biochemistry*, 1–14. https://doi.org/10.1007/s11010-023-04809-w

Loh, K., Zhang, L., Brandon, A., Wang, Q., Begg, D., Qi, Y., Fu, M., Kulkarni, R., Teo, J., Baldock, P., Brüning, J. C., Cooney, G., Neely, G., & Herzog, H. (2017). Insulin controls food intake and energy balance via NPY neurons. *Molecular Metabolism*, *6*(6), 574–584. https://doi.org/10.1016/j.molmet.2017.03.013

Lorenzo, I., Serra-Prat, M., & Yébenes, J. C. (2019). The role of water homeostasis in muscle function and frailty: A review. *Nutrients*, *11*(8), 1857. https://doi.org/10.3390/nu11081857

MacDonald, A. J. (2015). *Assessment of muscle wasting* [Dissertation, Edinburgh Medical School]. http://hdl.handle.net/1842/16455

Mahesh, M., Mahantesh, M., Vijayasree, K., & Kulkarni, V. (2018). Clinical profile of hypernatremic dehydration in neonates with special emphasis to acute kidney injury. *Journal of Pediatric Critical Care*, *5*(5), 26. http://doi.org/10.21304/2018.0505.00421

Margaritelis, N. V., Theodorou, A. A., Kyparos, A., Nikolaidis, M. G., & Paschalis, V. (2019). Effect of body composition on redox homeostasis at rest and in response to exercise: The case of underfat women. *Journal of Sports Sciences*, *37*(14), 1630–1637. https://doi.org/10.1080/02640414.2019.1578450

Mauvais-Jarvis, F., Clegg, D. J., & Hevener, A. L. (2013). The role of estrogens in control of energy balance and glucose homeostasis. *Endocrine Reviews*, *34*(3), 309–338. https://doi.org/10.1210/er.2012-1055

Mehmood, S. (2017). *Prediction of protein solubility in Escherichia coli and experimental verification* [Doctoral dissertation, University of Management & Technology]. http://hdl.handle.net/123456789/3458

Min, R., & van der Knaap, M. S. (2018). Genetic defects disrupting glial ion and water homeostasis in the brain. *Brain Pathology*, *28*(3), 372–387. https://doi.org/10.1111/bpa.12602

Minegishi, S., Luft, F. C., Titze, J., & Kitada, K. (2020). Sodium handling and interaction in numerous organs. *American Journal of Hypertension*, *33*(8), 687–694. https://doi.org/10.1093/ajh/hpaa049

Møller, J. B., Pedersen, M., Tanaka, H., Ohsugi, M., Overgaard, R. V., Lynge, J., Almind, K., Vasconcelos, N. M., Poulsen, P., Keller, C., Ueki, K., & Kadowaki, T. (2014). Body composition is the main determinant for the difference in type 2 diabetes pathophysiology between Japanese and Caucasians. *Diabetes Care*, *37*(3), 796–804. https://doi.org/10.2337/dc13-0598

Mosler, S., Relizani, K., Mouisel, E., Amthor, H., & Diel, P. (2014). Combinatory effects of SI RNA- induced myostatin inhibition and exercise on skeletal muscle homeostasis and body composition. *Physiological Reports*, *2*(3), e00262. https://doi.org/10.1002/phy2.262

Nicholls, J., Chin, J., Williams, T., Lenton, T., O'Flaherty, V., & McGrath, J. (2023). On the potential roles of phosphorus in the early evolution of energy metabolism. *Frontiers in Microbiology*, *14*. https://doi.org/10.3389/fmicb.2023.1239189

Nogueira, E. C., Porto, L. G. G., Nogueira, R. M., Martins, W. R., Fonseca, R. M., Lunardi, C. C., & de Oliveira, R. J. (2016). Body composition is strongly associated with cardiorespiratory fitness in a large Brazilian military firefighter cohort: The Brazilian firefighters study. *The Journal of Strength & Conditioning Research*, *30*(1), 33–38. https://doi.org/10.1519/JSC.0000000000001039

Öhrnell Malekzadeh, B. (2017). *Insulin-coated titanium implants-a potential therapy for local bone regeneration* [Dissertation, University of Gothenburg, Sahlgrenska Academy]. http://hdl.handle.net/2077/51877

Ørtenblad, N., Westerblad, H., & Nielsen, J. (2013). Muscle glycogen stores and fatigue. *The Journal of Physiology*, *591*(18), 4405–4413. https://doi.org/10.1113/jphysiol.2013.251629

Pardo, M. M. C., Crujeiras, A. B., Amil, M., Aguera, Z., Jiménez-Murcia, S., Baños, R., Botella, C., de la Torre, R., Estivill, X., Fagundo, A. B., Fernández-Real, J. M., Fernández-García, J. C., Fruhbeck, G., Gómez-Ambrosi, J., Rodríguez, R., Tinahones, F. J., & Casanueva, F. F. (2014). Association of irisin with fat mass, resting energy expenditure, and daily activity in conditions of extreme body mass index. *International Journal of Endocrinology, 2014*, 857270. https://doi.org/10.1155/2014/857270

Prado, M. M. C., Maia, L. M. M., Ormsbee, M., Sawyer, M. B., & Baracos, V. E. (2013). Assessment of nutritional status in cancer – the relationship between body composition and pharmacokinetics. *Anti-Cancer Agents in Medicinal Chemistry (Formerly Current Medicinal Chemistry-Anti-Cancer Agents), 13*(8), 1197–1203. https://www.ingentaconnect.com/content/ben/acamc/2013/00000013/00000008/art00007

Riaz, S. (2014). Obesity as a risk factor for diabetes mellitus in the local population of Pakistan. *Universal Journal of Clinical Medicine, 2*(3), 58–64. https://doi.org/10.13189/ujcm.2014.020302

Robinson, S. (2021). Diet and health. In *Priorities for health promotion and public health: Explaining the evidence for disease prevention and health promotion* (pp. 200–232). Routledge.

Rosenbaum, M., & Leibel, R. L. (2016). Models of energy homeostasis in response to maintenance of reduced body weight. *Obesity, 24*(8), 1620–1629. https://doi.org/10.1002/oby.21559

Salman, M. M., Kitchen, P., Halsey, A., Wang, M. X., Törnroth-Horsefield, S., Conner, A. C., Badaut, J., Iliff, J. J., & Bill, R. M. (2022). Emerging roles for dynamic aquaporin-4 subcellular relocalization in CNS water homeostasis. *Brain, 145*(1), 64–75. https://doi.org/10.1093/brain/awab311

Sandberg, C., Crenshaw, A. G., Christersson, C., Hlebowicz, J., Thilén, U., & Johansson, B. (2021). Despite reductions in muscle mass and muscle strength in adults with CHD, the muscle strength per muscle mass relationship does not differ from controls. *Cardiology in the Young, 31*(5), 792–798. https://doi.org/10.1017/S1047951120004709

Service, R. F. (2015). Protein power. *Science, 349*(6246), 372–373. https://doi.org/10.1126/science.349.6246.372

Shore, R. M., & Chesney, R. W. (2013). Rickets: Part I. *Pediatric Radiology, 43*, 140–151. https://doi.org/10.1007/s00247-012-2532-x

Singh, A. (2016). Indispensable role of protein in cancer. *Journal of Practical Biochemistry and Biophysics, 1*(1). https://www.researchgate.net/profile/Anju-Singh-15/publication/316560587_Indispensable_Role_of_Protein_in_Cancer/links/5904450d0f7e9bc0d58d9967/Indispensable-Role-of-Protein-in-Cancer.pdf

Sladek, C. D., & Johnson, A. K. (2013). Integration of thermal and osmotic regulation of water homeostasis: The role of TRPV channels. *American Journal of Physiology-Regulatory, Integrative and Comparative Physiology, 305*(7), R669–R678. https://doi.org/10.1152/ajpregu.00270.2013

Strzelczyk, M., Gimbut, M., & Łochyńska, M. (2023). Nuts of fibrous hemp cannabis sativa L.-concentrated power of nutrients. *Journal of Natural Fibers, 20*(1), 2128967. https://doi.org/10.1080/15440478.2022.2128967

Szczuko, M., Pokorska-Niewiada, K., Kwiatkowska, L., Nawrocka-Rutkowska, J., Szydłowska, I., & Ziętek, M. (2022). Level of potassium is associated with saturated fatty acids in cell membranes and influences the activation of the 9 and 13 HODE and 5 HETE synthesis pathways in PCOS. *Biomedicines, 10*(9), 2244. https://doi.org/10.3390/biomedicines10092244

Tang, S. Y., & Alliston, T. (2013). Regulation of postnatal bone homeostasis by TGFβ. *BoneKEy Reports, 2*. https://doi.org/10.1038%2Fbonekey.2012.255

Tee, C. C. L., Cooke, M. B., Chong, M. C., Yeo, W. K., & Camera, D. M. (2023). Mechanisms for combined hypoxic conditioning and divergent exercise modes to regulate inflammation, body composition, appetite, and blood glucose homeostasis in overweight and obese adults: A narrative review. *Sports Medicine, 53*(2), 327–348. https://doi.org/10.1007/s40279-022-01782-0

Thanigaivel, S., Chandrasekaran, N., Mukherjee, A., & Thomas, J. (2016). Seaweeds as an alternative therapeutic source for aquatic disease management. *Aquaculture, 464*, 529–536. https://doi.org/10.1016/j.aquaculture.2016.08.001

Turk, S. A., van Schaardenburg, D., Boers, M., de Boer, S., Fokker, C., Lems, W. F., & Nurmohamed, M. T. (2018). An unfavorable body composition is common in early arthritis patients: A case control study. *PLoS One*, *13*(3). https://doi.org/10.1371/journal.pone.0193377

Vigh-Larsen, J. F., Ørtenblad, N., Spriet, L. L., Overgaard, K., & Mohr, M. (2021). Muscle glycogen metabolism and high-intensity exercise performance: A narrative review. *Sports Medicine*, *51*(9), 1855–1874. https://doi.org/10.1007/s40279-021-01475-0

Waitt, A. E., Reed, L., Ransom, B. R., & Brown, A. M. (2017). Emerging roles for glycogen in the CNS. *Frontiers in Molecular Neuroscience*, *10*, 73. https://doi.org/10.3389/fnmol.2017.00073

Wang, Z. M., Pierson, R. N., Jr., & Heymsfield, S. B. (1992). The five-level model: A new approach to organizing body-composition research. *The American Journal of Clinical Nutrition*, *56*(1), 19–28. https://doi.org/10.1093/ajcn/56.1.19

Weber, D. R., Leonard, M. B., & Zemel, B. S. (2012). Body composition analysis in the pediatric population. *Pediatric Endocrinology Reviews*, *10*(1), 130–139. https://www.ncbi.nlm.nih.gov/pmc/articles/PMC4154503/

Yilmaz, U. C. A. N. (2013). Effects of different types of exercises on body composition in young men and women. *Life Science Journal*, *10*(3). http://www.lifesciencesite.com/lsj/life1003/269_20467life1003_1799_1805.pdf

Zemel, B., & Barden, E. (2004). Measuring body composition. In R. C. Hauspie, N. Cameron, & L. Molinari (Eds.), *Methods in human growth research* (Vol. 39, pp. 141–176). Cambridge University Press.

Zhang, R. H., Guo, Z. H., Zhang, Q., Zha, G. H., Cao, C. X., Fan, L. Y., & Liu, W. W. (2023). Determination of human serum total protein via electrophoresis titration and capacitively coupled contactless conductivity detection. *Chinese Journal of Chromatography*, *41*(8), 707–713. https://doi.org/10.3724/sp.j.1123.2023.04015

13

ENERGY PRODUCTION AND UTILIZATION

Nguyen Tra Giang and Oliver Napila Gomez

The requisite motor control and energy regulation skills allow people to carry out physical activities. Kinetic fitness, a term coined in the USFD Framework, refers to efficiently utilizing the energy generated by the cardiovascular and musculo-skeletal systems. For strength, power, and endurance to work together, kinetic fitness – supported by the anaerobic lactic, phosphocreatine, and aerobic energy systems, respectively – is essential. Differentiating between the several kinds of muscle fibers provides evidence of their function in enabling various muscu-lar actions. The human body contains various muscle fiber types, such as slow-twitch oxidative, fast-twitch glycolytic, and slow-twitch oxidative. Motor unit recruitment relies on intricate synchronization, and they are essential for efficient muscle contractions. Motor unit recruitment is impacted by task complexity and weight as well. Muscular fitness is also greatly affected by gender and body composition variations over life. A firm grasp of the kinetic fitness system and its parts is imperative to create successful training programs and encourage physical wellness in general.

Outcomes

By the end of this chapter, you will be able to:

- explain the concept of kinetic fitness, mainly its function in energy production and utilization and movement
- explore the physiological underpinnings of force production, the interaction between mass and acceleration, and practical ways for testing and strengthen-ing muscle strength

DOI: 10.4324/9781003502937-15

- investigate the concept of muscular power, stressing its importance in actions that require quick force generation
- investigate muscular endurance, with a focus on its involvement in extended contractions against resistance
- relate the concept of motor unit recruitment in coordinating muscles for varied tasks.

The system functions for skill

For review, flexibility, muscular strength, and muscular endurance are three aspects of muscle fitness that belong to the same category as cardiorespiratory fitness and body composition, according to what we know about health-related fitness so far (Blais, 2018; Cibulka & Barron, 2017). The risk of cardiovascular illness increases in children with poor cardiorespiratory fitness and muscular strength since these factors predict cardiovascular health in adults. In addition, the organization of HRF has included muscle power (Corbin & Le Masurier, 2014; Ahmed, 2015). When assessing health and disease, musculoskeletal fitness measures are crucial (Hsu et al., 2021). There is a correlation between the results of simple, noninvasive field musculoskeletal fitness testing and the health of youthful bones and muscles (Janz et al., 2022).

Nonetheless, our idea has progressed within the USFD structure. Two system functions for skill (movement and energy regulation) work together for energy production and utilization, making it possible to execute skills. We have coined the term "kinetic fitness" to characterize the unique fitness function that results from utilizing the kinetic energy produced by the musculoskeletal and cardiorespiratory systems (see Figure 13.1).

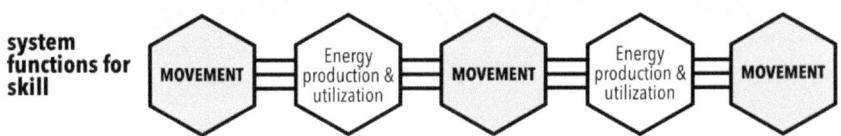

FIGURE 13.1   Energy production and utilization – shared by movement and energy regulation

Notice that in Figure 13.1, energy production and utilization are shared by two grouped system functions (movement and energy regulation. This implies that the function is primarily for skills to accomplish tasks.

Additionally, we recognize the role of coordination as the core component of the system functions for skill in synthesizing explosive strength (muscular power) and sustained exertion of muscular force (muscular endurance) (Kiely, 2017). Moreover, it is essential to remember that the motor control components (balance, flexibility, reaction time, speed control, and reactive agility) still play critical roles in effective and efficient strength and movement (Fort-Vanmeerhaeghe et al., 2016). Specifically, they contribute to the management and quality of strength execution suitable to the requirement of a specific task (Ojanen et al., 2020).

Muscular strength

The ability to move the joints freely is a hallmark of flexibility, yet the production of muscular force and energy expenditure are necessary for many activities. The development of muscular strength is antecedent to force (Narici et al., 2003). According to Newton's second law of motion, the product of mass and acceleration is force, $F = ma$. The mass of the body, or its capacity to increase speed, needs to be proportional to the force that the muscles produce. The amount of force that the muscles must provide is directly proportional to the product of the object's acceleration (in m/s^2) and its mass (in kg). According to this law of motion, an enormous amount of force is required to move a heavy body. Additionally, lifting, pushing, pulling, or moving a heavyweight requires tremendous force (Tamir, 2015).

Force gives the ability to grasp, push, pull, or lift a heavy object, requiring strength – the ability to move the body or an item with force measures muscular strength, a fitness component (Suchomel et al., 2018). A person's maximum force production is theoretically their muscular strength (Roberts & Petersen, 2023). The highest weight a person can lift for one repetition (also known as 1RM) is what we notice in terms of performance since force is equal to the object's mass multiplied by its acceleration (Taber et al., 2016).

Practical methods of determining the heaviest load capacity are precarious, especially for untrained and inexperienced individuals (DiStasio, 2014). Hence, existing muscular strength assessments focus on estimating maximum force using strength exercises with reduced load for safety (also known as submaximal strength exercises). Meanwhile, the physiological aspect of muscle contraction and force production is discussed to offer new perspectives on muscular strength.

Force production

A skeletal muscle has thousands of muscle cells (called muscle fibers) bundled together by connective tissues. According to Powers and colleagues (2021),

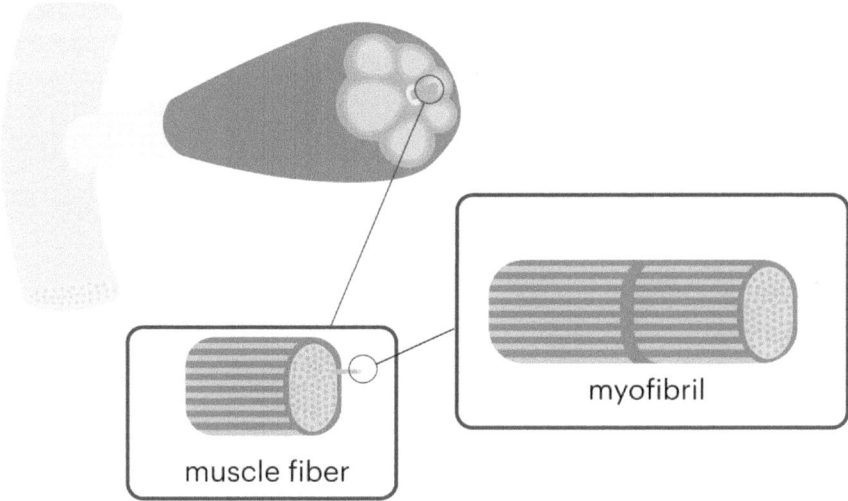

FIGURE 13.2   The myofibrils

the muscle cells are unique for their striated and cylindrical structure, generating force when they contract. On a cellular level, the sliding filament theory explains how muscle contractions convert adenosine triphosphate (ATP) into mechanical energy (Cooper, 2000). Muscle fibers contain segmented myofibrils. Each segment is called a sarcomere, the basic unit of the muscle fiber. Each sarcomere contains bundled protein filaments called myosin (thick filament) and actin (thin filament). Sarcomere contraction generates force. Inside the sarcomere, the myosin and actin overlap. The head of the myosin hydrolyzes ATP into adenosine diphosphate (ADP) and inorganic phosphate (IP). ATPase helps as a catalyst for ATP hydrolysis. Subsequently, the energy released from the hydrolyzed ATP (ADP+IP) invigorates the myosin to prepare it to form a cross-bridge with the actin.

The two proteins, tropomyosin and troponin, operate as barriers, obstructing actin's binding sites and preventing it from interlacing with myosin. Myosin can attach to actin because calcium (Ca^{2+}) binds with tropomyosin and troponin, revealing the binding sites. Myosin and actin weave together to separate ADP from inorganic phosphate. Muscular force is generated by cutting the inorganic phosphate. Because of this, it is known as a power stroke. Ultimately, the ADP separates from the myosin (Wakabayashi, 2015).

With every contraction of a sarcomere, force is generated. Nevertheless, actions involving strength differ. To comprehend different tasks that entail strength, it is necessary to include ATP, energy systems, and the many types of skeletal muscle fibers in this discussion. The two mixed-type components of

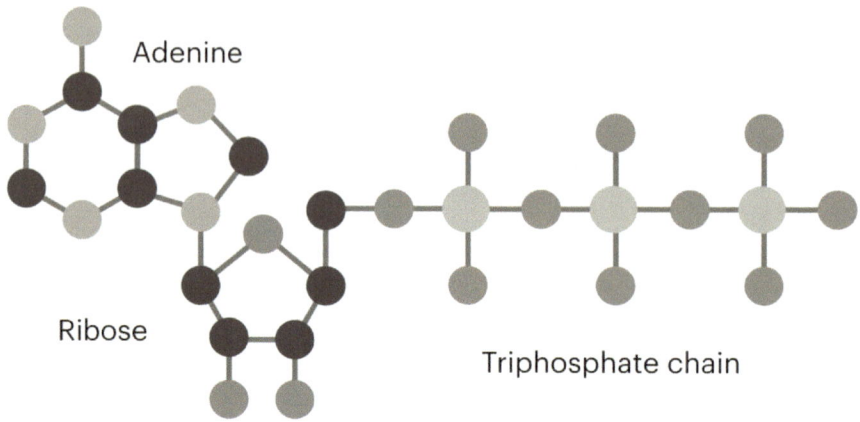

Adenine

Ribose

Triphosphate chain

FIGURE 13.3   Adenosine triphosphate

muscle strength, which are power and endurance, are better understood in light of the information presented here (Hargreaves & Spriet, 2020).

The role of adenosine triphosphate (ATP)

With every power stroke in the sarcomere, muscles can generate force, an essential precursor for muscular strength. It is necessary to understand where this energy comes from, which powers muscular contractions – adenosine triphosphate (ATP).

ATP is an energy-carrying molecule in all living cells metabolically processed from glucose, a simple sugar from carbohydrates. The digestive system digests and absorbs glucose from food. Glucose becomes glycogen stores in the liver and skeletal muscles through glycogenesis if not used as energy. When the body becomes active, a reverse metabolic process called glycolysis converts glycogen stores back into glucose for immediate energy requirement. The net upshot of glycolysis per glucose molecule includes two ATP, two pyruvate, and two NADH or nicotinamide adenine dinucleotide (NAD) + hydrogen (H) (Chandel, 2021).

Strength and anaerobic lactic energy system

In an environment with insufficient oxygen, the purpose of pyruvate is to neutralize acidosis so that the working muscle can last longer. The pyruvate bonds with two H^+ to form lactate. They exit from the cell and travel to the liver. This process reduces acidosis caused by the build-up of H^+ in the working muscle tissues (Wang et al., 2018; Semler & Singer, 2019).

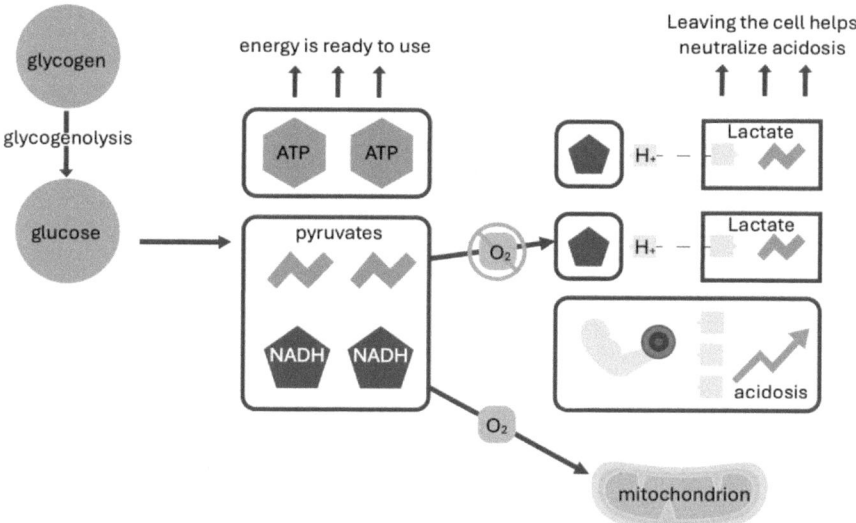

FIGURE 13.4   The anaerobic lactic energy system

In short, the ATP produced from glycolysis fuels muscular contraction. At the same time, the escape of lactate from the muscle cells is why people can endure anaerobic strength-related tasks such as the repeated lifting of heavyweights. This pathway is called the anaerobic lactic energy system.

Muscular strength works with the anaerobic lactic energy system to sustain strength-related tasks. The muscles do not use oxygen to generate ATP when gripping, pushing, pulling, or lifting heavy objects. Instead, the muscles rely on ATP and lactate to defuse the build-up of H^+.

Muscular power

The capacity to swiftly produce maximum force is a measure of muscular power, often known as explosive strength. Explosive motions like jumping, throwing, and sprinting rely on the brain's ability to coordinate elements such as muscle strength, speed control, and other senses (see Figure 13.5, for example). The capacity of the nervous system to assemble and activate motor units in a synchronized and coordinated fashion is essential for the quick production of force by the muscles.

Power and the phosphocreatine energy system

Some strength-related tasks need rapid contraction. Aside from changing the sarcomere's length, the increased contraction velocity can also increase force (Blazevich & Blazevich, 2017). Relating the velocity of shortening muscle length

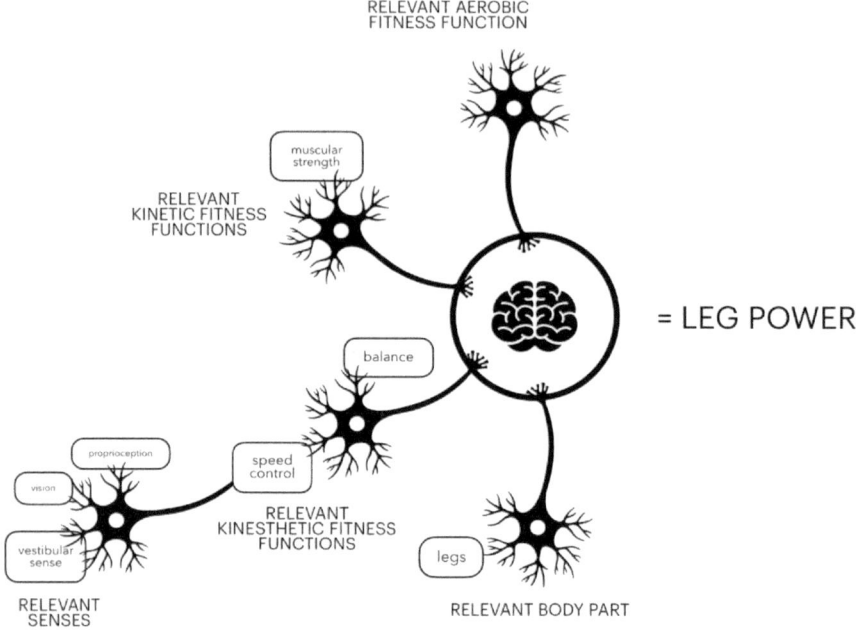

RELEVANT AEROBIC
FITNESS FUNCTION

muscular
strength

RELEVANT
KINETIC FITNESS
FUNCTIONS

= LEG POWER

balance

proprioception

vision

speed
control

vestibular
sense

RELEVANT
KINESTHETIC FITNESS
FUNCTIONS

legs

RELEVANT
SENSES

RELEVANT BODY PART

FIGURE 13.5   Leg power – a product of coordination

to force can yield a hybrid of kinetic (force) and kinesthetic fitness (speed) – muscular power.

In the anaerobic lactic energy system, anaerobic glycolysis takes ten seconds to three minutes to convert glucose into ATP, pyruvate, and NADH without oxygen. However, the demand for ATP production is more urgent than ten seconds for muscular power. The energy system that can produce immediate ATP this fast is the phosphocreatine energy system (Guimarães-Ferreira, 2014).

Creatine is a molecule naturally synthesized in the liver. It travels through the bloodstream and enters skeletal muscle fibers. The enzyme creatine kinase in the mitochondria catalyzes phosphorylation to produce creatine phosphate. Creatine phosphate enters the myofibrils, where used ATP drops an ADP. Another creatine kinase in the sarcomere catalyzes the transfer of phosphate from creatine phosphate to bond with ADP, producing ATP for immediate energy. The creatine molecule returns to the mitochondria for reuse as needed (Bonilla et al., 2021).

Power demands a rapid rate of force development (RFD), the ability to produce maximum force quickly in every muscle contraction (McLellan et al., 2011). The phosphocreatine energy system allows creatine phosphate to donate one phosphate molecule to convert ADP to ATP in the sarcomere immediately after a power stroke. However, although the body can produce creatine phosphate independently, it is limited and can only be used for up to ten seconds.

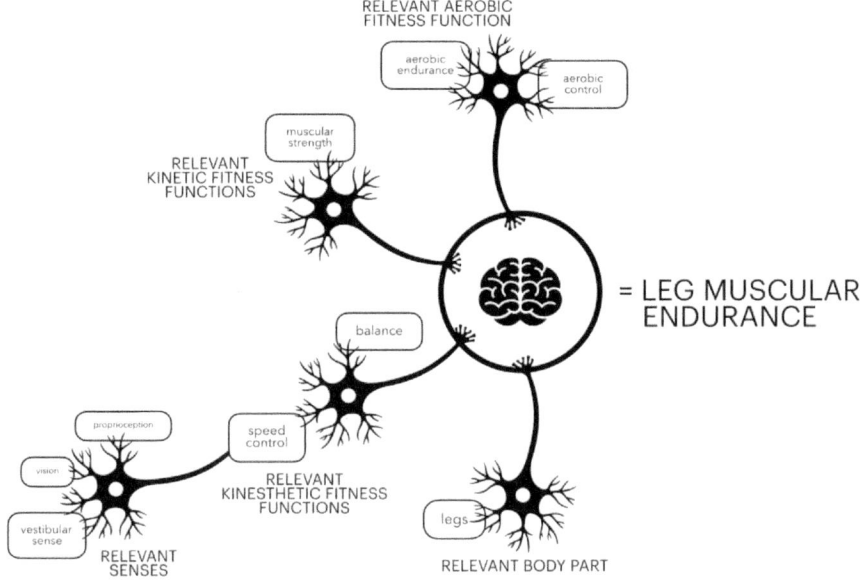

FIGURE 13.6   Leg muscular endurance – product of coordination

Hence, the activities involve explosive strength and speed, such as sprinting, throwing, and jumping.

Muscular endurance

The maximum time the anaerobic lactic energy system can work without oxygen is estimated to be from ten seconds to three minutes, depending on the performer's fitness level.

However, until the anaerobic threshold is reached – the limit beyond which the burning sensation generated by H^+ buildup may be tolerated – some strength-related tasks may continue longer (Wasserman, 2015). The contractions may become less intense while the body transitions from an anaerobic to an aerobic energy system (Swanwick & Matthews, 2018). At this stage, an oxygenated environment is utilized to make ATP, which enables muscles to contract for longer durations, resulting in endurance.

Endurance and the aerobic energy system

The pathway for the aerobic energy system begins at glycolysis. Glycogen turns into glucose. Then, glucose converts into two ATP, two pyruvate, and two NADH. With oxygen, these molecules enter the mitochondrion, the cell's powerhouse, where oxidative phosphorylation occurs (Morelli et al., 2020). Pyruvate converts into acetyl coenzyme A, an essential substance for the citric acid cycle (also known as Kreb's cycle). The citric acid cycle generates two ATP, eight NADH, two flavin adenine dinucleotide (FADH$_2$), and the by-product, carbon dioxide (Mahundi & Manwa, 2015). The NADH and FADH$_2$ are essential for the electron transport chain, which generates 34 ATP and the by-product, water (Cogliati et al., 2021).

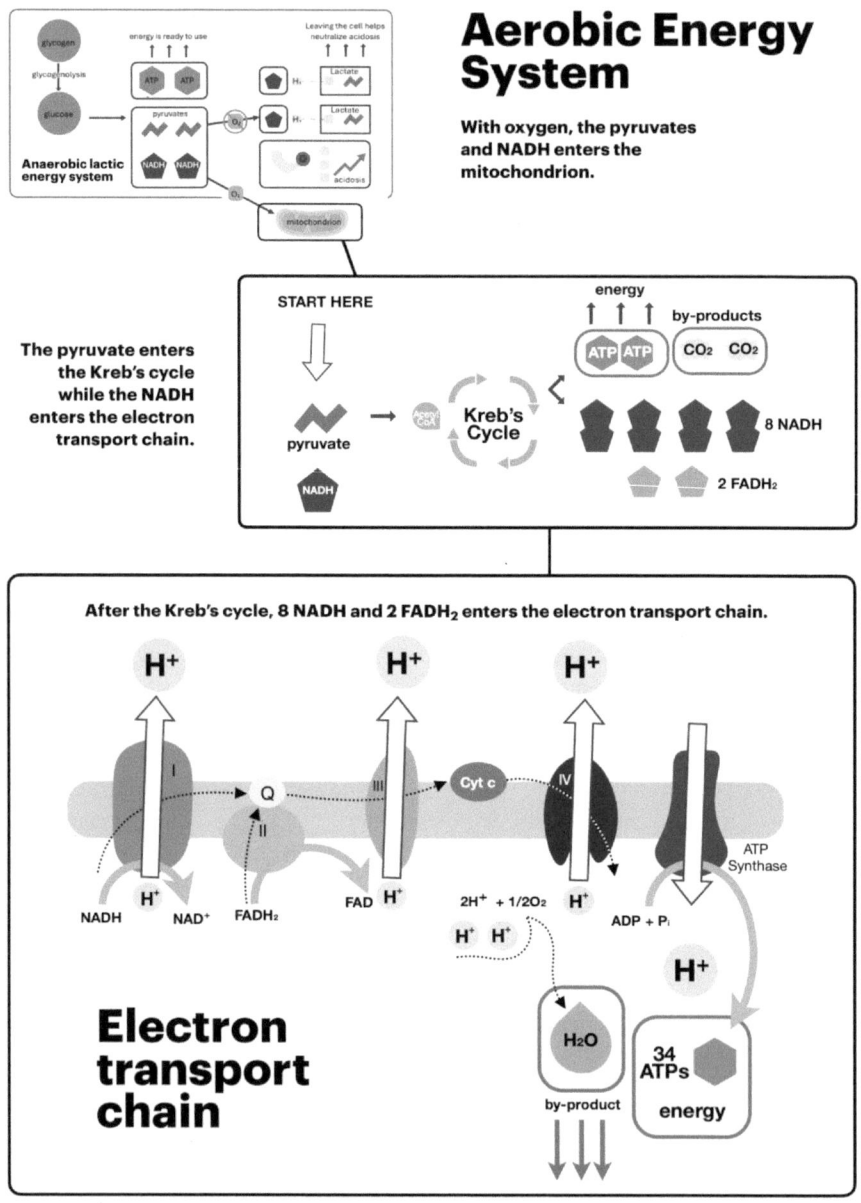

FIGURE 13.7 The aerobic energy system

Moreover, H⁺ does not build up in the mitochondrion. Instead, they play a vital role in the production of ATP through ATP synthase (Garcia-Bermudez et al., 2015). The aerobic energy system can sustain prolonged muscular contraction with oxygen at intensities lower than anaerobic levels. Activities such as running, cycling, swimming, mountain climbing, wall climbing, and other activities classified under aerobic activities require muscular endurance. Muscular endurance is the ability of the muscles or muscle group to generate force through a contraction for an extended period without easily tiring. Force moves the body or a heavy object.

Muscular contractions without oxygen can endure for a short period to produce force until the anaerobic threshold is reached. Thus, we call this anaerobic muscular endurance. Increasing the acceleration of moving an object may yield a similar effect.

As previously mentioned, muscular endurance is a hybrid function because oxygen supports the efficiency of muscular endurance. In an oxygenated environment, the muscles contract until their aerobic threshold, the margin between aerobic and anaerobic intensity when pyruvate begins to collect the hydrogen ions that are starting to build up. We call this type of endurance – aerobic muscular endurance – the ability of the muscles to endure contraction for an extended period with oxygen until reaching the aerobic threshold.

The interrelatedness of the kinetic fitness system functions

It is interesting to learn that muscular strength, power, and endurance are somehow related to the energy systems of the body:

- muscular strength works with the anaerobic lactic energy system
- muscular power works with the phosphocreatine energy system and
- muscular endurance works with the aerobic energy system.

Another compelling way to differentiate the three components involves the classification of the muscle fibers – slow-twitch and fast-twitch muscle fibers.

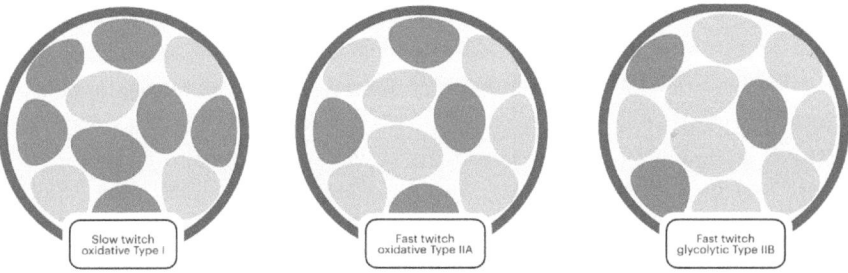

FIGURE 13.8   Types of muscle fibers

Slow twitch (Type I), called slow-twitch oxidative, is a fatigue-resistant muscle fiber. They contain abundant mitochondria and myoglobin, making the muscles reddish because they store iron and oxygen (Shenkman & Sharlo, 2021). Type I muscle fibers support the framework and flexibility of the body. These muscle fibers are responsible for slow and controlled movements intended for lifestyle activities such as rising and getting out of bed, preparing meals in the kitchen, getting ready for school or work, walking to a destination, and running errands (Jin et al., 2022). They maintain the body's upright posture and contribute to balance (Shenkman & Sharlo, 2021).

Fast-twitch oxidative (Type IIA) muscle fibers are used when the intensity of the activity increases. These muscle fibers are nearly the same as slow oxidative because they are rich in mitochondria and myoglobin but contract faster to generate force (Mishra et al., 2015). Fast-twitch oxidative muscle fibers are also called intermediate fibers because they possess the characteristics of slow-twitch oxidative and fast-twitch glycolytic muscles (Type IIB). They utilize glycogen through the aerobic energy system pathway. However, because fast-twitch oxidative muscle fibers generate force, they may become exhausted after a long work period, depending on the muscles' fitness level.

Type IIA muscle fibers sustain muscular endurance and aerobic fitness. These muscle fibers are responsible for movements demanding quick muscular contractions to generate force for aerobic activities (Plotkin et al., 2021). Running, swimming, rowing, climbing, and biking use Type IIA muscle fibers (Mitchell et al., 2018).

Moreover, the body uses the fast-twitch glycolytic muscle fibers (Type IIB) with anaerobic activities. These muscle fibers appear white because they contain fewer mitochondria and myoglobin. They contract quickly to generate force without oxygen. They metabolize glycogen for energy in approximately ten seconds up to three minutes for strength tasks. The fast-twitch glycolytic muscles utilize creatine phosphate for energy for immediate and abrupt power tasks. Because these muscle fibers do not use oxygen, they quickly become fatigued.

Type IIB muscle fibers support muscular strength. These muscle fibers are responsible for movements that demand quick muscular contractions to generate force intended for anaerobic activities. Resistance, weight training, and body-weight exercises use Type IIB muscle fibers to enhance muscular strength (Serrano et al., 2018).

Moreover, the kinesthetic fitness speed controlled by the nervous system can influence the quick muscular contraction of Type IIB muscle fibers (Reis et al., 2015) through rapid ATP phosphorylation from ADP and creatine phosphate. As a result, Type IIB muscle fiber combines force and speed to produce explosive strength, also called muscular power. Examples of activities that use muscular power include sprinting, jumping, and throwing. Ballistic training or jumping with weights and throwing heavy objects improves muscular power. Plyometrics or plyometric training also builds muscular power (Koh et al., 2018).

Motor unit recruitment – the link with kinesthetic fitness

Skeletal muscle fibers are voluntary because the nervous system controls their contraction. Each muscle fiber linked with a motor neuron is called a motor unit. Depending on the task, the nervous system recruits a specific type and number of muscle fibers to do the work (Celichowski & Krutki, 2019). With lifestyle activities, motor unit recruitment activates Type I muscle fibers (slow-twitch oxidative). Type IIA muscle fibers (fast-twitch oxidative) are activated at the aerobic level to support Type I muscle fibers. For anaerobic strength-related tasks, motor unit recruitment involves Type IIB muscle fibers (fast-twitch glycolytic), and the two muscle fibers are already working. Motor unit recruitment is the sequential engagement of motor units to add contracting muscles, leading to increased force production and muscular strength (Lai et al., 2018).

For tasks that involve weights and resistance, motor unit recruitment activates adjacent muscle groups successively to augment muscular contraction, raise force production, and increase muscular strength. If the weight exceeds the capability of a specific group of muscles, the motor unit recruitment activates other muscle groups (Steele & Fisher, 2018). However, suppose the object's weight is less than the strength capability of the same specific group of muscles. In that case, some motor units disengage so that force production concurs with the object's weight. Notice that the illustration in Figure 13.9 shows different objects that engage motor unit recruitment sequentially based on their weights.

Figure 13.9 provides a visual representation of the operationalization of successive motor unit recruitment in response to various weights and tasks, shedding light on the intricate coordination of muscles involved in different activities. Let us discuss each scenario:

a. **Holding a pen.** In this scenario, the task involves holding a lightweight pen, which primarily engages the motor units within the thumb and index

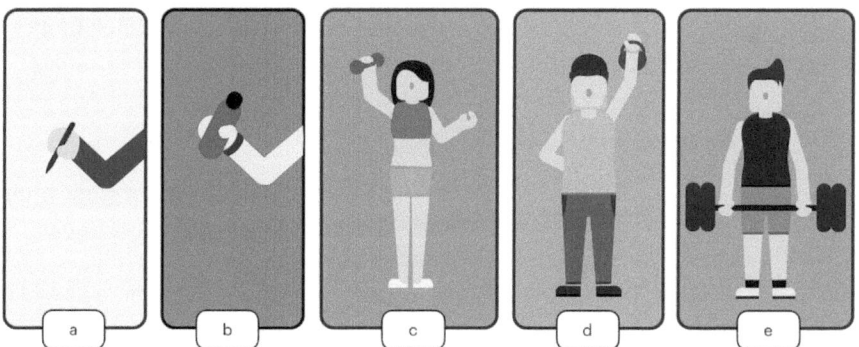

FIGURE 13.9   Successive motor unit recruitment with various weights

fingers. These motor units are typically composed of slow-twitch oxidative muscle fibers well suited for tasks requiring fine motor control and sustained contractions.

b. **Holding/gripping a water bottle**. When holding a water bottle, the task becomes slightly demanding. Additional motor units are recruited from adjacent muscle groups, including the middle, ring, pinky fingers, and palm. This expanded motor unit recruitment allows for a secure grip, accommodating the weight and shape of the water bottle.

c. **Holding and lifting a dumbbell**. Moving to a dumbbell involves a substantial motor unit recruitment pattern. Apart from the motor units responsible for handgrip, muscles spanning the wrist up to the midsection of the upper arm are activated. This recruitment facilitates the dumbbell's grip and lift, requiring strength and coordination.

d. **Holding and lifting a kettlebell**. The kettlebell represents a significant step up in terms of weight and, consequently, motor unit recruitment. When lifting a kettlebell, motor units in the deltoid and shoulder muscles are brought into action. This recruitment extends the involvement of muscles beyond the arm, engaging the shoulder region.

e. **Holding and lifting a barbell**. Finally, lifting a barbell is a complex task that necessitates recruiting motor units from various muscle groups. These include those responsible for handgrip and muscles in the back, chest, trunk, and even legs, depending on the specific lifting technique and the weight of the barbell. The engagement of these diverse muscle groups is essential for maintaining balance and control during barbell lifts, making it a comprehensive full-body exercise.

Figure 13.9 illustrates how motor unit recruitment adapts to the weight and complexity of tasks, emphasizing the importance of muscle coordination and strength in performing different activities. This insight into motor unit recruitment can be valuable for athletes, fitness enthusiasts, and healthcare professionals seeking to understand the mechanics of physical tasks and tailor training programs accordingly.

Factors that affect kinetic fitness functions

Aside from the type of muscle fibers and the energy systems, body composition can also affect muscular fitness, particularly the predominance of lean muscle tissues. Enormous muscle mass means many muscle fibers can contract to generate strength, power, and endurance. Likewise, weight training can help build muscle mass and strength. In addition, the quality of muscle fibers between boys and girls is theoretically the same during childhood. Children's muscle mass is premature. At puberty, the male sex hormone testosterone influences the body's ability to build muscle mass. Hence, muscular fitness can be influenced significantly by gender differences during adolescence. Muscle mass declines as people age (Goldspink, 2012; Keller & Engelhardt, 2014). When women reach the menopausal stage, the female sex hormone estrogen begins to drop, causing a decline in muscle mass and strength (Maltais et al., 2009).

Energy production and utilization and task performance

Task performance can be better understood by looking at the relationship between energy production and utilization through kinetic fitness. Physical activities are challenging because they require the efficient coordination of power, strength, and endurance, all of which are supported by distinct energy systems and types of muscle fibers. This knowledge is crucial in promoting physical fitness in general and creating effective training programs.

Research on the intricate relationship between energy production, use, and job performance is crucial to improving our health and fitness knowledge. The USFD Framework's description of "kinetic fitness" captures this dynamic by highlighting the significance of using the energy produced by the circulatory and musculoskeletal systems (Ahmed, 2015; Kiely, 2017). Performing physical tasks efficiently requires coordinating three distinct energy systems: anaerobic lactic, phosphocreatine, and aerobic. Each system contributes to muscle power, endurance, and strength (Corbin & Le Masurier, 2014; Hsu et al., 2021; Ojanen et al., 2020).

The capacity to generate force, as outlined by Newton's second law of motion, is intimately related to muscular strength, an essential part of this system (Narici et al., 2003; Tamir, 2015). A corresponding amount of muscular force is required for this kind of force production, which is, in turn, proportional to the mass and speed of the moving body or objects. Also, the sliding filament theory explains how muscles contract physiologically, which shows how ATP is involved in the contraction of muscle fibers and the inherent connection between energy utilization and strength (Cooper, 2000; Powers et al., 2021).

Furthermore, particular energy systems are highly related to muscle power and endurance. Rapid ATP production, essential for explosive actions such as jumping or running, depends on the phosphocreatine energy system, which depends on muscular strength (McLellan et al., 2011; Guimarães-Ferreira, 2014). Conversely, the aerobic energy system promotes muscular endurance, defined as the capacity to maintain force generation over long periods. This system's efficient ATP generation in an oxygen-rich environment allows running or cycling for extended periods (Morelli et al., 2020; Swanwick & Matthews, 2018).

The fact that humans possess a wide variety of muscle fiber types – including intermediate fast-twitch oxidative, slow-twitch oxidative, and fast-twitch glycolytic – adds to the complexity of kinetic fitness. Various physical activities call for different kinds of fibers because each one is optimized for a specific energy system. Anaerobic energy systems depend on fast-twitch fibers, which are vital for strength and power tasks, and slow-twitch oxidative fibers, which are vital for endurance and low-intensity activities (Shenkman & Sharlo, 2021; Jin et al., 2022; Mishra et al., 2015).

Summary

This chapter explored the complexities of kinetic fitness, emphasizing its critical role in energy production, utilization, and movement. It starts with the basics of muscular strength, addressing the physiological mechanics of force production and the link between mass and acceleration. There is a discussion of practical ways for testing and improving physical strength.

The chapter then changes its emphasis to muscular power, highlighting its importance in activities that require quick force creation. It presents the phosphocreatine energy system as a crucial aspect of muscle power maintenance. Muscular endurance is another thoroughly investigated component, emphasizing its significance in extended contractions against resistance. The chapter discusses the contribution of the aerobic energy system to muscle endurance and distinguishes it from anaerobic muscular endurance.

The notion of motor unit recruitment is covered, demonstrating how the nervous system coordinates muscle contractions for different tasks. Practical examples and visual aids can help in understanding how various activities activate motor units based on weight and complexity, highlighting the necessity of muscular coordination and strength in physical tasks. The relationship between muscle fibers, energy systems, and body composition is studied throughout the chapter, providing a comprehensive understanding of how these components influence kinetic fitness. Gender differences, as well as age-related variations in muscle mass and strength, are addressed.

Review questions

1. What are the three essential functions of muscle fitness addressed in this chapter, and why are they important for energy regulation and movement?
2. Describe the link between force generation, mass, and acceleration related to muscle strength.
3. What practical approaches are utilized to determine an individual's muscular strength, particularly when determining maximum force is difficult?
4. Explain the anaerobic lactic energy system's involvement in sustaining strength-related tasks and how it varies from other energy systems.
5. What role does the phosphocreatine energy system play in muscular power, and what activities rely significantly on it?

6. Define muscular endurance and discuss how the aerobic energy system helps to support prolonged muscle contractions.
7. What elements, such as muscle mass, gender, and age-related changes, can influence an individual's physical fitness?
8. Define motor unit recruitment and how it relates to strength-based tasks.
9. Give examples of how motor unit recruitment responds to changing task weights and complexities, as shown in the chapter.
10. What role does the interaction of muscle fibers, energy systems, and body composition play in an individual's total kinetic fitness, and why is this knowledge essential in skill execution and energy regulation?

Discussion questions

1. How can an understanding of the multiple energy systems (anaerobic lactic, phosphocreatine, and aerobic) be utilized to maximize performance in various sports and physical activities in real-world scenarios? Please provide detailed instances.
2. Muscular strength is frequently linked with sports such as weightlifting, but how can people with various fitness goals incorporate strength training into their workout routines for practical health benefits? Make suggestions for developing strength-training programs.
3. Discuss how coordination, control, and motor unit recruitment might help you perform complex movements efficiently. How may this information be used to enhance athletic performance or daily activities?
4. As people age, their muscle mass and strength tend to drop. What practical techniques may be used to combat the age-related deterioration in muscular fitness and retain functional independence as people age?
5. Consider the significance of muscle endurance in sports such as long-distance running or cycling. How can people enhance their muscle endurance, and what measures can they take to avoid tiredness during prolonged physical exertion?

References

Ahmed, T. A. E. (2015). Improving musculoskeletal fitness and the performance enhancement of basketball skills through neuromuscular training program. *Journal of Human Sport and Exercise, 10*(3), 795–804. http://www.redalyc.org/articulo.oa?id=301047714005

Blais, A. (2018). *Looking at the physical and psychosocial outcomes after participation in a community physical activity program among children with congenital heart disease* [Doctoral dissertation, Université d'Ottawa/University of Ottawa]. http://dx.doi.org/10.20381/ruor-21540246

Blazevich, A., & Blazevich, A. J. (2017). *Sports Biomechanics: The basics: Optimising human performance*. Bloomsbury Publishing.

Bonilla, D., Kreider, R., Stout, J., Forero, D., Kerksick, C., Roberts, M., & Rawson, E. (2021). Metabolic basis of creatine in health and disease: A bioinformatics-assisted review. *Nutrients, 13*(4). https://doi.org/10.3390/nu13041238

Celichowski, J., & Krutki, P. (2019). Motor units and muscle receptors. In *Muscle and exercise physiology* (pp. 51–91). Academic Press. https://doi.org/10.1016/B978-0-12-814593-7.00004-9

Chandel, N. (2021). Glycolysis. *Cold Spring Harbor Perspectives in Biology, 13*(5), 1–11. https://doi.org/10.1101/cshperspect.a040535

Cibulka, N. J., & Barron, M. L. (2017). *Guidelines for nurse practitioners in ambulatory obstetric settings.* Springer Publishing Company.

Cogliati, S., Cabrera-Alarcon, J., & Enríquez, J. (2021). Regulation and functional role of the electron transport chain supercomplexes. *Biochemical Society Transactions, 49*(6), 2655–2668. https://doi.org/10.1042/BST20210460

Cooper, G. M. (2000). *The cell: A molecular approach* (2nd ed.). Sinauer Associates. https://www.ncbi.nlm.nih.gov/books/NBK9961/

Corbin, C. B., & Le Masurier, G. C. (2014). *Fitness for life* (6th ed.). Human Kinetics.

DiStasio, T. J. (2014). *Validation of the Brzycki and Epley equations for the 1 repetition maximum back squat test in division I college football players.* Southern Illinois University. https://opensiuc.lib.siu.edu/cgi/viewcontent.cgi?referer=&httpsredir=1&article=1744&context=gs_rp

Fort-Vanmeerhaeghe, A., Romero-Rodriguez, D., Lloyd, R., Kushner, A., & Myer, G. (2016). Integrative neuromuscular training in youth athletes. Part II: Strategies to prevent injuries and improve performance. *Strength and Conditioning Journal, 38*(4), 9–27. https://doi.org/10.1519/SSC.0000000000000234

Garcia-Bermudez, J., Sánchez-Aragó, M., Soldevilla, B., Arco, A., Nuevo-Tapioles, C., & Cuezva, J. (2015). PKA phosphorylates the ATPase inhibitory factor 1 and inactivates its capacity to bind and inhibit the mitochondrial H(+)-ATP synthase. *Cell Reports, 12*(12), 2143–2155. https://doi.org/10.1016/j.celrep.2015.08.052

Goldspink, G. (2012). Age-related loss of muscle mass and strength. *Journal of Aging Research, 2012.* https://doi.org/10.1155/2012/158279

Guimarães-Ferreira, L. (2014). Role of the phosphocreatine system on energetic homeostasis in skeletal and cardiac muscles. *Einstein, 12*(1), 126–131. https://doi.org/10.1590/S1679-45082014RB2741

Hargreaves, M., & Spriet, L. (2020). Skeletal muscle energy metabolism during exercise. *Nature Metabolism, 2,* 817–828. https://doi.org/10.1038/s42255-020-0251-4

Hsu, C. Y., Chen, L. S., Chang, I. J., Fang, W. C., Huang, S. W., Lin, R. H., Ueng, S. W. N., & Chuang, H. H. (2021). Can anthropometry and body composition explain physical fitness levels in school-aged children? *Children, 8*(6), 460. https://doi.org/10.3390/children8060460

Janz, K. F., Baptista, F., Ren, S., Zhu, W., Laurson, K. R., Mahar, M. T., Pavlovic, A., & Welk, G. J. (2022). Associations among musculoskeletal fitness assessments and health outcomes: The Lisbon study for the development and evaluation of musculoskeletal fitness standards in youth. *Measurement in Physical Education and Exercise Science, 26*(4), 297–305. https://doi.org/10.1080/1091367X.2021.2000414

Jin, S., Lee, G., Kim, J., Kim, C., Choo, Y., Cho, W., Han, E., Hwang, Y., Kim, Y., & Jeong, H. (2022). Effect of porcine whole blood protein hydrolysate on slow-twitch muscle fiber expression and mitochondrial biogenesis via the AMPK/SIRT1 pathway. *International Journal of Molecular Sciences, 23*(3). https://doi.org/10.3390/ijms23031229

Keller, K., & Engelhardt, M. (2014). Strength and muscle mass loss with aging process: Age and strength loss. *Muscles, Ligaments and Tendons Journal, 3*(4), 346–350. https://www.ncbi.nlm.nih.gov/pmc/articles/PMC3940510/

Kiely, J. (2017). The robust running ape: Unraveling the deep underpinnings of coordinated human running proficiency. *Frontiers in Psychology, 8*. https://doi.org/10.3389/fpsyg.2017.00892

Koh, H., Ørtenblad, N., Winding, K., Hellsten, Y., Mortensen, S., & Nielsen, J. (2018). High-intensity interval, but not endurance, training induces muscle fiber type-specific subsarcolemmal lipid droplet size reduction in type 2 diabetic patients. *American Journal of Physiology. Endocrinology and Metabolism, 315*(5), e872–e884. https://doi.org/10.1152/ajpendo.00161.2018

Lai, A., Biewener, A., & Wakeling, J. (2018). Metabolic cost underlies task-dependent variations in motor unit recruitment. *Journal of the Royal Society Interface, 15*(148). https://doi.org/10.1098/rsif.2018.0541

Mahundi, P., & Manwa, L. (2015). Energy nutrient metabolism: The inter-conversions and the chain reaction leading to oxidative-phosphorilation and production of adenosine tri-phosphate (ATP). *Journal of Emerging Trends in Educational Research and Policy Studies, 6*(5), 383–390. https://hdl.handle.net/10520/EJC183950

Maltais, M. L., Desroches, J., & Dionne, I. J. (2009). Changes in muscle mass and strength after menopause. *Journal of Musculoskeletal and Neuronal Interactions, 9*(4), 186–197. https://pubmed.ncbi.nlm.nih.gov/19949277/

McLellan, C. P., Lovell, D. I., & Gass, G. C. (2011). The role of rate of force development on vertical jump performance. *The Journal of Strength & Conditioning Research, 25*(2), 379–385. http://doi.org/10.1519/JSC.0b013e3181be305c

Mishra, P., Varuzhanyan, G., Pham, A., & Chan, D. (2015). Mitochondrial dynamics is a distinguishing feature of skeletal muscle fiber types and regulates organellar compartmentalization. *Cell Metabolism, 22*(6), 1033–1044. https://doi.org/10.1016/j.cmet.2015.09.027

Mitchell, E., Martin, N., Bailey, S., & Ferguson, R. (2018). Critical power is positively related to skeletal muscle capillarity and type I muscle fibers in endurance-trained individuals. *Journal of Applied Physiology, 125*(3), 737–745. https://doi.org/10.1152/japplphysiol.01126.2017

Morelli, A., Ravera, S., & Panfoli, I. (2020). The aerobic mitochondrial ATP synthesis from a comprehensive point of view. *Open Biology, 10*(10). https://doi.org/10.1098/rsob.200224

Narici, M. V., Maganaris, C. N., Reeves, N. D., & Capodaglio, P. (2003). Effect of aging on human muscle architecture. *Journal of Applied Physiology, 95*(6), 2229–2234. https://doi.org/10.1152/japplphysiol.00433.2003

Ojanen, T., Häkkinen, K., Hanhikoski, J., & Kyröläinen, H. (2020). Effects of task-specific and strength training on simulated military task performance in soldiers. *International Journal of Environmental Research and Public Health, 17*(21). https://doi.org/10.3390/ijerph17218000

Plotkin, D., Roberts, M., Haun, C., & Schoenfeld, B. (2021). Muscle fiber type transitions with exercise training: Shifting perspectives. *Sports, 9*(9). https://doi.org/10.3390/sports9090127

Powers, J., Malingen, S., Regnier, M., & Daniel, T. (2021). The sliding filament theory since Andrew Huxley: Multiscale and multidisciplinary muscle research. *Annual Review of Biophysics, 50*(1), 373–400. https://doi.org/10.1146/annurev-biophys-110320-062613

Reis, F., Haro, A., Bacurau, A., Hirabara, S., Wasinski, F., Ormanji, M., Moreira, J., Kiyomoto, B., Bertoncini, C., Brum, P., Curi, R., Bader, M., Bacurau, R., Pesquero, J., & Araújo, R. (2015). Deletion of kinin b2 receptor alters muscle metabolism and exercise performance. *PLoS ONE, 10*(8). https://doi.org/10.1371/journal.pone.0134844

Roberts, T., & Petersen, J. (2023). An ambitious study finds the limits of force production in human skeletal muscles. *The Journal of Physiology, 601*(10), 1695–1696. https://doi.org/10.1113/JP284655

Semler, M., & Singer, M. (2019). Deconstructing hyperlactatemia in sepsis using central venous oxygen saturation and base deficit. *American Journal of Respiratory and Critical Care Medicine*, *200*(5), 526–527. https://doi.org/10.1164/rccm.201904-0899ED

Serrano, N., Colenso-Semple, L., Lazauskus, K., Siu, J., Bagley, J., Lockie, R., Costa, P., & Galpin, A. (2018). Extraordinary fast-twitch fiber abundance in elite weightlifters. *PLoS One*, *14*(3). https://doi.org/10.1371/journal.pone.0207975

Shenkman, B., & Sharlo, K. (2021). How muscle activity controls slow myosin expression. *Journal of Evolutionary Biochemistry and Physiology*, *57*, 605–625. https://doi.org/10.1134/S002209302103011X

Steele, J., & Fisher, J. (2018). Effort, discomfort, group iii/iv afferents, bioenergetics, and motor unit recruitment. *Medicine and Science in Sports and Exercise*, *50*(8), 1718–1718. https://doi.org/10.1249/MSS.0000000000001605

Suchomel, T., Nimphius, S., Bellon, C., & Stone, M. (2018). The importance of muscular strength: Training considerations. *Sports Medicine*, *48*, 765–785. https://doi.org/10.1007/s40279-018-0862-z

Swanwick, E., & Matthews, M. (2018). Energy systems: A new look at aerobic metabolism in stressful exercise. *MOJ Sports Med*, *2*(1). https://doi.org/10.15406/mojsm.2018.02.00039

Taber, C., Bellon, C., Abbott, H., & Bingham, G. (2016). Roles of maximal strength and rate of force development in maximizing muscular power. *Strength and Conditioning Journal*, *38*(1), 71–78. https://doi.org/10.1519/SSC.0000000000000193

Tamir, A. (2015). Newton's 2nd law. In *Industrial engineering and management*. OMICS Publishing Group. https://doi.org/10.4172/2169-0316.1000150

Wakabayashi, T. (2015). Mechanism of the calcium-regulation of muscle contraction – in pursuit of its structural basis. *Proceedings of the Japan Academy. Series B, Physical and Biological Sciences*, *91*(7), 321–350. https://doi.org/10.2183/pjab.91.321

Wang, Y., Huang, Y., Yang, J., Zhou, F., Zhao, L., & Zhou, H. (2018). Pyruvate is a prospective alkalizer to correct hypoxic lactic acidosis. *Military Medical Research*, *5*(13). https://doi.org/10.1186/s40779-018-0160-y

Wasserman, K. (2015). The anaerobic threshold measurement to evaluate exercise performance. *The American Review of Respiratory Disease*, *129*(2P2), S35–S40. https://doi.org/10.1164/ARRD.1984.129.2P2.S35

PART III

Real-world application of the USFD Framework

Unveiling the principles and potential of the USFD Framework to real-life success

14

THE ROLE OF WELLNESS IN USFD

Oliver Napila Gomez and Nguyen Tra Giang

This chapter provides an overview of wellness as part of the USFD Framework. The framework has also included mental health and considered wellness a standalone construct that underpins and improves general fitness. The chapter explores different dimensions of well-being: physical, emotional, intellectual, spiritual, social, and occupational aspects to show how it is dynamic and multifaceted. The key issues concerning wellness within the USFD Framework include self-awareness and competence, individual preferences and motivation, and personal choice for fitness engagement. This chapter also focuses on cultural diversity regarding well-being, emphasizing that wellness is a positive force toward healthy living. The chapter also deals with the multidimensionality of wellness, underscoring the intricate workings of human health and the need for balanced growth in all areas to ensure healthier living. In addition, it examines wellness as a dynamic state whereby lifestyle choices may lead to deteriorating, stagnant, or progressive states. Self-awareness and competence are pivotal in promoting health since they help individuals make positive steps toward better health.

Outcome

By the end of this chapter, you will be able to

- describe the multifaceted character of wellness about the USFD Framework, emphasizing its significance in promoting holistic well-being
- investigate the dynamic nature of well-being within the USFD, such as how it might develop, plateau, or degrade over time as a result of individual decisions and lifestyles

DOI: 10.4324/9781003502937-17

- explain the importance of self-awareness as the cornerstone of well-being and how competence supplements it by allowing individuals to make proactive efforts toward enhancing their health and wellness
- understand how aligning wellness goals with personal values can lead to sustainable habits by analyzing the influence of personal preferences, choices, and intrinsic and extrinsic motivation in developing wellness practices
- discuss the value of cultural sensitivity and diversity in wellness efforts and the necessity for flexibility and adaptability as individuals progress through their health journey within the USFD Framework

Does the USFD Framework still include wellness?

Embracing the principles of holistic well-being within its framework, the Unified Systems Fitness Design (USFD) reflects its comprehensive character. With an eye on fostering the ever-present complementarity of roles supporting health and skill development, USFD has widened its focus to include mental health. It is critical to outline the unique function of wellness as a separate construct in this chapter to support and enhance the overall fitness paradigm in the USFD Framework.

The USFD Framework changed the way we think about health. In this chapter, we explore the perspective of the USFD Framework on wellness, covering topics such as the multifaceted and dynamic nature of wellness, the significance of self-awareness and competence, the part played by individual preferences, motivational factors, and the role of personal choice in ensuring wellness adherence, and health philosophies. These components will aid in elucidating the specific role of wellness in our framework for attaining optimum well-being.

Definition of wellness

The National Wellness Institute (2020) thoroughly comprehends well-being by elucidating numerous essential dimensions. Being healthy involves taking control of life and consciously reaching full potential. It covers a lot of ground, including mental and spiritual well-being, lifestyle, and environmental factors. At its core, wellness is a positive force that promotes an optimistic outlook and the maintenance of a long and healthy life span. It is an all-encompassing concept that considers cultural variety and various aspects of well-being. Ultimately, being healthy is all about making the most of what you have right now.

Multidimensionality of wellness

Holistic health and quality of life, according to Hettler's 1976 dimensions of wellness, include many different aspects, highlighting the complex nature of human health and happiness. General health is affected by how these interrelated characteristics interact and are incorporated into everyday life. A happier, healthier existence is possible when we work to achieve harmony and growth in all areas. Achieving wellness in all three areas is a never-ending journey that calls for introspection, hard work, and a dedication to bettering oneself (Hettler, 1976).

Physical wellness

Physical well-being includes overall health and fitness, emphasizing the value of preventative self-care and good dietary and lifestyle choices. It comprises doing what is best for health regarding exercise, diet, and general way of life (Badawi et al., 2017). The capacity to carry out normal functions and deal with the stresses of everyday life is an indicator of physical wellness (Tint et al., 2018). Cardiovascular fitness, flexibility, strength, and food choices all fall under this aspect of health, which aims to decrease the risk of illnesses and increase overall vitality (Bankimbhai & Kapse, 2019). Physical well-being is all about actively and consistently preserving well-being through good living practices. It is about completing daily tasks without feeling too tired or stressed (Johnson, 2017). It stresses the need to eat well, stay flexible, strengthen, and improve cardiovascular fitness (Canfield, 2018).

Emotional wellness

Emotional wellness, in its most basic definition, refers to a person's ability to deal with and overcome emotional difficulties in life, identifying and accepting feelings must be emotionally healthy, therefore controlling emotions and constructively reacting to them. Building emotional resilience is learning to deal with stressful situations, maintaining a positive outlook on life, and generally being a good person. A high level of emotional wellness allows individuals to handle difficult situations effectively, keep their emotions in check, and cultivate positive relationships. Strong self-esteem, which includes a solid sense of self-identity and good self-regard, is the bedrock of this aspect of wellness (Salonen, 2017). Being emotionally healthy is a never-ending journey that includes self-awareness, expressing feelings, and managing them effectively (Venasse et al., 2018). It also includes positively expressing, controlling, and integrating emotions like optimism (Raj et al., 2022).

Intellectual wellness

The ability to take in, organize, and apply new knowledge is at the heart of being intellectually healthy, contributing to physical health. It includes a dedication to learning new things throughout life, developing critical thinking and problem-solving capacity, and encouraging creativity. This quality is essential for doing things that challenge the brain, keeping curiosity alive, and looking for ways to improve oneself intellectually and personally.

According to multiple sources, a sense of intellectual wellness stems from enjoying mentally challenging pursuits (Zainab & Naz, 2017; Salonen, 2017; Fredhoi, 2015). It is also part of engaging in creative and mental activities and successfully utilizing knowledge resources (Bankimbhai & Kapse, 2019). A state of intellectual well-being is when a person is self-aware enough to realize creative capacities, and ambitious enough to seek learning opportunities (Halloran, 2017). Also, it has to do with how much time a person spends thinking about things that make them intelligent and creative (Avci, 2017).

Spiritual wellness

A person's spiritual health includes their values, sense of purpose, and life's meaning. Religion is just one facet: how people organize their values and beliefs to reason uprightly and feel connected to something bigger than themselves. The understanding of a profound connection – through religion, nature, or personal philosophy – and introspection and self-awareness are encouraged by this component.

When people talk of spiritual wellness, they often mean different things. One interpretation is that it represents a person's intimate relationship with a transcendental force, such as God or a higher power (Leventhal, 2016). To be spiritually healthy involves embracing ideas of completeness and significance and working toward finding a purpose in life (Paramananda, 2015) or creating them. Integrating the ideals with those of society and the divine steadily and harmoniously is also relevant (Duyan et al., 2021).

Aside from seeking an essential life purpose, being spiritually well includes living life to the fullest and offering and receiving love, joy, and peace (Ford, 2015). Integral to spiritual wellness are compassion, forgiveness, selflessness, tolerance, and love (Kuru, 2022). Having a positive outlook on life's meaning and purpose, which indicates knowing what life is about, is what it is about in the end (Fredhoi, 2015).

Social wellness

The ability to form and maintain meaningful relationships with other people signifies social wellness. This aspect includes communicating effectively, empathizing with others, and belongingness to social and communal networks.

Social wellness thrives through relationships with friends and family, active participation in social activities, and community involvement (Priebe, 2018).

Connectivity, quality of relationships, and social engagements all play a role in an individual's social well-being (Raj et al., 2022). It indicates a constructive trend toward harmony and unity in the relationships among people, communities, and the natural world (Ford, 2015).

Additionally, social wellness encompasses receiving and providing help to others (Canfield, 2018). Two aspects of social support include relying on loved ones and making a difference (Zainab & Naz, 2017; Salonen, 2017). The perception of having support available from family and friends when needed and being a valued provider of support are essential aspects of social wellness (Fredhoi, 2015).

Occupational wellness

Occupational wellness is exemplified by people actively involved in and happy with what they do for a living. A sense of purpose, meaning, and fulfillment in everyday activities goes beyond fulfilling professional tasks. The capacity to achieve professional and personal fulfillment in a chosen sector while preserving a balanced life is a hallmark of occupational wellness.

Different definitions highlight different parts of well-being in the workplace. It entails dealing with stress at work, maintaining positive connections with coworkers, and balancing work and leisure time (Kuye et al., 2022). Enjoying what they do for a living and being grateful for its impact on others are the keys to a healthy workplace (Fatima et al., 2020). It can be about using unique abilities to do work, which gives them a personally satisfying experience, whether with payment or without (Caingcoy, 2021).

In other words, being healthy at work means doing the job properly in a setting that makes people happy individually and collectively. Occupational wellness is not based on monetary compensation, but on the joy and fulfillment people get from their job (Hoeger & Hoeger, 2012).

Wellness as a dynamic state

The USFD embraces wellness as a dynamic state, aligning with our perpetual complementation theory, as various external factors constantly threaten the interrelationship between the system functions for health and skill. Recognizing the constant changes individuals experience, the USFD acknowledges three possible trajectories within this dynamic perspective – deterioration, stagnation, and progression.

- **Deterioration** – Unhealthy lifestyles such as poor nutrition, sedentary lifestyles, chronic stress, and destructive behaviors can lead to the deterioration of wellness over time (Padilla & Mayo, 2018).

- **Stagnation** – Characterized by a lack of proactive efforts to enhance well-being, this state is when a person adheres to existing habits and routines, neither actively pursuing wellness nor experiencing declining health (de Wind et al., 2017).
- **Progression** – Adopting positive choices and healthy habits like regular exercise, balanced nutrition, stress management, and other wellness-promoting behaviors can encourage individuals to progress toward a higher level of wellness (Rippe, 2018).

Everyday decisions and ways of living are inextricably bound up with wellness as an ongoing process. These decisions may affect a person's health over time, stressing that their level of wellness is greatly affected by their deliberate decisions and not just by their genes or environment (Janecka, 2017).

Ensuring health and wellness by making deliberate and well-informed decisions is a personal duty. Wellness can be achieved through deliberate choices and actions (Cathomas et al., 2019). The dynamic character of wellness highlights the ability to adapt and persevere in adversity. Resilience – the capacity to recover quickly from adversity – is seen as fundamental to wellness, emphasizing that general health need not be defined by adversity.

Viewing wellness as a continuous process encourages people to think about their health and well-being in the grand scheme. Achieving long-term wellness requires dedication and perseverance, even while there may be quick wins with short-term strategies. This view aligns with the idea that being healthy is an unending process that involves changing and adapting throughout life (Vaziri et al., 2023).

Principles of wellness in the USFD Framework

We developed five principles of wellness based on the USFD Framework, which are comprehensive and dynamic strategies for holistic and inclusive health and wellness practices based on introspection and skill development. These principles rest on the premise that people's awareness, competence, philosophies, beliefs, preferences, and motivations impact their decisions and actions about their wellness journey and commitment.

USFD wellness principle 1: awareness (I know!)

Self-awareness is a critical aspect of wellness (Hettler, 1976), the ability of an individual to reflectively recognize and understand their physical and mental health. Individuals can establish and enhance their overall wellness by cultivating self-awareness.

Meanwhile, aligning with the framework's focus on dynamic wellness and perpetual complementation, the USFD Framework developed four aspects of awareness that are vital for achieving holistic well-being.

1. **Physical activity awareness and movement system functions.** We linked grouped system functions for movement and physical activity awareness in the USFD Framework. Everyone should be aware of how active they are, whether it be through regular exercise, walking around the block, or even just sitting around all day. This knowledge lays the groundwork for encouraging physical fitness, an enduring asset to general wellness. Observing their activity patterns makes it possible to determine if an individual is getting enough exercise. When people are conscious of the need to improve their physical health, they can make the changes required to increase their daily physical activity.

2. **Dietary awareness and energy regulation system functions.** Regulating energy is associated with dietary awareness. It entails keeping track of eating habits, including what a person eats, how much, and how often. People can evaluate the dietary quality of their food when they understand their dietary requirements. People can find places to improve and make educated nutrition decisions when they understand how food choices affect energy levels and general health. Dietary awareness supports energy regulation by providing the body's needs to sustain physiological health and skill components.

3. **Emotional awareness and physiological health system functions.** Within the physiological health function, the USFD Framework incorporates emotional awareness. Awareness of how mental and emotional emotions might influence physical health is critical. Knowing what causes stress, how people naturally feel when stressed, and how stress affects the body's physiological systems are all parts of this awareness. Individuals can actively manage stress and foster emotional wellness by knowing the links between emotions and physical health. Managing stress favors general health and improves the capacity to engage in physical activity efficiently, so being mindful of emotions may complement physiological health.

4. **Awareness of destructive behaviors and homeostasis system functions.** Homeostasis is associated with the awareness of harmful activities. People must understand the long-term effects of harmful habits like smoking, drinking excessive alcohol, abusing substances, or engaging in dangerous activities that affect internal balance in the body. This awareness should encourage people to seek better options that improve their health. Refraining from harmful habits allows people to contribute to the body's internal balance (homeostasis) and lessen the likelihood of negative consequences.

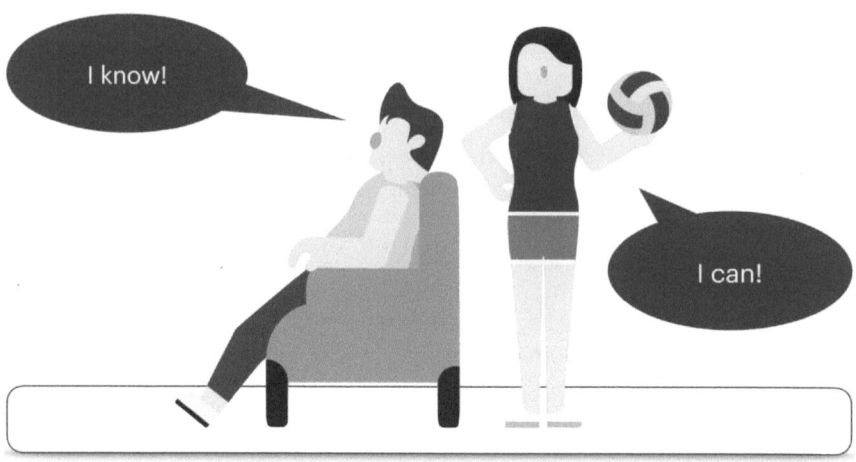

FIGURE 14.1   Awareness and competence for wellness

USFD wellness principle 2: competence (I can!)

We affirm that self-awareness and competence are the cornerstones of wellness. While being aware of oneself is the first and most significant step, it is also crucial to note that competence, which emphasizes taking the initiative to improve and sustain personal health, goes hand in hand with awareness.

When it comes to health, competence means being able to take responsibility for health proactively and successfully. Rather than stopping at awareness, it entails actively using knowledge and abilities to bring about significant transformations. To be competent, a person must know what needs doing and have the capacity and drive to implement that knowledge.

Competence and self-awareness are seen as complementary qualities within the USFD. Practicing self-awareness is mindful living, aiming to help people pay attention in the here and now. It entails being mindful of mental, emotional, and bodily conditions. Cultivating an awareness of the present moment allows everyone to gain insight into their mental and physical health, stress levels, eating patterns, and physical activity levels.

Being competent means being able to turn self-awareness into proactive measures. It entails learning to make intelligent choices and putting wellness plans into action. For instance, knowing how to include regular physical activity into a routine, creating realistic fitness goals, and sticking to them after learning the adverse outcomes of an inactive lifestyle.

Aside from identifying problem areas, wellness is also about having the skills to fix them. It promotes the idea that people should be proactive in their wellness by taking the initiative to improve physical, emotional, and mental health.

Individuals can establish and actively pursue wellness objectives with a healthy dose of self-awareness and competence.

USFD wellness principle 3: preference and personal choice (I want!)

Every one of us naturally leans toward certain activities or pursuits. Regarding free time, people have different preferences; some like reading, drawing, hiking, or playing an instrument. Recognized in USFD is the fact that specific individuals may despise competitive sports. The concept of personal choice is foundational to making sense of the dynamic wellness scene in the USFD.

Achieving wellness is not a destination but rather a process, and each person has the power to take an active role on their path to health. At its core, the USFD is based on the principle that people should use their discretion to investigate various wellness possibilities and choose approaches that suit their interests and general health. Critical aspects of preference and personal choice within the USFD Framework include:

1. **Active engagement in wellness** – Wellness is something we actively pursue. A person's path to wellness should include physical activity and healthy eating but also emotional and mental health, strong relationships, and the ability to cope with stress.
2. **A rich plethora of wellness options** – The USFD Framework acknowledges that people can access various wellness alternatives. People nowadays have many options for improving their health, including different types of exercise, diets, and ways to deal with stress.
3. **Personalization** – Belief in the profound personal nature of well-being is fundamental to the USFD Framework. The path to wellness is subjective and depends on the individual's values, goals, and preferences. Individuals are given the power to customize their wellness approach according to their unique requirements and goals.
4. **Exercising judgment** – The ability to make informed decisions about health is central to the USFD Framework, suggesting that people think carefully about the wellness options that are accessible to them, weigh the pros and cons, and then make a well-informed decision.
5. **Empowerment through personal choice** – People are likely to take charge of their health and well-being when given agency in making decisions about it. It allows people to do what makes them happy, according to their principles and goals.
6. **Respect for individual preferences** – The USFD is about creating a space where people's preferences are valued. As a result, it promotes inclusivity and helps individuals on their paths to well-being by acknowledging that what helps some may not help others.

7. **Flexibility and adaptability** – Individual decisions about health are dynamic, mirroring the idea of wellness as an unending journey. People are free to try new things regarding their health, adjust to new situations, and develop new preferences. Embracing personal wellness choices promotes a state of flexibility and adaptability. As people go through their journeys and face ever-changing challenges, they can change, adapt, and improve their wellness strategies.

USFD wellness principle 4: motivation (I must!)

As a motivating factor that impacts people's decisions and actions, motivation is essential to the USFD Framework. It acknowledges that people's dedication to living healthily and improving their general well-being can originate from various places. It is crucial for people starting their wellness journey to understand these drivers.

Motivation can be categorized into two primary types within the USFD Framework, aligned with existing theories of motivation (Ryan & Deci, 2000):

1. **Intrinsic motivation.** A person's intrinsic or internal motivation comes from their inner drive and pleasure from engaging in healthy actions. It is marked by an authentic, intrinsic motivation to participate in health-promoting pursuits. Intrinsic motivators encompass (a) enjoyment from physical activity engagement, (b) achievement of wellness goals, (c) feeling better in various aspects of life – physically, emotionally, and mentally, and (d) a sense of autonomy and the desire to make choices.
2. **Extrinsic motivation.** External factors and rewards incentivize individuals to engage in wellness-related activities. These motivators originate outside the individual and encompass (a) receiving praise, acknowledgment, or recognition from others for wellness efforts, (2) tangible rewards, such as prizes, monetary incentives, or gifts, (c) competitive settings, whether in sports, fitness challenges, or group activities, and (d) the expectations and support of peers, family members, or colleagues.

While internal and external forces might drive people, motivations might change over time. An example of intrinsic motivation would be a person who starts exercising to win a prize but eventually develops a true passion for fitness.

Moreover, wellness is not a one-size-fits-all concept. We recognize diversity and that motivating factors for one person may differ for others. Hence, the USFD Framework promotes motivation-based personalization strategies, enabling individuals to recognize and maximize their distinct drive sources. In addition, long-term inspiration is highly valued. Intrinsic motivation typically results in long-lasting wellness behaviors, but extrinsic rewards may offer short-term motivation. People are likely to commit to their health in the long run if encouraged to enjoy making healthy choices for their own sake.

To stay motivated, it is best to set wellness objectives aligning with what we genuinely value and what interests us. This promotes wellness by encouraging people to engage in pursuits that are meaningful to them on a personal level. When these two things are in harmony, it is like a rocket ship taking people on their health journey.

USFD wellness principle 5: philosophies and beliefs (I believe!)

People's ideas and beliefs matter when making decisions and taking actions that promote wellness. Individuals' perspectives on health are significantly impacted by their deeply held beliefs, cultural standards, and personal principles, as the USFD acknowledges. We need to look at various ideas and viewpoints to understand the complexities of the wellness journey.

Several critical aspects of philosophies and beliefs within the USFD Framework include:

1. **Cultural norms** – Cultural traditions and conventions shape health and wellness perspectives. People's food habits, levels of physical exercise, and perspectives on mental health reflect their cultural values. Hence, their general health may be affected by their cultural background.
2. **Spirituality** – Dietary restrictions, fasting, and the search for inner peace are all aspects of wellness that are influenced by a person's religious and spiritual beliefs. Many people place a high value on making wellness decisions that align with their religious views.
3. **Personal values** – Personal values heavily impact wellness decisions, including family, community, environmental sustainability, and ethical considerations. What matters most to a person regarding their health, fitness, and diet is their values.
4. **Personal health philosophies** – An individual's approach to well-being is shaped by their personal health philosophy, which may include holistic health, preventive medicine, or alternative therapies. These ideologies influence decisions about healthcare and wellness.
5. **Critical examination of wellness decisions** – We encourage people to think deeply about whether their values and principles align with their health goals and examine their decisions, ensuring that they align with their values and goals through this introspection.
6. **Adaptability** – The USFD promotes a growth mindset, allowing people to change beliefs in response to new facts or experiences. Being open-minded allows for self-improvement and progress on the path to wellness.

7. **Cultural sensitivity** – The USFD recognizes and honors various cultural practices and beliefs to foster cultural sensitivity and inclusion. It promotes the idea that people should value cultural diversity for what it is and adjust their health habits appropriately.
8. **Discouraging rigid adherence** – It is not encouraged to be overly committed to an ideology, arguing that, instead, a holistic view of health is flexible enough to respond to people's unique situations.

Individuals can customize their wellness strategy by evaluating philosophies and beliefs to align with their values and objectives. This process empowers people to make deliberate decisions that align with their values.

Moreover, the USFD acknowledges the complex relationship between philosophy and beliefs and other aspects of health, such as exercise, nutrition, and stress reduction. It stresses the importance of consistently motivating oneself to make health-conscious choices by aligning beliefs with wellness goals. The USFD promotes deliberate decision-making by examining how values and beliefs impact their health choices. The importance of intentionally choosing choices that align with underlying values is underscored.

Lastly, the beliefs and values underpinning wellness must be flexible, as it is an unrelenting process. Perspectives on well-being can change when people experience personal growth and transformation.

Summary

Wellness includes physical, emotional, intellectual, spiritual, social, and occupational components of an individual's well-being. The USFD considers well-being a dynamic state that is influenced by everyday decisions and lifestyle, and it acknowledges that it can grow, stagnate, or degrade over time. Hence, the role of wellness is essential and multifaceted in the USFD. Within the USFD, self-awareness is regarded as the foundation of well-being, allowing individuals to comprehend their physical and psychological well-being. Competence is also essential, emphasizing the practical use of information and abilities to effect substantial changes in well-being.

Furthermore, personal preferences and choices are recognized, allowing individuals to personalize wellness plans to their interests and values. Motivation is recognized as a driving element behind wellness choices, whether intrinsic (motivated by personal satisfaction) or extrinsic (influenced by external influences). Inclusivity and cultural sensitivity are encouraged, as cultural norms, beliefs, and values substantially impact wellness decisions. The USFD promotes ongoing growth in well-being, encouraging people to think long-term, take responsibility for their health, and be resilient in the face of adversity.

Through wellness, the USFD can help individuals actively engage in their wellness journey, make informed decisions connected with their values, and pursue a holistic and dynamic path to well-being via wellness.

Review questions

1. What are the main wellness components described in the USFD Framework, and how do they contribute to overall well-being?
2. How does the USFD perceive well-being as a dynamic state, and what three paths does it recognize in this dynamic perspective?
3. What role does self-awareness play in the USFD Framework, and why is it considered the cornerstone of wellness?
4. Using the USFD Framework, explain the concept of competence in the context of wellness. What does it have to do with self-awareness?
5. Why is it necessary for the USFD to promote personal choices and preferences in wellness decisions?
6. What are the two main types of motivation described in the USFD Framework, and how do they influence people's commitment to living a healthy lifestyle?
7. How does the USFD enable people to discover intrinsic satisfaction in making healthy choices, and why is long-term motivation emphasized?
8. According to the USFD Framework, how do an individual's philosophy and values influence their wellness choices? Why is it critical to assess and connect these beliefs with wellness objectives?
9. What role do cultural sensitivity and inclusivity play in the USFD's wellness strategy, and how does it influence individuals' wellness decisions?
10. How does the USFD encourage a long-term outlook on well-being and resilience in adversity? What are the essential wellness lessons from the USFD Framework?

Discussion questions

1. How can individuals use the self-awareness and competence concepts mentioned in the USFD Framework to create practical gains regarding physical health and overall well-being in their daily lives?
2. How may personal preferences and choices be included in a tailored wellness strategy, and how does this approach result in sustainable and pleasurable wellness practices?
3. What strategies can people use to harness intrinsic motivation for their wellness journey, and how can they gradually shift away from extrinsic motivators and toward self-generated sources of drive?

4. How can cultural sensitivity and inclusivity be included in wellness practices to ensure that people from all walks of life can access and benefit from health initiatives?

5. How does the USFD Framework encourage people to adjust and develop their wellness practices as they progress? What are some real-world instances of adapting to changing circumstances and shifting tastes in the quest for happiness?

References

Avci, M. (2017). *Total wellness of Turkish international students in the US: Perceptions and inherent growth tendencies*. St. Mary's University.

Badawi, H. F., Dong, H., & El Saddik, A. (2017). Mobile cloud-based physical activity advisory system using biofeedback sensors. *Future Generation Computer Systems, 66*, 59–70. https://doi.org/10.1016/j.future.2015.11.005

Bankimbhai, T. M., & Kapse, S. (2019). *Employee wellness: A study of the banking sector in Gujarat* [Doctoral dissertation, Gujarat Technological University]. http://gtusite circulars.s3.amazonaws.com/uploads/Full%20Thesis_743374.pdf

Caingcoy, M. E. (2021). University-wide extension project: Its impact on holistic wellness of third agers and contribution to development goals. *International Journal of Engineering, Science and Information Technology, 1*(1), 1–9. https://doi.org/10.52088/ijesty.v1i1.34

Canfield, I. L. (2018). *The impact of social support and stigmatization upon the wellness of females diagnosed with a substance use disorder* [Doctoral dissertation, Florida Atlantic University]. https://www.proquest.com/openview/a5baa5449e884f7a2304c8509b06bb56/1?pq-origsite=gscholar&cbl=18750&diss=y

Cathomas, F., Murrough, J., Nestler, E., Han, M., & Russo, S. (2019). Neurobiology of resilience: Interface between mind and body. *Biological Psychiatry, 86*(6), 410–420. https://doi.org/10.1016/J.BIOPSYCH.2019.04.011

de Wind, A., Boot, C., Sewdas, R., Scharn, M., Heuvel, S., & Beek, A. (2017). Do work characteristics predict health deterioration among employees with chronic diseases? *Journal of Occupational Rehabilitation, 28*, 289–297. https://doi.org/10.1007/s10926-017-9716-z

Duyan, V. E. L. İ., Kiliç, C., & Pak Güre, M. (2021). The Turkish adaptation of the spiritual wellness inventory manevi iyilik hali envanteri'ni türkçeye uyarlama çalışması. *Ankara Universitesi Ilahiyat Fakultesi Dergisi, 62*(2). http://doi.org/10.33227/auifd.968816

Fatima, T., Tabassum, M. F., Khan, S. U., Mahmood-ul-Hassan, S., & Karim, R. (2020). Wellness impact on the performance of young female athletes. *Ilkogretim Online, 19*(4), 5462–5470. https://doi.org/10.17051/ilkonline.2020.04.764952

Ford, S. B. (2015). *Getting to the heart of our students: First-year students and their wellness* [Master's thesis, University of Nebraska]. https://digitalcommons.unl.edu/cehsedaddiss/226/

Fredhoi, C. (2015). *The importance of positive and negative well-being in older people; associations with psychosocial factors, cortisol and cognitive performance* [Doctoral dissertation, University of Westminster]. https://bit.ly/46eaD7U

Halloran, T. (2017). *The impact of a workplace wellness program on employees in a university setting*. http://hdl.handle.net/10342/6150

Hettler, B. (1976). *The six dimensions of wellness model* (pp. 1–2). National Wellness Institute.

Hoeger, W. W. K., & Hoeger, S. A. (2012). *Principles and labs for fitness and wellness* (12th ed.). Wadsworth Cengage Learning.

Janecka, I. (2017). Health, health care, and systems science: Emerging paradigm. *Cureus*, *9*(2). https://doi.org/10.7759/cureus.1030

Johnson, C. (2017). *The fitness tourist: Goal content of exercisers in the wellness tourism industry* [Doctoral dissertation, Arizona State University]. https://www.proquest.com/openview/fb7e32a2b392eab0cdad1eab4430ac14/1?pq-origsite=gscholar&cbl=18750

Kuru, H. (2022). *Designing and evaluating a need-based employee wellness program* [Doctoral dissertation, Middle East Technical University]. https://hdl.handle.net/11511/96381

Kuye, J., Akinyemi, P. A., Olanrewaju, O., Emmanuel, O. N., & Olusola, F. (2022). Occupational wellness and its determinants among cocoa farmers in South-West Nigeria. *Texila International Journal of Public Health*, *10*(1), 1–9. https://doi.org/10.21522/TIJPH.2013.10.01.Art013

Leventhal, B. (2016). *The role of spiritual wellness as a predictor of employment satisfaction in addiction treatment professionals* [Doctoral dissertation, Capella University]. https://www.proquest.com/openview/b3733109351302ffa4d9ef15768fcd3b/1?pq-origsite=gscholar&cbl=18750

National Wellness Institute. (2020). *NWI's six dimensions of wellness*. https://national-wellness.org/resources/six-dimensions-of-wellness/

Padilla, R., & Mayo, A. (2018). Clinical deterioration: A concept analysis. *Journal of Clinical Nursing*, *27*(7–8), 1360–1368. https://doi.org/10.1111/jocn.14238

Paramananda, S. (2015). Meditation: The key to overall wellness. *The International Journal of Religion and Spirituality in Society*, *5*(4), 109. https://www.proquest.com/openview/5246348c584faac72383aee4480b95dd/1?pq-origsite=gscholar&cbl=5529393

Priebe, D. R. (2018). *Does perceived wellness influence employee work engagement? Examining the effects of wellness in the presence of established individual and workplace predictor variables* [Doctoral dissertation, The Ohio State University]. http://rave.ohiolink.edu/etdc/view?acc_num=osu152330257997838

Raj, M., Jimenez, F. E., Rich, R. K., Okland, K., Roy, L., Opollo, J., Rogers, J., & Brittin, J. (2022). Influence of evidence-based design strategies on nurse wellness. *HERD: Health Environments Research & Design Journal*, *15*(4), 233–248. https://doi.org/10.1177/19375867221110915

Rippe, J. (2018). Lifestyle medicine: The health promoting power of daily habits and practices. *American Journal of Lifestyle Medicine*, *12*(6), 499–512. https://doi.org/10.1177/1559827618785554

Ryan, R. M., & Deci, E. L. (2000). Self-determination theory and the facilitation of intrinsic motivation, social development, and well-being. *American Psychologist*, *55*(1), 68. https://psycnet.apa.org/doi/10.1037/0003-066X.55.1.68

Salonen, T. A. (2017). *Promoting wellness to a rural area through recreation facility and programming*. https://repository.stcloudstate.edu/pess_etds/10

Tint, A., Hamdani, Y., Sawyer, A., Desarkar, P., Ameis, S. H., Bardikoff, N., & Lai, M. C. (2018). Wellness efforts for autistic women. *Current Developmental Disorders Reports*, *5*, 207–216. https://doi.org/10.1007/s40474-018-0148-z

Vaziri, N., Bonnett, M., Kennedy, M., & Garstka, T. (2023). *Linking community resilience to health and wellness* [Technical Report]. The University of Kansas. https://doi.org/10.61152/pvtk9816

Venasse, M., Edwards, T., & Pilutti, L. A. (2018). Exploring wellness interventions in progressive multiple sclerosis: An evidence-based review. *Current Treatment Options in Neurology*, *20*, 1–14.

Zainab, N., & Naz, H. (2017). Daily living functioning, social engagement and wellness of older adults. *Psychology, Community & Health*, *6*(1). https://doi.org/10.23668/psycharchives.2312

15

PERPETUAL COMPLEMENTATION THEORY AND THE BRAKE MECHANISM

Nguyen Tra Giang and Oliver Napila Gomez

The perpetual complementation theory stresses the need for curative and preventative actions to preserve the intricate relationship between health and skill system functions. Preventive medicine has long been led by physical education teachers who have stressed the need to take preventative actions to avoid health problems. Safeguarding physiological health and homeostasis through preventative actions like regular physical exercise, maintaining a healthy diet, and refraining from engaging in dangerous behaviors is possible. Curative medicine, on the other hand, is proactive in preventing illness and resolving imbalances once they have occurred. To maintain the perpetual complementation between system functions for health and skill, guarantee sustained participation in physical activities, and achieve optimal overall wellness, comprehending the interaction between preventative and curative approaches is essential. Preventive measures are like armor against harm; curative actions are like bandages for existing health problems; this never-ending cycle of prevention and cure keeps people fit and performing at their best.

Outcome

By the end of this chapter, you will be able to:

- explore how the perpetual complementation theory conceptualizes preventative measures to keep the body's health and skill system functions in balance.
- discover how medicine has evolved through time to prioritize health promotion above disease treatment.

DOI: 10.4324/9781003502937-18

- investigate how changes in a system function for health or skill can affect task performance.
- assess how the perpetual complementation theory can be used to create comprehensive fitness and PE programs
- examine how the brake mechanisms can slow down or stop the perpetual complementation cycle in fitness
- find ways to mitigate the brake mechanisms to restore the perpetual complementation cycle and promote health and fitness.

Perpetual complementation theory and preventive medicine

The phrase "preventive medicine" pops up often in our work as fitness and PE program directors. To differentiate ourselves from healthcare providers whose primary focus is on curing sickness, physical educators have always maintained an emphasis on prevention.

It is essential to talk about curative and preventative measures in this chapter because threats to the perpetual complementation between the system functions for health and skill are just looming around the corner.

Maintaining general health requires consistent physical activity through exercises. To that end, preventive medicine has long promoted the benefits of exercise to enhance physiological health. In addition, preventative medicine emphasizes maintaining a healthy physiological state, eating a balanced diet, and refraining from dangerous habits. Protecting against disturbances to physiological health and equilibrium, these actions, like medicine, serve as preventative measures.

We acknowledge the possibility of unexpected diseases, illnesses, physiological issues, and imbalances. In these cases, curative medications are necessary to bring about a return to health and equilibrium inside the body. Doctors and other medical experts play an essential and unique role in society. Patients must recover before engaging in physical activity or exercise to ensure a never-ending cycle of health–skill perpetual complementation. To better grasp preventive and curative medicine, let us explore the interplay between the two in the following section, highlighting the importance of taking a comprehensive view of health and wellness.

Preventive vs. curative medicine

With the relentless pursuit of scientific understanding and the ever-present desire to alleviate human suffering, the history of medicine has been a narrative of continual progress. The medical field has transformed tremendously from classical humoral pathology to modern iatro-technology and molecular medicine. Nevertheless, the distinction between curative and preventive medicine has impacted the field. This section delves into the various preventive and curative medicine aspects by exploring their respective historical contexts, contemporary importance, and the continuing disagreement over their roles in healthcare.

Preventive medicine: a proactive approach

Preventive medicine is an all-encompassing approach to better health that aims to stop adverse health outcomes before they begin. It encompasses a range of strategies to encourage individuals to lead healthier lives, including personalized illness prediction, focused treatment, and early intervention (Hirooka, 2022). Preventive medicine aims to restrict the progression of diseases before they become severe health issues by focusing on early identification and preventative actions (Demirci et al., 2023).

Preventive medicine is part of the medical profession mainly focused on preventing illnesses and promoting individual health (Reijonsaari, 2013). It is proactive, as it focuses on early detection and action. It involves implementing measures to ward against disease development, highlighting the importance of this approach in preserving good health (Kim et al., 2020).

In the long term, preventive medicine can enhance health outcomes by lowering healthcare costs and disease burden through early identification and elimination of risk factors. However, particular challenges associated with preventative medicine must be considered, especially when dealing with long-term health conditions, notwithstanding the advantages that may be gained.

Curative medicine: addressing established diseases

Curative medicine focuses on treating already existing disorders, in contrast to preventive medicine's emphasis on proactive efforts to maintain health. A wide range of care, restoration, and improvement actions are included in curative medicine to heal diseases and alleviate suffering (Lifshitz, 2020). Many people go to curative medicine for help when sick (Obidigbo, 2021).

When it comes to healthcare, the function of curative medicine is crucial. It provides life-saving therapies and interventions in response to patients' urgent needs. When people are sick and need to get well, curative medicine is what they turn to. Nevertheless, it goes beyond just treating acute illnesses; it also includes managing chronic disorders, relieving symptoms, and improving quality of life generally.

Preventive and curative medicine: complementary approaches

From philosophical, economic, and practical standpoints, the superiority of preventative medicine over curative care is indisputable. Disease prevention is fundamentally more desired and cost-effective than disease treatment (Lifshitz,

2020). The viability of comprehensive preventive medicine, however, remains a difficulty, mainly when dealing with chronic disorders. As a result, curative medicine continues to be relevant and complementary to preventative care, addressing individuals' needs when they become ill.

The perpetual complementation in the USFD Framework

Figure 15.1 shows the interdependent and complementary nature of the health and skill system and its paired and grouped system functions. Note that in this model, energy production and utilization and body function regulation are seen as "pure" functions because the former is a paired system function for health and the latter with skill. A few others, such as metabolic rate, aerobic regulation, motor regulation, and body composition, are common to the health and skill systems.

There is a clear separation of purpose between the two system functions – health and skill – in the context of paired system functions. Let us explore each system function.

Body function regulation and energy production and utilization

Body function regulation is a paired system function that primarily serves to maintain health, and the idea of perpetual complementation becomes clear when we go into this topic. On the one hand, regarding homeostasis, body function regulation keeps vital signs normal, ensures steadiness (not dizziness), and promotes stable mental health. The apparent threats that disrupt body function

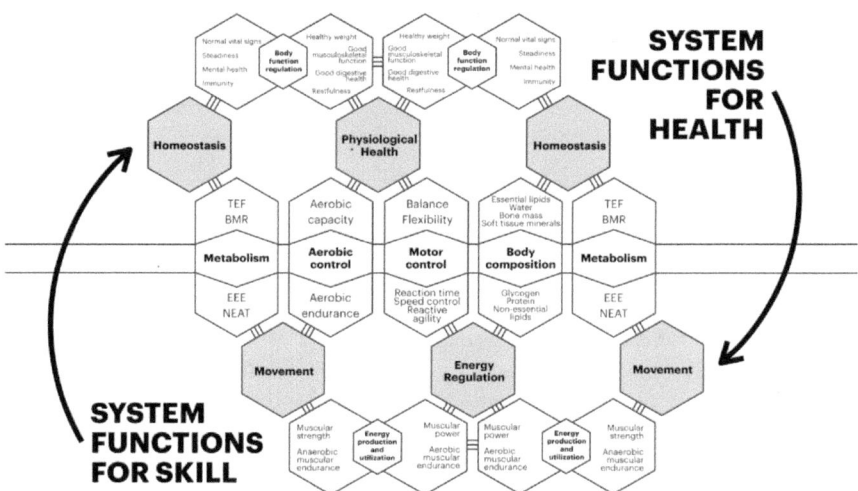

FIGURE 15.1 The big picture of the perpetual complementation

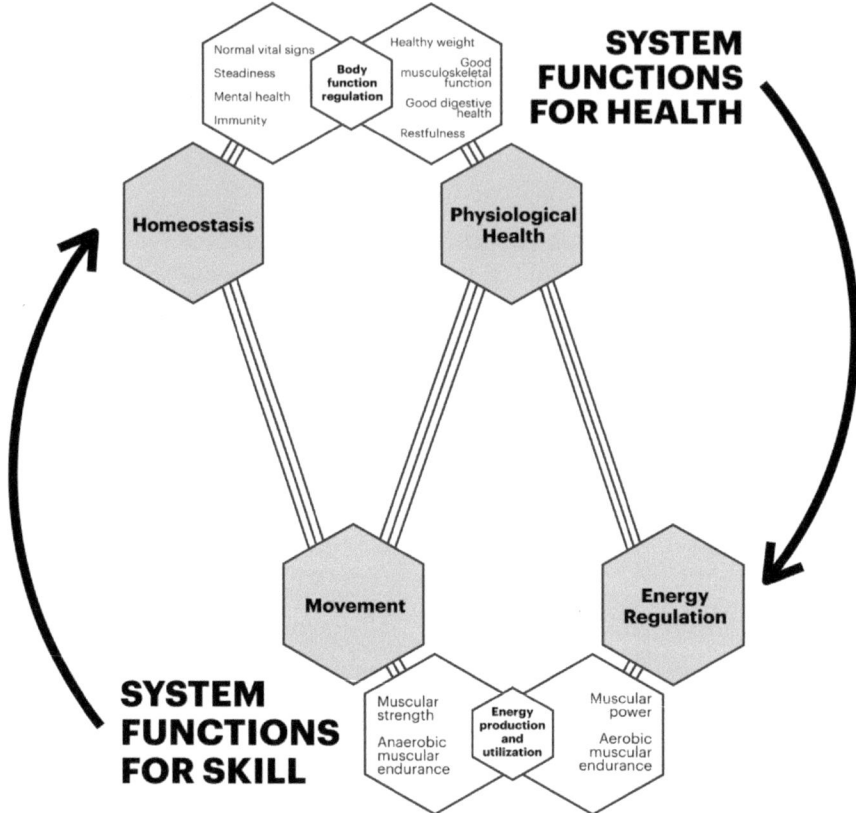

FIGURE 15.2 Perpetual complementation between body function regulation and energy production and utilization

regulation for homeostasis include stress, infections, environmental changes (such as temperature and humidity), poor nutrition, hormone imbalance, injury, chronic health conditions, side effects of medication, and psychological problems (such as anxiety and depression), among others.

On the other hand, regulating body function takes on a new dimension when seen through the perspective of physiological health as it becomes linked with getting and staying at a healthy weight, improving mobility in the muscles and joints, easing indigestion, and helping to have a good night's sleep. Properly managing bodily functions is crucial to the flourishing of these aspects of physiological health as diseases, poor nutrition, a sedentary lifestyle, environmental factors, stress, sleeping disorders, substance abuse, injury, aging, and genetics can threaten it.

Moreover, perpetual complementation emphasizes how interrelated system functions are for health and skill. In this context, the two grouped system functions of movement and energy regulation – energy production and utilization – emerge as critical system functions for skill. Muscle strength and anaerobic muscular endurance are functions of energy production and utilization, crucial for the efficient performance of skill-based physical tasks within the context of movement. Threats to the perpetual complementation concerning energy production and utilization for movement function include nutrient deficiency, metabolic disorders like diabetes, breathing problems that cause insufficient oxygen supply, injuries, neuromuscular disorders like Parkinson's disease, endocrine disorders such as thyroid dysfunction, heart failure, and stroke, among others.

Meanwhile, muscular power and aerobic muscular endurance are components of the context of energy regulation that facilitate deft energy management throughout a range of tasks. However, loss of muscle mass (atrophy), sarcopenia, inadequate protein intake, sedentary lifestyle, chronic diseases (cancer or AIDS), neuromuscular disorders, injury, overtraining, and joint inflammation are some of the threats that affect energy production and utilization for movement function.

While regular physical activity participation and safe workouts promote health, keeping physiological health and homeostasis in check ensures continued involvement in physical efforts. The system functions for health and skill play essential roles in this process. Ultimately, the necessity of both health and skill in achieving overall physical well-being and performance is reinforced by the fact that they complement each other continuously.

However, threats serve as brake mechanisms that disrupt the perpetual complementation cycle. Note that in the USFD Framework, we think of perpetual complementation as gears for the proper functioning of the human body to perform its purpose. The brake mechanisms slow down or stop the perpetual complementation temporarily or permanently, which may adversely affect physical fitness. Hence, preventive measures for avertable brake mechanisms and curative measures for an existing health condition (for example) are critical to restoring the disrupted fitness gears.

Metabolism

Two separate but interrelated components of metabolism – health and skill – are essential to our physiological processes. We initially come across basal metabolic rate (BMR) when we think about metabolic system activities for health. BMR is the bare minimum needed to keep vital body systems going when at rest. It represents the number of calories our body needs to stay alive in a sedentary state. Another system process concerning health is the thermal effect of food (TEF). The energy that is used up when food is broken down and processed is explained by this effect. Our bodies can carry out essential tasks and make good use of nutrients when basal metabolic rate (BMR) and the thermal effect of food work in tandem to promote good health through homeostasis.

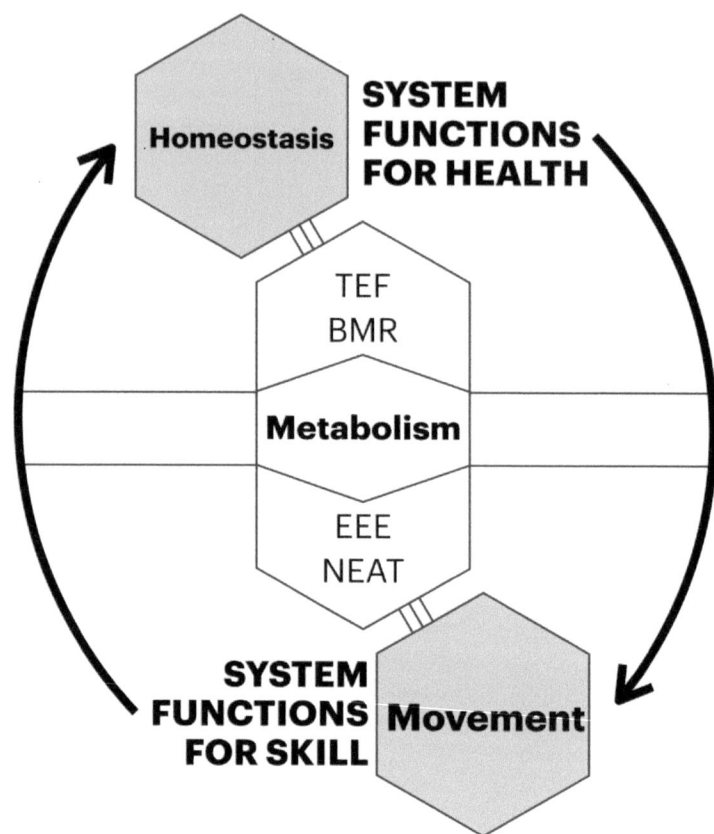

FIGURE 15.3   Perpetual complementation in metabolism

Exercise energy expenditure (EEE) and non-exercise activity thermogenesis (NEAT) are metabolic system processes involved in the system function for skill, particularly concerning movement. Energy expenditure during exercise and training can be measured using EEE. Sports and fitness enthusiasts must know the energy required to participate in their hobbies. NEAT includes the energy used for typical, everyday motions like fidgeting, standing, and walking. Anyone looking to maximize their physical performance and efficiently control their energy consumption must pay close attention to these skill-related metabolic processes.

Moreover, metabolic processes for homeostasis and movement can be threatened by poor diet, sedentary lifestyle, medications, genetics, stress, sleeping disorders, toxins, aging, and chronic diseases, among others. These constitute the brake mechanisms for the perpetual complementation in metabolism. When metabolic processes for homeostasis and movement are disturbed, metabolism may become problematic (either too slow or too fast), resulting in problems with health, skill, and performance of assigned tasks.

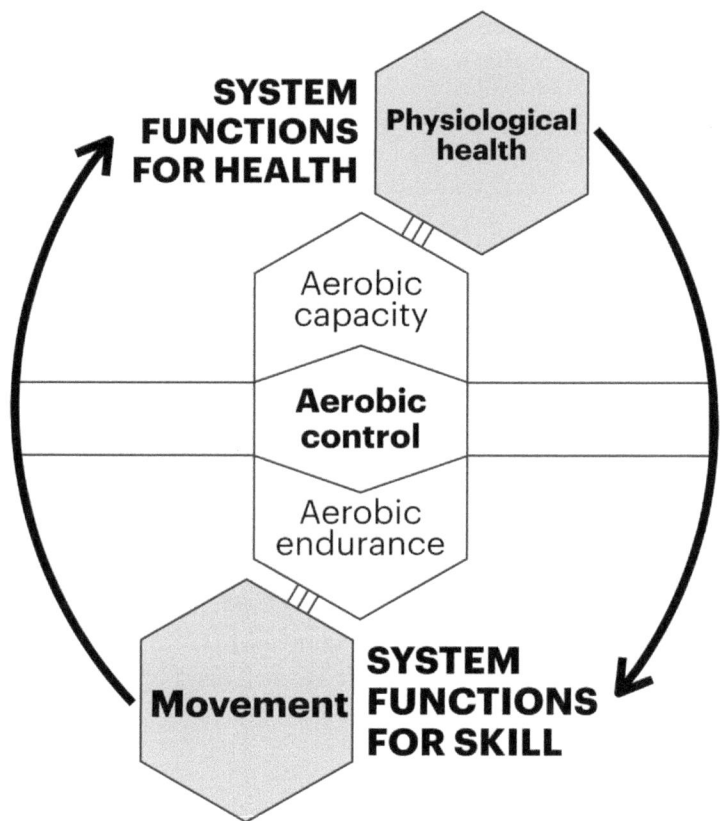

FIGURE 15.4   Perpetual complementation in aerobic control

Aerobic control

Likewise, we can look at aerobic control from a health and skill perspective. Aerobic capacity is a crucial concept, the maximum amount of oxygen a person can use while engaging in aerobic activities. It is the measure of general health and cardiorespiratory fitness. Maintaining an excellent aerobic capacity depends on sustaining vital daily activities and lowering the risk of chronic diseases. At the same time, aerobic capacity may complement movement.

Aerobic endurance surfaces when we explore the system functions related to skill in aerobic control. A person's aerobic endurance can be defined as their capacity to maintain aerobic activity for a long time. It is an essential skill in endurance sports and other activities that need stamina. To succeed at sports requiring prolonged efforts, like long-distance running or cycling, fitness enthusiasts and athletes concentrate on increasing their aerobic endurance. People can improve their performance in some fitness and athletics regions by working on their aerobic endurance, which may complement physiological health.

However, smoking, chronic stress, lack of sleep, obesity, air pollution, chronic diseases, and medication, among others, constitute the brake mechanisms for the perpetual complementation of aerobic capacity and endurance. When a person's ability to manage breathing and heartbeat is disturbed by the brake mechanisms, the health condition, quality, and efficiency of task performance are affected. Hence, management of the brake mechanisms through preventive and curative measures is necessary.

Motor control

Motor control, which includes movement and body control coordination, is also essential for health and skill-related functions. We have flexibility and balance when it comes to health. Preventing falls and injuries, especially in older persons, requires the capacity to maintain bodily stability and equilibrium, which is

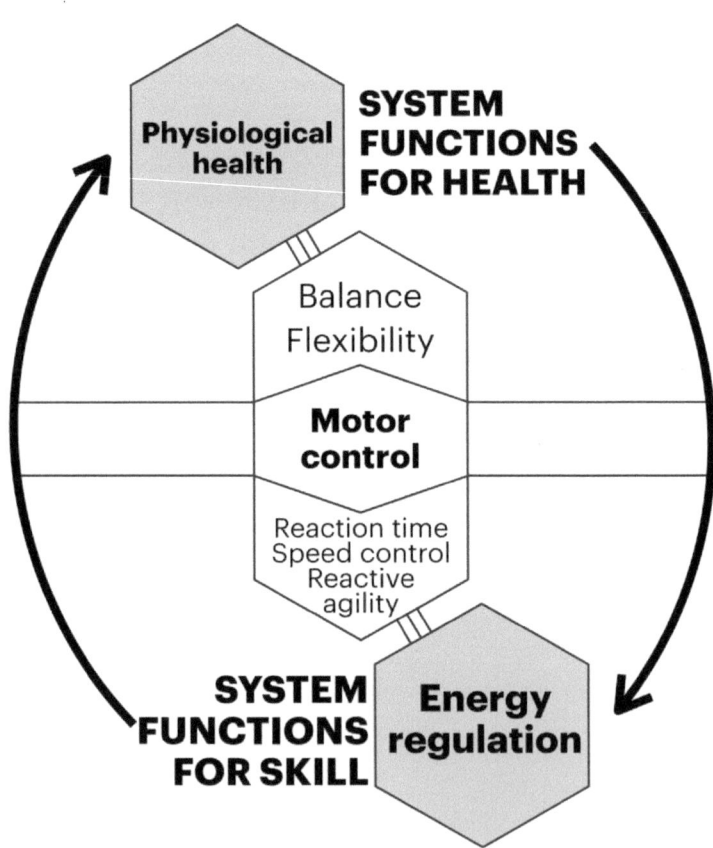

FIGURE 15.5 Perpetual complementation in motor control

known as balance. Conversely, mobility at joints is what we mean when discussing flexibility. Because it facilitates mobility and lessens the likelihood of musculoskeletal issues, it adds to general health. Additionally, balance and flexibility support the system function for skill.

The system functions for skill, including reaction time, speed control, and reactive agility support skills in the motor control context. A person's reaction time measures how quickly they react to certain stimuli. The capacity to control speed is a crucial skill in many kinds of athletics and other physical pursuits. Sports that need quick movements in response to the environment necessitate reactive agility, which is the ability to change directions quickly and easily overcome obstacles. Sports and emergencies necessitate thinking and coordinating movements rapidly, which are also crucial for health.

However, the brake mechanisms of motor control in the perpetual complementation include neurological disorders, brain and spinal cord injuries, muscle weakness and fatigue, poor coordination, musculoskeletal disorders, joint inflammation and pain, and alcohol or drug use, among others. When motor control is disrupted by, for example, brain and spinal injuries, the necessity for curative measures and rehabilitation is imperative to help keep the perpetual complementation mechanism running again. However, the time required for rehabilitation depends on the enormity of the injury.

Body composition

Finally, body composition demonstrates how different components are distributed throughout the body, which are essential for system functions for health and skill. When considering health, water, essential fats, bone mass, and soft tissue minerals perform vital body processes for internal balance. They play a role in maintaining health, and simultaneously support the system functions for skill.

Glycogen, protein, and nonessential lipids are the structural support of the system functions for skill within the body composition context. To fuel physical activities and endurance, glycogen is stored in the liver and muscles as an energy reserve. Muscle growth, healing, and general skill performance are all impacted by protein. Nonessential lipids may contribute to skill performance, especially in endurance-based activities, and can also be an energy supply for longer-duration activities. Optimizing health and skill sets necessitates balancing these factors for physical preparedness for various situations.

Nonetheless, poor nutrition and overeating, a sedentary lifestyle, hormonal imbalance, genetics, age, stress, medication, lack of sleep, and thyroid conditions, among others, may disturb the perpetual complementation between body composition system functions, health, and skill. In this case, preventive and curative measures are essential to put the gears of perpetual complementation back to work.

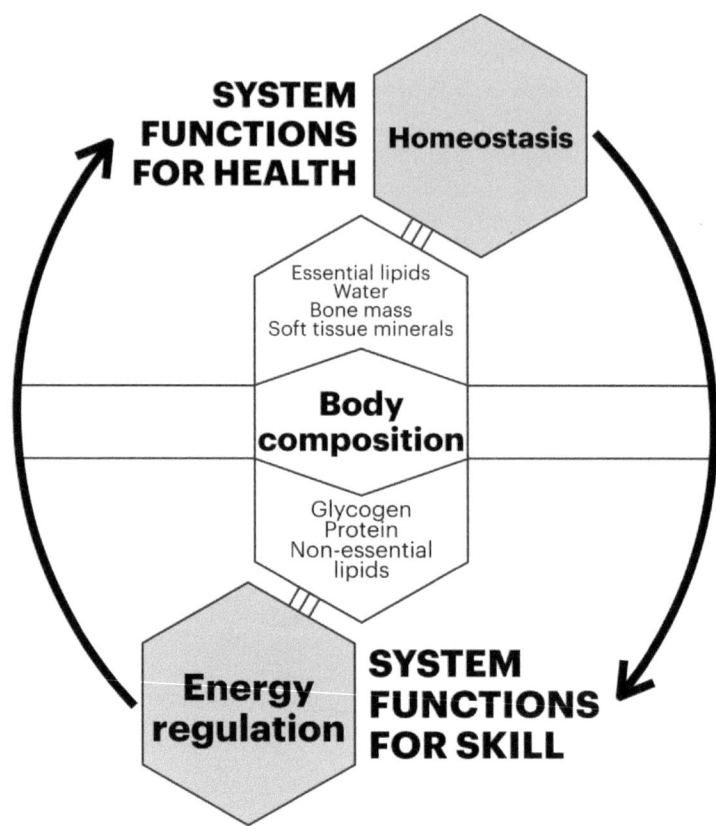

FIGURE 15.6   Perpetual complementation in body composition

Summary

The chapter stresses the importance of taking precautions to avoid problems by contrasting preventive medicine's proactive with curative medicine's reactive approach, stressing the need for a holistic view of health and wellness.

On the one hand, preventive medicine aims to halt the beginning or course of diseases before they become severe, and it is defined by customized illness prediction, focused treatment, and early intervention. This method stresses the need for early detection and intervention to reduce health risks and keep everyone healthy. Curative medicine, on the other hand, seeks to treat long-term illnesses by restoring health and reducing suffering through care, restoration, and improvement measures.

Differentiating between preventative and curative medicine highlights how they work hand in hand in healthcare. Acute health demands and chronic condition management still require curative medicine despite the widespread praise for preventive medicine for its attractiveness and cost-effectiveness.

Integral to the USFD Framework's perpetual complementation theory is the idea that the health and skill systems' operations are mutually supportive and reliant on one another. It emphasizes how threats, called brake mechanisms, to the body's energy production and utilization, metabolism, body function regulation, aerobic control, motor control, and body composition can upset the equilibrium between system functions for health and skill processes.

Disruptions to homeostasis and movement can impact general physical well-being, and threats to the body's ability to regulate and produce energy include stress, illnesses, poor nutrition, and injury. Similarly, metabolic process disturbances brought on by unhealthy eating, lack of exercise, and long-term health conditions may influence health and skills. Cigarette smoking, excess body fat, and chronic stress all lower aerobic control, which in turn lowers cardiorespiratory fitness and endurance, which impacts general health and the ability to accomplish tasks.

Furthermore, difficulties with physical functioning might arise due to impairments in coordination and movement caused by threats to motor control, such as neurological illnesses and weak muscles. Moreover, changes in body composition due to aging, hormone imbalances, or lousy eating might impact physical readiness and performance in different settings.

This chapter stresses the significance of preventative and curative measures when protecting the ongoing mutual support of health and skill system functions. The efficient operation of the body's complex systems depends on people minimizing these risks to their health and performance.

Review questions

1. How does preventative medicine vary from curative care, and what is its focus?
2. Explain the importance of preventative medicine and its proactive approach to health maintenance.
3. When it comes to long-term health issues, what are some of the obstacles to preventative medicine?
4. Describe how curative medicine helps with health problems and why it is crucial.
5. How can healthcare that focuses on both prevention and cure work together?
6. Discuss how the USFD Framework's idea of perpetual complementarity affects health and skill.
7. In body function regulation, energy production, and utilization, brake mechanisms interrupt the perpetual complementation cycle.
8. In terms of physical fitness, what are some threats to energy production and utilization for movement?

9. Describe the brake mechanisms that interrupt perpetual complementation in the context of metabolism and explain its relevance to health and skill.
10. Explain how aerobic capacity and endurance relate to general health, and name some risks that might compromise aerobic control.

Discussion questions

1. In light of the perpetual complementation theory, consider preventive measures. In what ways can preventative measures help keep the body's skills and health systems in harmony?
2. Historically, medicine has shifted its focus from treating illness to preventing it. What are the continuing arguments about preventative and curative medicine responsibilities, and how has this change affected healthcare practices?
3. Using the perpetual complementation theory as a framework, examine the relationships between the health and skill functions. How does a change in one part, like energy production and utilization, influence the performance of tasks?
4. In order to create holistic fitness and PE programs, it is essential to consider the real-world implications of the perpetual complementation theory. In what ways may teachers use this model to encourage the growth of healthy habits and competent abilities in students of all ages?
5. How can brake mechanisms interrupt the perpetual complementation cycle in fitness? Discuss how stress, poor diets, sedentary lifestyles, and chronic diseases affect the interdependent system functions for health and skill. Explore ways to mitigate these brake mechanisms and restore the cycle to improve fitness and health.

References

Demirci, Ü., Mert, A., & Kaptanoğlu, A. (2023). Developing a scale to make suggestions to overweight people for efficient weight loss and weight management. *Cyprus Journal of Medical Sciences, 8*(2). https://doi.org/10.4274/cjms.2022.2022-25

Hirooka, Y. (2022). Shifting the emphasis from presymptomatic states to preemptive medicine: Increasing the scope of medical ultrasound. *Journal of Medical Ultrasonics, 49*(4), 759–759. https://doi.org/10.1007/s10396-022-01268-6280

Kim, S., Kang, S., Kim, J., Lee, D., Kim, S., Lee, J., Jang, K. I., Oh, Y. S., Rah, J. C., Huh, M. S., Paek, S. H., & Choi, J. W. (2020). Closed-loop neuromodulation for Parkinson's disease: Current state and future directions. *IEEE Transactions on Molecular, Biological and Multi-scale Communications, 7*(4), 209–223. https://doi.org/10.1109/TMBMC.2020.3036756

Lifshitz, A. (2020). Rhetorics of cure. *Gaceta Medica de Mexico, 156*(6), 484–485. http://dx.doi.org/10.24875/GMM.M21000458

Obidigbo, J. C. (2021). An overview of Igbo traditional medicine. *Ochendo: An African Journal of Innovative Studies, 2*(1). https://acjol.org/index.php/ochendo/article/view/3534

Reijonsaari, K. (2013). *Co-creating health-examining the effects of co-creation in a lifestyle intervention service targeting physical activity* [Doctoral dissertation, Aalto University]. http://urn.fi/URN:ISBN:978-952-60-5132-1

GLOSSARY

2C Model   A two-compartment model of body composition that divides the body into fat mass and fat-free mass, simplifying the assessment of body composition for health and fitness evaluation.

3C Model   The three-compartment model further splits fat-free mass into lean body mass (including muscle and organs) and bone mineral content, providing a more detailed analysis of body composition.

4C Model   A four-compartment model that divides body composition into fat mass, bone mineral content, total body water, and protein, offering a comprehensive assessment of body composition and metabolic health.

Aerobic Capacity   The maximum rate at which an individual can consume oxygen during intense physical activity, a critical indicator of cardiorespiratory fitness and physical performance.

Aerobic Control   The capacity to regulate one's breathing and heart rate during physical activity, optimizing cardiorespiratory function for both health and performance.

Aerobic Control (NC)   The capacity of the respiratory centers in the brainstem to regulate heart rate and breathing during rest and exercise, reflecting effective management of aerobic capacity and endurance.

Aerobic Endurance   The ability to perform moderate- to high-intensity physical activity for extended periods without undue fatigue, essential for sustained physical performance.

Aerobic Energy System   A long-duration energy system that produces ATP through oxidative phosphorylation in the presence of oxygen, supporting sustained physical activities and muscular endurance.

Aerobic Respiration   A process by which cells convert glucose and oxygen into energy, carbon dioxide, and water, primarily supported by the cardiorespiratory system during sustained physical activity.

Aerobic Threshold   The exercise intensity at which the body starts to produce lactate at a faster rate than it can be removed, marking the transition from aerobic to anaerobic metabolism.

Agility The ability to change direction and position quickly and effectively while maintaining balance, involving both reactive agility and controlled agility.

Anaerobic Lactic Energy System An energy pathway that supports high-intensity, short-duration activities by generating ATP through glycolysis in the absence of oxygen, producing lactate as a by-product.

ATP (Adenosine Triphosphate) The primary energy carrier in cells, essential for muscle contraction and other cellular functions, with its availability and regeneration crucial for muscular strength, power, and endurance.

Awareness in Wellness The recognition and understanding of one's physical, emotional, and overall health status, emphasizing the importance of self-knowledge as a foundation for wellness.

Balance The ability to maintain the body's center of mass over its base of support, critical both in health-related contexts (e.g., preventing falls in the elderly) and skill-related fitness (e.g., in athletic performance).

Balance The capacity to maintain the body's center of gravity within its base of support, crucial for stability during both static and dynamic situations.

Basal Metabolic Rate (BMR) The rate at which the body uses energy while at rest to maintain vital bodily functions such as breathing and maintaining normal body temperature.

Body Composition The ratio of different types of body tissue (fat, muscle, bone) in an individual's body, affecting metabolic rate and health.

Body Composition Refers to the proportions of fat, bone, water, and muscle in human bodies. It is crucial for assessing health, nutritional status, and physical performance.

Body Composition (ME) The regulation of tissue proportions in the body, influenced by the endocrine and musculoskeletal systems, highlighting the importance of maintaining a healthy balance between lean mass and fat mass.

Body Function Regulation The collaborative effort of the nervous and endocrine systems to ensure optimal organ function and physiological equilibrium, essential for overall health.

Body Function Regulation (NE) The collaborative function of the endocrine and nervous systems in controlling various physiological processes and maintaining internal stability.

Bone Mass The quantity of bone tissue in the body, significant for providing structural support, protecting organs, and storing minerals like calcium and phosphorus.

Bone Mineral Content The amount of mineral (calcium and phosphorus) in bone tissue, providing structural strength to bones and serving as a vital component in assessing overall health and risk for conditions like osteoporosis.

Brain Function The central organ of the human nervous system responsible for processing sensory information, regulating bodily functions, and executing movements.

Brake Mechanisms Factors or conditions that disrupt or impede the normal functioning of the body's perpetual complementation system, affecting the balance between health and skill system functions. These mechanisms can temporarily or permanently halt progress in physical fitness, necessitating preventive or curative measures to restore balance and functionality. Examples include injuries, chronic diseases, poor nutrition, sedentary lifestyles, and environmental stressors.

Cardiorespiratory Component Measures the efficiency of the heart, lungs, and vascular system in supporting sustained physical activity and overall cardiorespiratory health.

Cardiorespiratory System Comprises the cardiovascular and respiratory systems, working together to supply oxygen to and remove carbon dioxide from the body, supporting energy production for physical activity.

Competence in Wellness The ability to apply knowledge and skills to improve personal health and well-being, highlighting the importance of taking proactive steps towards wellness based on self-awareness.

Conceptual Definition A broader definition of a concept that encompasses its fundamental characteristics and theoretical basis, without focusing solely on measurable indicators.

Construct An abstract concept that represents a theoretical collection of attributes, such as physical fitness, which is operationalized through measurable indicators for study and application.

Coordination The process through which the body's systems work together to perform movements accurately and effectively, involving precise control and synchronization of different body parts.

Coordination Impairments Conditions caused by neurological disorders affecting the brain's ability to coordinate movements, leading to decreased balance, clumsiness, or difficulty performing precise motions.

Cultural Sensitivity in Wellness Acknowledgment and respect for cultural differences in wellness practices and beliefs, emphasizing the importance of incorporating diverse cultural perspectives into wellness strategies.

Curative Medicine Involves treating and managing existing diseases with the goal of curing or significantly improving the condition of the patient, including the use of medications, surgeries, and other treatments to address symptoms and underlying causes.

Elements of Coordination Components that contribute to the smooth execution of movements, including senses, body parts, and energy regulation, essential for performing tasks efficiently.

Emotional Wellness The ability to successfully handle life's stresses and adapt to change and difficult times. It highlights the importance of awareness, acceptance, and healthy expression of one's emotions.

Endocrine System A collection of glands that produce hormones regulating metabolism, growth and development, tissue function, sexual function, reproduction, sleep, and mood, among other things.

Energy Production and Utilization (CM) The combined capability of the cardiorespiratory and musculoskeletal systems to produce energy for movement and physical activity through efficient oxygen delivery and usage.

Energy Regulation Another grouped system function in USFD, emphasizing the body's ability to manage energy production and consumption effectively for physical activity.

Energy Regulation (MCE) The integrated function of musculoskeletal, cardiorespiratory, and endocrine systems in managing energy generation and consumption, crucial for high-level physical activity, metabolism, and maintaining healthy body composition.

Essential Fats Fatty acids that the body cannot synthesize and must be obtained through the diet, crucial for various physiological functions including cell membrane integrity and hormone production.

Exercise Energy Expenditure (EEE) The amount of energy expended during physical activity, contributing significantly to total daily energy expenditure.

Fairness Impartial and just treatment without favoritism or discrimination, especially in the context of including diverse populations in fitness concepts and applications.

Fitness The capacity of being in harmony with physical, mental, and social environments, highlighting health, skills, and task suitability.

Flexibility The range of motion available at a joint or group of joints, affecting movement efficiency and risk of injury.

Genes   Units of heredity that dictate the development, growth, and functioning of the body, including the influence on body structure, function, and susceptibility to certain health conditions.

Glycogen   A vital glucose storage molecule found in organs like the liver and brain, playing a key role in energy regulation, especially during high-intensity exercise and cognitive functions.

Health-related Fitness (HRF)   Components of fitness that contribute to the operation of bodily functions and overall health, including body composition, cardiorespiratory fitness, flexibility, strength, and endurance.

Health-Ability-Task Suitability (HATS) Framework   A conceptual model emphasizing the interrelation of health, ability, and task suitability in defining fitness.

Heart Rate Reserve (HRR)   The difference between a person's resting heart rate and maximum heart rate, used to determine exercise intensity levels.

Holistic Approach   Considering the whole of something or someone and not just a part; in physical fitness, it emphasizes the interdependence of various components for overall health and performance.

Homeostasis   The ability of the body to maintain a stable internal environment despite changes in external conditions, regulated by various body systems including the endocrine and nervous systems.

Hormonal Regulation   The control of metabolic processes through the action of hormones, which regulate various physiological functions and influence overall health.

Hormones   Biochemical substances produced by various glands in the body, playing a pivotal role in regulating physiological functions and influencing overall health.

HRF–SRF Model   A previously established model that categorizes fitness components into health-related and skill-related groups, now considered within the broader context of USFD.

Hydrogen Ion Buildup   Accumulation of hydrogen ions in muscles during high-intensity exercise, leading to acidosis and muscle fatigue, affecting aerobic and anaerobic performance.

Immunity   The body's defense mechanism against infections and diseases, highlighting the importance of a robust immune system for physiological health and task performance.

Inclusion   The practice or policy of providing equal access to opportunities and resources for people who might otherwise be excluded or marginalized, such as those having physical or mental disabilities or belonging to other minority groups.

Inclusive Assessment   An evaluation strategy that accommodates diverse populations by considering individual differences, cultural norms, lifestyles, and geographical locations in physical fitness assessments.

Intellectual Wellness   Encourages creative and stimulating mental activities. It involves one's openness to new ideas, a capacity to think critically, and a desire to learn and grow.

Irisin   A hormone produced by muscles during exercise, involved in energy regulation by promoting the browning of white fat cells and improving metabolic health.

Karvonen Formula   A method to calculate target heart rate zones for exercise based on an individual's age, resting heart rate, and maximum heart rate.

Kinesthesia   The sense of movement and body position, relying on the coordinated function of the central nervous system, proprioceptive system, and vestibular system for physical activity and balance.

Kinesthetic Fitness   The ability to control movements efficiently for health enhancement and performance, focusing on motor control functions.

Kinetic Fitness   A term introduced within the USFD Framework that characterizes the fitness function resulting from the utilization of kinetic energy produced by the musculoskeletal and cardiorespiratory systems for performing skills and tasks efficiently.

Lean Body Mass   Refers to the total weight of one's body minus all the weight due to fat mass, including weight of muscles, bones, organs, and water, crucial for understanding metabolic health and physical fitness.

Lifestyle Behaviors   Activities and habits, including diet and physical activity, that significantly impact body functions, health conditions, and overall physiological health.

Locomotor Movements   Movements that involve transporting the body from one location to another, requiring synchronization between limbs and coordination between different parts of the body.

Manipulative Movements   Activities that involve handling or manipulating objects using the body or implements as extensions, requiring coordination of sight, proprioception, and movement for successful execution.

MC Model   The multi-compartment model expands upon the 4C model by including additional components like glycogen and nonessential lipids, for a detailed and nuanced understanding of body composition and its impact on metabolic functions.

Mental Health   A critical aspect of physiological health, encompassing emotional, psychological, and social well-being, and significantly influenced by the body's regulatory functions.

Metabolic Balance   The regulation of the body's metabolic processes, including energy production and utilization, nutrient synthesis, and waste elimination, primarily influenced by the endocrine system.

Metabolic Disorders   Conditions that affect the body's metabolism, leading to health problems such as obesity, diabetes, and cardiovascular diseases.

Metabolism   The complex network of cellular processes in the body that convert food into energy, necessary for growth, reproduction, and maintaining life.

Metabolism (CE)   The regulation of energy production and utilization, influenced by the interaction between the cardiorespiratory and endocrine systems, affecting metabolic rate and overall energy efficiency.

Morphologic Component   Pertains to physical characteristics such as body mass, height, percentage of body fat, and overall body composition.

Motivation for Wellness   The internal and external drivers that encourage individuals to adopt and maintain healthy behaviors, distinguishing between intrinsic (internal) and extrinsic (external) motivation.

Motor Component   Assesses balance, coordination, and proprioceptive abilities as key elements of physical performance.

Motor Control   The process by which humans use their brain to activate and coordinate the muscles and limbs involved in the performance of a motor skill.

Motor Control (NM)   The coordinated function of the musculoskeletal and nervous systems in generating and controlling movement, crucial for physical activities and workouts.

Motor Unit Recruitment   The process by which the nervous system activates specific muscle fibers (motor units) to generate the required force for various tasks, highlighting the coordination of muscles involved in different activities.

Movement   A grouped system function under USFD that consolidates traditional fitness components related to motor control, aerobic capacity, and muscular fitness.

Movement (NMC)   A grouped system function that encompasses motor control, energy production and utilization, and aerobic control, reflecting the body's capability for effective and efficient task performance.

Muscular Component   Involves attributes related to muscle strength, endurance, and overall muscular health.

Muscular Endurance   The capacity of a muscle or muscle group to continuously exert force over an extended period, enabling prolonged physical activity without fatigue, supported by the aerobic energy system.

Muscular Power   The ability to exert maximum force in the shortest possible time, often associated with explosive actions like jumping or sprinting, relying on rapid ATP production via the phosphocreatine energy system.

Muscular Strength   The ability of a muscle or group of muscles to generate force in a specific effort, crucial for performing tasks that require lifting, pushing, or pulling objects.

Musculoskeletal System   An organ system that enables humans to move using the muscular and skeletal systems, including bones, muscles, cartilage, tendons, ligaments, joints, and other connective tissue.

Nervous System   A complex network of nerves and cells that carry messages to and from the brain and spinal cord to various parts of the body, coordinating body functions and movements.

Neurological Disorders   Medical conditions that affect the nervous system, leading to coordination impairments and affecting an individual's ability to perform movements and tasks efficiently.

Nonessential Lipids   Lipids that the body can produce and are not required to be obtained from the diet, important for storing energy and contributing to adiposity when in excess.

Nonessential Fats   Fats produced by the body and not required to be obtained from diet, playing roles in energy storage, hormone production, and cellular structure, impacting overall metabolic health.

Non-exercise Activity Thermogenesis (NEAT)   The energy expended for everything we do that is not sleeping, eating, or sports-like exercise, such as walking, standing, and fidgeting.

Non-locomotor Movements   Movements performed in place without changing the location, requiring coordination for precise and synchronized execution, often involving balance and body positioning.

Occupational Wellness   The personal satisfaction and enrichment derived from one's work. It involves engaging in work that provides personal satisfaction and enrichment and is consistent with one's values, goals, and lifestyle.

Operational Definition   A way to define a construct by relating it to measurable indicators, allowing for assessment and quantification of abstract concepts.

Paired Systems Matrix   A methodological tool within the USFD that examines the interdependent nature of physiological systems by analyzing the primary functions of two combined systems to reveal complex mechanisms of physical abilities.

Perpetual Complementation   A concept within the Unified Systems Fitness Design (USFD) that emphasizes the continuous interaction and mutual support between health and skill system functions, highlighting the importance of maintaining a balance between physical fitness components for optimal well-being.

Philosophies and Beliefs in Wellness   The underlying values, beliefs, and worldviews that shape an individual's approach to wellness, recognizing the influence of personal, cultural, and spiritual factors on health decisions.

Phosphocreatine Energy System   An immediate energy system that provides ATP for short, explosive efforts by breaking down creatine phosphate stored in muscles, crucial for activities requiring muscular power.

Physical Fitness   A state of health and well-being, and the ability to perform aspects of sports, occupations, and daily activities without undue fatigue.

Physical Literacy   The ability, confidence, and desire to be physically active for life, encompassing a wide range of physical activities and the development of fundamental movement skills.

Physical Wellness   Involves maintaining a healthy body and seeking care when needed. Physical health is attained through exercise, eating well, getting enough sleep, and paying attention to the signs of illness and getting help when needed.

Physiological Fitness   Refers to the effective operation of the body's systems, including anatomical, muscular, circulatory, nervous, and glandular systems, to facilitate physical activity and achieve optimal physical fitness.

Preference/Personal Choice in Wellness   The empowerment and autonomy of individuals to make decisions that align with their personal values and preferences in pursuit of wellness, emphasizing the role of individual agency.

Preventive Medicine   Focuses on preventing diseases and maintaining health through proactive measures, such as vaccinations, lifestyle changes, and regular screenings to identify and mitigate risk factors before diseases develop.

Proprioception   The awareness of the position and movement of the body, mediated by proprioceptors in muscles, tendons, and joints, essential for coordinating movements and maintaining balance.

Proprioceptive System   Sensory feedback system that provides information on the position and movement of the body's parts, essential for balance and coordinated movement.

Protein   Essential macronutrients that serve as building blocks for body tissues and play a crucial role in growth, repair, and overall physiological functions including energy regulation.

Range of Motion (ROM)   The full movement potential of a joint, usually its range of flexion and extension, important for flexibility and overall movement efficiency.

Reaction Time   The duration between the onset of a stimulus and the initiation of a motor response, indicating the speed of cognitive processing and motor output.

Reactive Agility   The ability to quickly change direction in response to unpredictable stimuli, integrating cognitive decision-making with physical agility for effective movement adaptation in dynamic environments.

Restfulness   The quality of sleep that contributes to physiological health, emphasizing the restorative aspect of sleep for overall well-being.

Sarcopenia   The loss of muscle mass and strength that occurs with aging, affecting metabolism, physical performance, and overall health.

Sensory Systems   The parts of the nervous system involved in receiving and processing sensory information from the environment, essential for coordinating movements and adjusting to changes.

Skill-related Fitness (SRF)   Components of fitness that enhance one's ability to perform specific physical activities, including power, speed, agility, balance, and reaction time.

Social Wellness   The ability to relate to and connect with other people in our world. It involves building and maintaining positive relationships that add value to our and others' lives.

Soft Mineral Tissues   Refer to the body's mineral content critical for maintaining physiological processes like muscle contraction, nerve transmission, and bone health.

Speed Control   The ability to regulate the speed of movement in response to task demands, focusing on precision rather than maximum speed.

Spiritual Wellness   A personal matter involving values and beliefs that provide a purpose in our lives. It can be achieved in many ways, including religion, meditation, yoga, or personal reflection.

Substrate Utilization   The process by which the body uses various nutrients (carbohydrates, fats, and proteins) for energy during metabolic activities.

System Functions for Health   Encompasses physiological health and homeostasis, highlighting the role of physical fitness in maintaining bodily functions and internal balance.

System Functions for Skill   Includes movement and energy regulation, focusing on the capacity for physical activity and the efficiency of energy utilization during exercise.

Systems Theory   A theoretical framework focusing on the interdependencies within systems, including the human body's subsystems, and their interactions with the environment.

Task Performance   The ability to efficiently complete tasks, directly influenced by the regulation of body functions and the maintenance of homeostasis for optimal physical and mental performance.

Thermal Effect of Food (TEF)   The increase in metabolic rate after ingestion of food, accounting for energy used in digestion, absorption, and distribution of nutrients.

Total Body Water   The sum of all fluids within the body, including intracellular and extracellular water, essential for physiological processes, metabolism, and maintaining homeostasis.

Transformative Worldview   A research approach that emphasizes social justice, challenges unequal power dynamics, and promotes equitable and inclusive practices in physical fitness.

Type I, IIA, IIB Muscle Fibers   Classifications of muscle fibers based on their contraction speed and fatigue resistance, with Type I being slow-twitch oxidative, Type IIA being fast-twitch oxidative, and Type IIB being fast-twitch glycolytic, each playing distinct roles in kinetic fitness and energy systems.

USFD Framework   A comprehensive model that integrates the interconnections within physiological systems, emphasizing the complex mechanisms underpinning physical abilities through the study of nervous, musculoskeletal, cardiorespiratory, and endocrine systems.

USFD Wellness Principles   A set of principles within the Unified Systems Fitness Design (USFD) Framework that guide individuals toward holistic well-being, including awareness, competence, preference and personal choice, motivation, and philosophies and beliefs.

Vestibular Sense   A system located within the inner ear that contributes to balance and spatial orientation by detecting changes in head movements and position, crucial for maintaining equilibrium.

Vestibular System   Part of the inner ear responsible for detecting head movements and maintaining balance and spatial orientation.

Visual System   The sensory system responsible for processing visual information, playing a significant role in balance and spatial orientation.

VO$_2$ Max   The maximum amount of oxygen an individual can utilize during intense or maximal exercise, serving as a key measure of aerobic fitness.

Water   Essential for life, playing a critical role in regulating body temperature, transporting nutrients, and removing waste, among other physiological processes.

Wellness   The act of practicing healthy habits on a daily basis to attain better physical and mental health outcomes, so that instead of just surviving, you're thriving.

INDEX

Note: Page numbers in *italics* indicate a figure and page numbers in **bold** indicate a table on the corresponding page.